THE HEALTHCARE INTERPRETER

A Textbook for Advanced Medical Interpreting

Applied Ethics, Terminology and Medical Specializations

Suzanna Reiss-Končar, MPH, CHI™

Published by Culture & Language Press, a division of Cross-Cultural Communications, LLC.

This book was previously published under the title *Healthcare Interpreting with Heart and Mind* (ISBN: 978-0-9966517-5-2).

Culture & Language Press
10015 Old Columbia Road, Suite B-215
Columbia, MD 21046
USA
+ 1 410-312-5599
www.cultureandlanguage.net
clp@cultureandlanguage.net

ISBN-13: 978-1-7332491-5-7

Suzanna Reiss-Končar's work is a masterfully complex resource. Each chapter marries an ethical principle with a medical specialty and performance-based practice. Deeply multi-dimensional and adaptable, it propels student-centered learning via transformative engagement, skill development and self-analysis. All in one. One chapter at a time. Students walk away knowing where they are and what remains to discover along their professional development continuum.

E. Zoe Schutzman, MA, NYS CCI, CHI™
Program manager, educator, specialist, CCHI commissioner
The University of New Mexico Hospital - Health Sciences Center

[This textbook] is a wonderful and practical book for healthcare interpreters who want to continue their education at their own pace after finishing initial training. The Reflect and Practice sections are handy tools to develop critical thinking skills.

Margarita Bekker, CoreCHI™, Russian interpreter, trainer,
CCHI commissioner emerita, former chair

A dynamic and timely contribution to healthcare interpreting, this textbook could complement an institution's diversity, equity and inclusion training for advanced medical interpreters. It would also support novice healthcare interpreters in learning how to navigate the profession with confidence while significantly expanding their medical glossaries.

Sara Juarez, MA, CHI™
Director of interpreting and translations programs
Durham Technical Community College

Reiss-Končar's book is a treasure trove of ideas and resources for interpreter trainers everywhere.

Heather Glass
Trainer and assessor

This book is written with knowledge, passion and love. Ms. Reiss-Končar explores the complexities interpreters must consider and sort out when interpreting in medical settings.

Chapter after chapter, with a pedagogical approach and quasi-surgical precision, she dissects the anatomy and soul of healthcare encounters, exposing the challenges they impose: from what is written or said to what is hinted or lies between the lines; from specialized terminology to colloquial or idiomatic expressions; from culture-bound beliefs and practices to differences in communication styles; from the review of ethical principles to ethical dilemmas.

In addition, the author suggests readings and study material. Highly recommended for both those relatively new to the field and the well-seasoned healthcare interpreter, as well as interpreter trainers.

Sylvana Fernández-Ellauri, hospital staff interpreter, UVA Health
Coauthor, Medical Terminology for Interpreters: An Instructor's Guide (2nd ed.)

Woolly Mammoth,
Volim te, ljubim te.

•

For my mother Ann.
For Doña Violeta.

•

For Shaíl,
Oči moje, vuk, light of my life.

Contents

"Of all the forms of inequality, injustice in healthcare is the most shocking and inhumane."

—Martin Luther King Jr.

"Healthcare without language access is no healthcare...It means life and death to patients."

—Alice Lai-Bitker

"It don't mean a thing if it ain't got that swing."

—Duke Ellington, Irving Mills

Read this first: Important information for you, the interpreter

Prepare yourself

Develop your skills as a medical interpreter and prepare for challenging encounters. Use this advanced textbook to boost your terminology, knowledge and decision-making skills. Coach yourself emotionally for the unexpected. Engage with the powerful role plays, practical exercises, readings and terminology lists; then immerse yourself in the extensive glossary.

Who should use this book?

Medical interpreters

Any medical interpreter of any language pair who has completed basic training (a minimum of 40 to 100 hours) can use this book. It supports seasoned hospital staff interpreters, bilingual employees who interpret and healthcare interpreters still new to the job.

Important points to consider:

- Any medical interpreter will find value in:
  - The drawings labeled in English (and Spanish).
  - The terminology lists with space for completion in the other working language.
  - The English glossary.
- Interpreters who interpret between Spanish and English will find translations for medical terms into Spanish.
- The book is helpful for both spoken- and signed-language interpreters. However, the author is a Spanish interpreter, and the role plays do not involve Deaf or hard-of-hearing patients.[1]
- While the focus is on U.S. healthcare, most of the problems and challenges found in this book apply to medical interpreting in almost any country, especially industrialized nations with complex healthcare systems.

Instructors of medical interpreting

Interpreter trainers and university or college instructors who teach medical interpreting (especially beyond entry level) will also find this book of value. It can be used by instructors:

- As a core textbook.

1 Note that in healthcare and other settings, spoken language interpreters may be called to work with a signed-language interpreter (or team) to interpret for members of a family with complex language needs (for example, a monolingual Spanish-speaking parent and a Deaf child who communicates in American Sign Language).

- As a reference book.
- As a source of ideas, scenarios and exercises for student practice.
- As a repository of some of the richest, most realistic role plays in the field.

The extensive appended glossary of English and English-Spanish medical terms is also valuable. More specific guidance for instructors on how to use this book is provided below.

Can I study this book by myself?

The Healthcare Interpreter is designed for class use or self-study. If you have a fellow interpreter as a "study buddy," this book will be a wonderful resource to help both of you study and practice together.

What is in this book?

Each chapter in this textbook focuses on a medical specialization. It launches with a role play and an analysis of the linguistic and cultural challenges; then the chapter takes a closer look at tough ethical decisions for interpreters and dives into practical activities and exercises. Each chapter concludes with a specialization-specific diagram with labeled medical terms, a blank version of the diagram where interpreters can fill in the missing words in both (or all) their working languages and a list of those terms.

An advanced glossary is included in Appendix 3.

Goals for the book

The primary goal for this book is to prepare healthcare interpreters for what they will face when they work in hospitals and clinics. In this way, they can become more accurate, confident and successful in the profession.

Most interpreters receive inadequate mentoring, shadowing, vetting and the kind of advanced training they need to work in hospitals and clinics. As a result, they are not adequately prepared for challenging encounters or advanced terminology and may freeze in the moment. To interpret hard news (for example, when a doctor informs parents that their child is dying) can come as a brutal shock for many interpreters. Some withdraw from a session or the profession because they cannot cope with such challenges.

This textbook supports the professional development and continuing education of professional interpreters.

Just as important, the author seeks to inspire interpreters to become impassioned contributors to actions that support patient safety, quality of care, health equity and social justice.

Finally, this guide can provide a helpful platform to discuss how language and communication barriers play out in health inequity. The author's cherished long-term goal is to contribute to meaningful strategies for change that can help to reduce, and perhaps one day eliminate, health disparities rooted in language barriers.

Most chapters also address cultural competence, language access and advocacy.

How do I use the book?

For self-study

How the book works

The Healthcare Interpreter prepares you for real-life challenges in hospitals and clinics. Each chapter addresses a medical specialty or service and opens with a complex clinical role play followed by a discussion of its linguistic, professional, ethical and cultural challenges. The next section addresses one of the U.S. national ethical principles and standards for healthcare interpreters followed by practical exercises. Each chapter closes with a medical diagram labeled in English and Spanish, a second diagram with blank labels (for interpreters to fill in) and a list of terminology related to that chapter.

Try to find a "study buddy"

This book will be easier to study if you can find one other interpreter to study with. We call that person your "study buddy." However, you can also study this book on your own.

Do the role play first

First, find two volunteers (not your "study buddy" if possible). Ideally, each person will speak at least one of your working languages. Ask them to record the role plays on a smartphone or recorder. Don't look at the role plays ahead of time but let your volunteers do so.

Ask your volunteers to read each role out loud for recording as follows:

- The person who plays the health professional reads the text in English.
- The person who plays the patient reads the text in either Spanish (using the Spanish-English version of the role play); English (if that person speaks no other working language); or your other working language (e.g., Twi, Arabic, Bengali, Mandarin, Russian, etc.).
    - In other words, if the person playing the patient speaks a language other than English or Spanish that you interpret, ask that person *to read the patient's text out loud in the other language during the recording* (not sight translating it word for word, but reading it out loud in the other language to give the same general meaning).

If you cannot find two volunteers, it is still helpful to do this recording with you as one of the volunteers and/or your "study buddy" (if you have one) as a volunteer.

Save these role play recordings somewhere where they will not be erased and you can easily find them later, such as a computer hard drive, on your smartphone or tablet or in the cloud. When you are ready to start each chapter, pull out a separate smartphone or recorder. As you listen to your previous recording for that role play, use another device to *record yourself interpreting what you hear into your other working language.*

(Spoken-language interpreters can record audio only if they wish, or on video; signed-language interpreters would need to record themselves on video.)

Once you start self-recording your interpretation of the role play, do not:

- Correct yourself.
- Look up words.
- Stop the recording until you finish the role play for any other reason than to interpret (or for an emergency).

Do, however:

- Relax! It's just an exercise. No one will see or hear you.
- Skip over (omit) any terms that you don't know.
- Try not to worry about anything you can't interpret. Take it easy. That's why you're doing this practice: to learn.

Follow the exercises

After you finish recording the role play for a chapter, if you have a "study buddy," listen to your own recording and to each other's recordings and give each other helpful feedback. Start with at least three aspects of the interpreting that were successful. Then give kind suggestions for improvement.

If you are studying alone, listen to your recording and note down any difficult terms or passages that you struggled with. Then read the whole chapter that follows that role play you recorded and do all the suggested exercises.

Interpret the role play again

This activity is very important. After you complete the reading and exercises in the chapter, go back to the same role play you recorded yourself interpreting for—*and do it again.*

Yes: even though you have just analyzed that role play in detail and you now know all the terms in it, *doing the role play a second—or third or fourth—time isn't redundant: it's beneficial.*

The scenarios in these role plays are rich and real, spanning sensitive topics, including human immunodeficiency virus/acquired immunodeficiency syndrome (HIV/AIDS), gender identity and genetics counseling. As you face difficult decisions in the role plays and then work through the exercises in each chapter, you will find value in executing the role plays a second time. In fact, do them again and again, as often as you wish. It is still helpful and beneficial practice.

For use in class

Here are a few suggestions for class use that the publisher has found helpful.

Allow four to five hours of class time per chapter

The publisher of this textbook is also a U.S. national training agency. At the time of publication, Cross-Cultural Communications has about 400 licensed trainers for its programs in 43 U.S. states;

Washington, DC; Guam; Puerto Rico and six other countries. (See www.cultureandlanguage.net for more information.)

We have discovered that each chapter in this book appears well suited to approximately a half-day's work in class. For university instructors who teach three hours at a time, it may be possible to assign some of that work, such as the role plays, to language labs or assignments where three interpreters meet in person or via an online videoconference platform to record the role plays live.

Launch with the role play

We recommend, after the class begins, that each session based on a single chapter of this textbook begin with the students or learners in groups of three (or more, depending on the role play) acting out the role play for that chapter.

Here are the reasons for this recommendation. Each chapter begins with a role play dialogue or script. The content of that scenario acts as a thematic anchor for the chapter. Role plays are a standard component in the training and education of medical interpreters. Such dialogues provide an opportunity for simulated, realistic practice in the appropriate modes of interpreting (consecutive, simultaneous and sight translation). Role play scripts in this book are set in authentic U.S.-based clinical encounters that target a particular area of healthcare and the human body.

In addition:

- Interpreters need advanced practice in simulated clinical settings and rarely get enough of it.
- Interpreters and students of interpreting tend to learn more from these chapters when they are first exposed to the challenges in the chapter by executing the role play before addressing the chapter's discussions, exercises, readings, applications and terminology practice.
- The emotional impact of these role plays can motivate learning and inspire compassion for all parties to the encounter as they work through the rest of the chapter.
- Role plays like these engage interpreters' minds, hearts, reason, professionalism, past learning and their sense of emotional connection to the work they perform.

Each role play comes in two versions: an English-English version (where, during live practice, the person who plays the patient or a patient's family member would be expected to sight translate the English text into the interpreter's other working language) and an English-Spanish version, where the text for the patient (and for any patient family members) is in Spanish.

How to execute role plays

With the exception of Chapter 10, all dialogues in this book are intended to be acted out by interpreters for practice. Here are a few guidelines to help make such practice more effective and beneficial.

First, wherever possible, try to ensure that all the participants share the same working languages and take turns playing the interpreter, regardless of skill level.

While practicing the role plays, participants who play the patient or provider (or family members of the patient) will ideally:

- Continue without stopping.
- Act out the scenario as *realistically* as possible. Inject emotion. Keep it real.
- NOT HELP THE INTERPRETER. Do not assist the person who plays the interpreter role by supplying a term when the interpreter gets "stuck" and can't remember what to say. (Remember: in real life, no one is there to help a medical interpreter!)
- Avoid speaking one sentence at a time. Don't help interpreters by making the exercise too easy. Speak at a normal rhythm.
- Avoid pausing for the interpreter: instead, allow the interpreter to manage the flow.
- Keep talking. Do not interrupt the dialogue to critique the interpreter, discuss a term or for any other reason but an emergency. Wait until the end to share comments.
- Note down, if you can, anything that the interpreter did well and any mistakes or terms that catch your attention.
- Try to allow extra time and give feedback at the end of the role play, offering the interpreter positive feedback first, then suggestions for improvement. After doing so, it can be helpful to discuss the challenging terms or regionalisms used.
- Avoid reading the footnotes while acting out the role plays. Read them and discuss them *before* or *after* acting out the role plays.

If necessary, one person could play both the patient and any family members present. One person can also play, as needed, both the health professional and the patient.

Those who play the interpreter in role plays should try to:

- Continue without stopping.
- Stay in character. (Don't say things like, "Oh, no, I forgot that term," or, "Sorry, let me start over.")
- Avoid panicking over unfamiliar words. Relax. Just keep going.
- Let go of mistakes. Ignore them. Continue. Your job in role plays is to practice and improve—to make mistakes and learn from them.
- Take notes, instead of interrupting the speakers, wherever possible.
- Increase your concentration:
    - Practice active listening.
    - Avoid eye contact.
    - Breathe from the abdomen—not from your chest or throat.
- Remember you are here to learn—not to be perfect.

Following these suggestions will greatly improve the quality of role play practice.

Debriefing

After each role play, it is helpful to debrief by asking participants how the practice went and what they felt. If language coaches can provide them with language-specific feedback at this time, so much the better.

Each role play includes specific medical terms and common vocabulary. The Spanish texts also offer a variety of regionalisms spoken by many immigrant populations in the United States. They reflect the varied sociolinguistic registers of both formally educated and low-literacy patients. The Spanish role plays include rural and urban varieties of Spanish from across Latin America. Thus, the Spanish text might be typical of language spoken in parts of México, El Salvador, Nicaragua, Perú and Cuba.

The English versions are intended to replicate the various registers, tones and linguistic complexity to the extent possible.

Students of any language pair are encouraged to share their knowledge of regionalisms with each other after practice sessions and discuss the valuable information in the footnotes to these role plays. However, *students will ideally avoid interrupting role play practice to discuss these issues—or anything else.*

Discussion questions

Questions about professional and ethical challenges are built into the dialogues, footnotes and suggested readings in addition to the guided exercises. Participants are encouraged to explore questions of race, class, sociolinguistics, gender and any other themes that emerge during practice or discussion, for all of these can influence interpreters' responses while interpreting.

Exercises

There is typically no time for a given group of interpreters or students to execute every exercise in the book in class. Therefore, it is helpful for instructors to choose which exercises and activities to conduct in class and which to hand out as assignments.

Practical exercises

This book offers exercises to reinforce the reader's, student's or training participant's understanding of the content and related best practices. For example, each chapter contains a section titled "Ethics and standards: Reflect and practice" with exercises based on *A National Code of Ethics for Interpreters in Health Care* (NCIHC, 2004) and *National Standards of Practice for Interpreters in Health Care* (NCIHC, 2005). These activities review specific ethical principles or standards and explore how to implement and act on them in real-life encounters.

Other exercises encourage the reader to reflect on or discuss controversial topics, examine interpreter behaviors or reflect on critical interpreting challenges and healthcare issues related to the chapter's theme.

Anatomy and physiology

Opportunities for interpreter skill-building in medical terminology and basic knowledge of human anatomy are included. Bilingually labeled anatomical drawings accompany the dialogues, except for Chapter 10, which addresses pharmacology and telephone interpreting.

Suggested readings

Together with the exercises, suggested readings introduce relevant topics, such as:

- Language barriers in healthcare
- Health disparities and disparities in access to quality care among minority populations
- The role of the interpreter
- Language access laws and requirements
- Patient advocacy
- Language access advocacy

Inclusion of these topics highlights the compelling links between medical interpreting, public health and social responsibility.

Conclude the class with a reiteration of the role play

The impact of having your class redo the role play after rich classroom discussions, practical exercises and work on medical terminology can be powerful. The use of the intervening time has laid the groundwork for a much more confident, accurate and emotionally prepared execution of the role play.

Even seasoned hospital interpreters have found repeating the role plays a powerful reinforcement and helpful for their professional development.

Appendices

Resources for medical interpreters

Appendix 1 lists practical resources that can help the novice or intermediate interpreter continue professional development. From websites to dictionaries and training programs, these resources are critically important for U.S.-based medical interpreters.

Language access resources

Appendix 2 includes a list of references and information about language access advocacy and resources relevant to U.S. interpreters in healthcare and the staff of U.S. healthcare organizations, including practitioners. Printable hands-on aids are included. Readers are encouraged to use them.

Glossaries

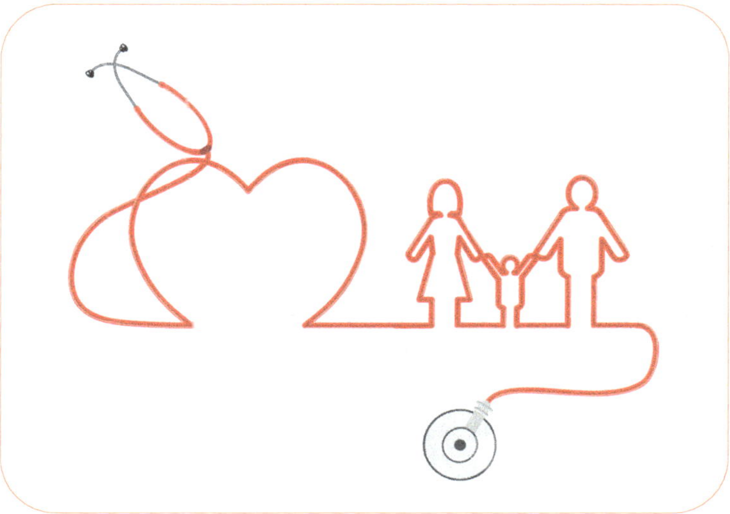

Appendix 3 offers an English-Spanish/Spanish-English glossary in addition to an English glossary that includes blank spaces for the non-Spanish interpreter to insert translations of each term into another language. This appendix may prove useful in preparing for role play practice. It can also add to the background knowledge of interpreters who study this textbook. It is intended to help interpreters make sure they know and understand the terms that a medical interpreter today is expected to master.

Training participants can, of course, add to this glossary with the support of peers, enriching their learning and helping to maximize the benefits of a training program based on this book.

Non-Spanish interpreters can find equivalent terms in their other working language(s), a powerful exercise to help them study these terms.

Medical terms: A study guide

Appendix 4 is a list of terms that any interpreter in a hospital or other complex clinical setting should be prepared to interpret. The purpose of the list is (a) to help interpreters test themselves to see if they know the terms in their other working language(s); (b) help interpreters who cannot use Appendix 3 because they are not Spanish-speaking to research and write down the translation of each term in this list in their non-English working language(s) to study and learn it.

Theoretical framework

The pedagogical or educational approach of this textbook supports listening, dialogue, reflection and action, all important elements of critical pedagogy as defined by the Brazilian educator, Paulo Freire. This book is intended to motivate critical thinking and to identify social contexts, root causes, challenges and outcomes that interpreters, as conscious participants, can help to shape or influence.

Many factors that contribute to health disparities are rooted in perceptions of language, ethnicity and race. Interpreters, consciously or unconsciously, hold their own perceptions. These perceptions may mirror or conflict with the views of others. As a result, this book encourages a view of healthcare interpreting within a broader context of social justice.

Although research does not yet appear to address this topic, it has become clear that in the United States, in contrast to many other countries and regions such as Canada and the United Kingdom, the profession of healthcare interpreting (like social work) is in many ways a social justice profession anchored within a public health perspective. Yet even in those countries that prohibit or discourage *patient advocacy* by healthcare interpreters, the social justice dimension of the work performed by interpreters is often nearly impossible for the interpreter to ignore and can be addressed through *language access advocacy*.

A note on *language access* advocacy

It's important to bear in mind that there are different definitions of "advocacy" depending on context. A chapter section from another textbook (*The Medical Interpreter: A Foundation Textbook for Medical Interpreting*, Section 5.3)[2] is reproduced before Chapter "Read This First: Important Information for You, the Interpreter"; it is a guide to *patient advocacy, in the individual medical encounter*. In public health, this context would be referred to as the "downstream" setting. Advocacy in this context occurs as a response, intervention, or strategy to mitigate negative impacts.

Patient Advocacy	Language Access Advocacy
During individual health encounter	**Outside individual health encounter**
Responsive	**Preventive**
"Downstream"	**"Upstream"**
Often addresses individual behaviors and actions	**Often addresses systemic, structural barriers and supports**
More controversial re: interpreter role	**Less controversial re: interpreter role**

There are other important forms of advocacy that can be practiced appropriately by interpreters and are urgently needed. What is *not* a focus of the reproduced section on advocacy is how interpreters can promote understanding, educate and shape informed policy through many venues to promote *language access advocacy, outside the individual medical encounter*, in the "upstream "setting. Advocacy in this context occurs as a prevention, intervention or strategy to improve structures, decrease barriers and support access to care.

These activities can occur appropriately in a wide range of venues, from participation on advisory councils, to contributing to provider educational training, to discussions with medical providers and administrators, to reporting and documenting incidents and systems that—because of language or national origin—allow for inequities in care, risks, threats or negative outcomes for patient health.

Both kinds of advocacy are urgently needed, but how and when advocacy takes place is key, and the truth is that advocacy in any form is not without risks.

Putting the interpreter's unique bilingual, bicultural perspective to maximum use for the benefit of improved language access is an opportunity. Anyone who is concerned for those unable to speak the language of service, and for equity in general, cannot afford to lose this opportunity.

Advocacy, in this context, is a matter of human dignity and of life and death.

2 Bancroft, M.A., García-Beyaert, S., Allen, K., Carriero-Contreras, G., & Socarrás-Estrada, D. (2016). *The Medical Interpreter: A Foundation Textbook for Medical Interpreting*. (M. A. Bancroft, Ed.). Columbia, Maryland: Culture & Language Press.

A note on *patient* advocacy

Interpreters can, and do, exert a certain amount of control in a health encounter. They sometimes intervene to address communication and access barriers while acting within their role. If such strategies fail, patient safety is at risk. Relevant U.S. state laws and requirements addressing medical interpreters permit advocacy; therefore, interpreters can also step out of their role to take action to protect patients and their health outcomes. Legal or professional ethical requirements and restrictions surrounding interpreter advocacy vary from country to country.

This book takes the view that healthcare interpreters *are obligated to prevent medical harm and point out inequities that could impact patient safety.* Whether one refers to taking such action as "intervening," "cultural mediation," "reporting critical incidents" or "advocacy," the action itself is often necessary and urgent.

Patient safety first. If the patient is allergic to a certain medication and the interpreter knows that information from another encounter, but the provider here is about to administer the medication—is it realistic or appropriate to expect the interpreter to stand by and say nothing? What if the surgeon is about to operate on the wrong limb?

To many interpreters, service providers, institutions and government agencies that regulate or oversee the activities of medical interpreters, the term *advocacy* can be seen as problematic, high-risk or even forbidden to interpreters. However, the interpreter's work and conduct often have a huge impact on the access of Limited English Proficient (LEP), Deaf and hard-of-hearing patients to services. It can also influence their quality of care, adherence to treatment plans and understanding of preventive health.

Interpreters are important partners in healthcare delivery. They play a powerful role in maintaining or shaping the status quo. Properly guided, they can help to reduce health inequities.

Does all this happen when someone is "*just*" an interpreter? How does perception of the interpreter's role influence their performance? Is the interpreter a neutral facilitator, a member of the treatment team, an institutional representative or a patient advocate? What are the limitations of the interpreter as a language access advocate (acting outside the encounter on the interpreter's own time) or as a patient advocate (acting before, during or after the encounter)? Do these different roles support the same or different ends? Are the two types of advocacy in conflict?

Step back a moment. What *is* advocacy? Is advocacy permitted? Should it be? If so, is advocacy more successful *inside* or *outside* a professional role or an institution? Is it more appropriate in the individual patient appointment or in a broader context?

To clarify the many questions that surround advocacy in healthcare interpreting, since it is a central theme in this book, as mentioned above, Section 5.3 of *The Medical Interpreter: A Foundation Textbook for Medical Interpreting* has been reproduced before Chapter 1, both as a thematic introduction and a clarification of what is understood by the author and the publisher of this textbook as patient advocacy.

Thus, this curriculum is intended not only to support the training and education of interpreters; but also to tackle the ever-evolving role of interpreters in healthcare. The author hopes that this book will encourage deeper and wider discussion of the interpreter's role in healthcare.

Acknowledgments

There are people whom without this book would never have happened. Of one thing I am sure; these words can't possibly reflect the depth of my gratitude.

Margarita Antonetti, words can't convey the value of your support, contribution and faith. Margarita so generously spent many Sundays with me, reading, reviewing and proofreading the Spanish and the English, discussing content and sharing her wisdom and her home; she offered unwavering encouragement even in the face of adversity and difficult times. She pulled in her husband Mikel De Sanctis, who was so generous with technical support, ideas and warmth. Thank you, *compañeros del año de la rata, son maravillosos.*

Marjory Bancroft at Cross-Cultural Communications, LLC, is my *chevalier* in shining armor. I had the honor of attending a training with her, "Healing Voices: Interpreting for Survivors of Torture, War Trauma and Sexual Violence." Her expertise, professionalism and accessible glow drew me to her with the idea of publishing this manual. From the start, Marjory responded with enthusiasm and encouragement. She and Michelle at Cross-Cultural Communications have been absolutely kind and supportive of my novice dip into these waters, educating and reassuring me all the way. Thanks for including me in your circle.

Thank you to my wonderful son Shaíl, who grew from a young boy to a young man during the course of this work, *volim te*. Thank you to my mother Ann, who taught me to love languages and explore the world, who babysat, listened and always encouraged me; *hvala ti mama, gde god da si.* Thank you to my sister Diana, for her support, for sharing her knowledge and experience in health provision and access, for her artistic inspirations and her encouragement. Thanks Becky, you are here too.

I am grateful to you, Rebecca Denison, for decades of friendship, family, wisdom and encouragement, for educating me and for your invaluable advice and contribution to this book. Thanks to Daniel Johnston for always being there to back me up.

Thank you to so many other friends, family and colleagues who have been so supportive all along the way, listening and understanding that interpreting is about social equity and healing. Thank you, Elizabeth Milos, for never giving up; to Wendi Felson and the University Professional and Technical Employees (UPTE) for standing up for us. Thank you, Rikki. Thank you, Lisa Gottreich, the Rhinos; Lorain Woodard, Lucia López, Andi Kuster; to Katie Spence, Susan Payne, Laurinda and Alex Ross, many thanks for your friendships and examples. A salute to the spark, Djohra Chaboub, Georgia Shreiber and Juliana Van Olpen.

I am grateful to the many friends and family not mentioned by name; to the excellent health providers, interpreter colleagues and social workers I have worked with and to the patients who shared their lives with yet another stranger and taught us at every encounter; to my colleagues on the National Council on Interpreting in Health Care (NCIHC) listserv.

To all of you, an enormous, heartfelt "Thank you. Gracias."

About the author

Suzanna Reiss-Končar worked as a staff medical interpreter for more than 20 years at the University of California, San Francisco Medical Center, a teaching hospital. She holds a bachelor of arts (BA) degree in community studies from the University of California at Santa Cruz, a master of public health (MPH) degree from San Francisco State University and a certificate in legal and medical interpreting from San Francisco State University. She obtained a California teaching credential and studied Serbo-Croatian in Belgrade and Spanish in Latin America. She is a Certified Healthcare Interpreter™ (CHI™).

Suzanna's past work experience spans immigration defense, community health initiatives and teaching in public schools. Her advocacy initiatives include establishing a hospital certification requirement for new-hire interpreters (Certification Commission for Healthcare Interpreters—CCHI—or National Board of Certification for Medical Interpreters—NBCMI), instituting language competency testing for healthcare providers and promoting compliance with language access laws. She also supports patient and provider education that links equity in healthcare provision to health and safety outcomes.

Advisory

Part of the beauty and the challenge of working as a medical interpreter is that you never know what you will encounter. There's so much that's interesting and sometimes unexpected.

For this reason, certain chapters in this book tackle important topics, such as human immunodeficiency virus/acquired immune deficiency syndrome (HIV/AIDS); sexually transmitted infections (STIs, which might develop into sexually transmitted diseases or STDs); sexual orientation; gender identity and intimate partner violence (domestic violence). These are topics that arise often in healthcare settings. However, if you or someone close to you has suffered trauma related to these issues, some of the dialogues in this book might be difficult for you to read or practice. Before going on, please take a moment to consider whether you are ready for such material.

If you are interested in interpreting for survivors of trauma, torture, child abuse, intimate partner violence (domestic violence) or sexual assault, please consider getting specialized training and preparation first. Also, look for training on how to protect yourself from vicarious trauma. It's real.

If you are *not* planning to do this kind of interpreting but *are* planning to interpret in hospitals and other healthcare settings, please *also* seriously consider specialized training and preparation about interpreting for trauma. In healthcare settings, you cannot always know in advance what you might be expected to interpret. The vast majority of medical interpreters will interpret traumatic content.

Back yourself up with information first. Then get support when you need it. For example, download the free training manual and workbook called *Breaking Silence: Interpreting for Victim Services* (Bancroft et al., 2016[3]). Practice the realistic role plays in the workbook (for example, about domestic violence and sexual assault). Don't ignore your own symptoms of vicarious trauma in real life, such as anxiety or nightmares about what you interpreted, or physical feelings, such as lightheadedness, nausea or shortness of breath that arise while you interpret. Check in with yourself from time to time. Take care of yourself.

If you feel disturbed or upset after an assignment, often you can find support services in the healthcare facilities where you interpret or the language service that sent you to the assignment. If no one is available to debrief you or support you, often someone can point you in the right direction. For service providers, such as health professionals and social workers, this kind of support is often routine. Seek it yourself.

[3] Available at https://static1.squarespace.com/static/5597f49ce4b07b7dda504921/t/5995f33b1e5b6c564a79fe40/1502999358619/Breaking+Silence+Training+Manual.pdf.

Guide to exercises

Embracing national ethics and standards

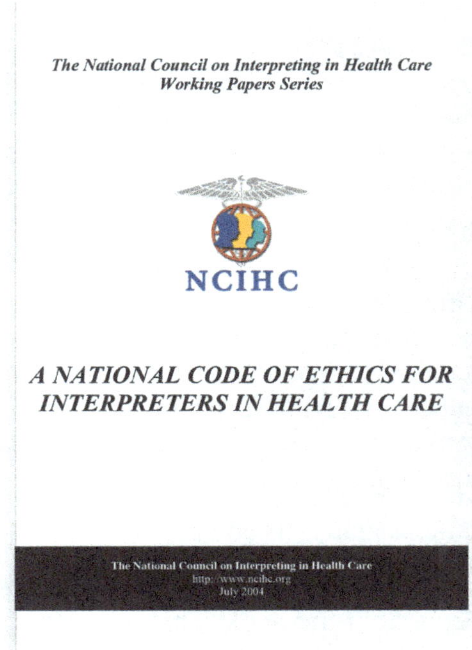

Whether you practice as an interpreter in the United States or another country, it is important to become familiar with the code of ethics and standards of practice that apply to you.

In the United States, interpreters are fortunate to have widely accepted national ethics and standards for interpreters in healthcare. They were developed and published by the National Council on Interpreting in Health Care (NCIHC). You can find these documents along with information about the collaborative process that led to their creation at www.ncihc.org.

NCIHC. (2004). *A National Code of Ethics for Interpreters in Health Care*

NCIHC. (2005). *National Standards of Practice for Interpreters in Health Care*

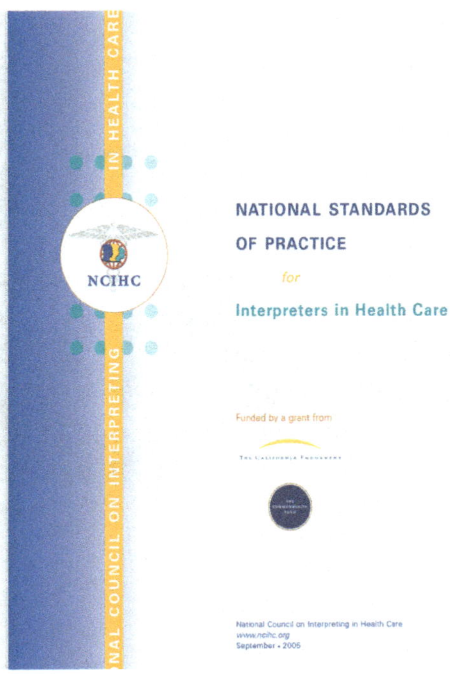

These U.S. national ethics and standards were the result of a national process with contributions from multiple stakeholders and experts, including interpreters, researchers, health professionals, policymakers, language services, interpreter service coordinators, trainers and educators, government agencies and others. The two documents are the product of a considerable amount of time, work, integrity and commitment. They are likely to evolve.

While codes of ethics and standards for interpreters around the world have much in common, many variations also exist. For purposes of the exercises in this training guide, please refer to the national ethics and standards published by NCIHC. To review ethics and standards for interpreters compiled from around the world, contact the publisher at clp@cultureandlanguage.net.

If you live in a country that has no national standards for medical interpreters, you can research various documents and decide which one seems best for you and your region. In many U.S. institutions and services today, medical interpreters are expected to know and adhere to the NCIHC national ethics and standards.

Disclaimer

This publication serves as a textbook and a resource for the training and education of interpreters. Although medical topics are addressed here, none of the content in this book should be used as, or considered to be, medical advice. This book is not intended to teach health professionals how to practice medicine. Many of the healthcare role plays and encounters included here are intended to be realistic to facilitate the training of interpreters, but such material does not constitute medical advice or medical opinions. **Do not use this textbook to make decisions about healthcare or treatment.**

All names used in the dialogues in this book are fictitious. Any resemblance between the characters in these materials and actual people, living or dead, is unintentional.

Note that the terms "medical interpreter" and "healthcare interpreter" are used synonymously throughout the book. They refer to any interpreter who interprets in healthcare settings for staff, patients and patients' families.

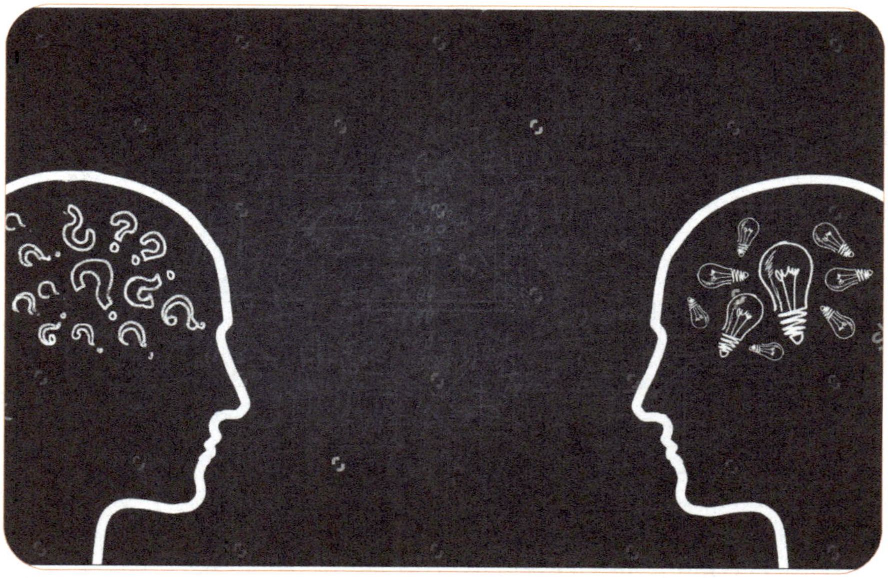

Guide to advocacy

The following excerpt is taken from Chapter 5 of a textbook called ***The Medical Interpreter: A Foundation Textbook for Medical Interpreting.*** (García-Beyaert, 2016, pp. 259-266). This excerpt should be used as basic guidance to inform the discussions in this book related to patient safety, quality of care and advocacy.

Advocacy and Medical Interpreters

Learning Objective
After completing this section, you will be able to:
Apply a decision-making protocol for advocacy to medical interpreting.

Overview

Should you advocate or not? This is a question that you will face often in the field. In general, there is no agreement about what advocacy even is–and far less agreement about whether interpreters (including medical interpreters) should perform it. Some U.S. hospitals forbid interpreters from advocating. According to national standards in Canada, interpreters are not permitted to advocate at all (HIN, 2007).

Still, in real life you will almost certainly run into situations where you will feel a desire to advocate. The goal of this section is to clarify the idea of advocacy and help you make effective decisions about whether or not to advocate and how to advocate if you choose to do so.

DEFINITION

Advocacy

Taking action or speaking up on behalf of a service user whose safety, health, well-being or human dignity is at risk, with the purpose of preventing harm.

Advocacy is understood as an action taken on behalf of an individual that goes beyond facilitating communication, with the intention of supporting good health outcomes. In general, advocacy means that a third party (in this case, the interpreter) speaks for or pleads the cause of another party, thereby departing from an impartial role.

NCIHC (2005, p. 11)

Learning Content

What is advocacy?

Defining advocacy

"Advocacy" is a fuzzy word. It means many different things. The authors of this textbook suggest a definition for advocacy in healthcare settings that you will find in the box on the right. NCIHC offers its own definition, which is the second definition (in italics) in the box on the right. Note that in the NCIHC definition, advocacy involves "departing from an impartial role." Because advocacy clashes with impartiality, many stakeholders across the country are not comfortable with the idea of suggesting that medical interpreters have to advocate.

Advocacy means stepping out of role

Interpreters, Ethics and Advocacy

It is important for medical interpreters to be aware that codes of ethics published by interpreting associations show differing approaches to advocacy. Some simply forbid it. For example, the AUSIT code from Australia (AUSIT, 2012) and the *National Standard Guide for Community Interpreting Services* (HIN, 2007) from Canada prohibit advocacy under the ethical principle of role boundaries.

In the United States, however, NCIHC and CHIA include advocacy among their ethical principles and standards for medical interpreters. After all, health professionals are often expected to advocate for patient safety. IMIA (2006) in its own code of ethics includes patient advocacy and intercultural mediation in the same ethical principle, suggesting that both actions are within the interpreter's role.

Advocacy is not part of your job

The NCIHC definition clearly shows that the interpreter who advocates steps out of role. The authors of this textbook agree. If you advocate, you are stepping out of your professional role as an interpreter.

As an individual interpreter, your role is limited to avoid interfering with the communication process of patient and provider.

Because advocacy involves taking actions beyond the interpreter role of transferring messages and enabling communication, only exceptional circumstances can justify advocacy on the part of the interpreter. You will have no choice if you encounter a serious risk to the safety, health, well-being or human dignity of the service user. You will have to advocate if that happens. But it also means that you will no longer be respecting professional ethics such as impartiality or role boundaries.

This section will help you clarify in your own mind what it means to "step out of role" and the potential consequences of doing so–for you and for others.

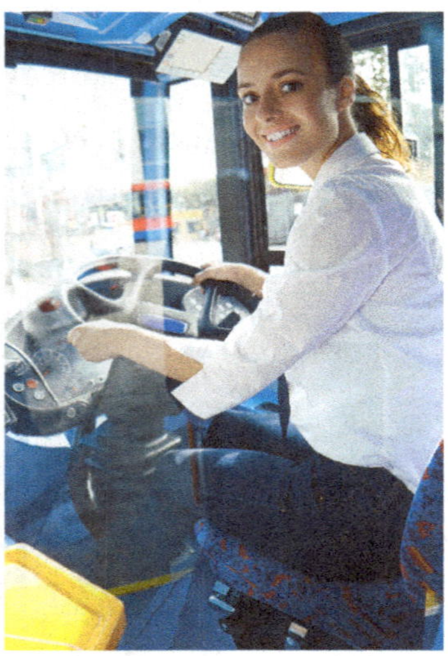

Advocacy can interfere with clear communication

Remember: provider and patient can only communicate effectively if they have communicative autonomy. To help parties be in control of their own communication process, your role is limited. Everyone at the encounter also needs to know what to expect of you. Take the example of the bus driver: for the bus system to work, every driver needs to follow their route and stick to the schedules. If interpreters start interfering with communication, providers and patients will be confused.

Since advocacy involves taking actions beyond the interpreter role of transferring messages and enabling communication, only exceptional circumstances can justify advocacy on the part of the interpreter. A serious risk to the safety, health, well-being or human dignity of the service user justifies advocacy, but that means you are breaching your professional ethics. When acting as an interpreter, avoid taking on an advocacy role.

Advocacy presents an ethical dilemma

When advocacy is necessary

It is worth repeating: when acting as an interpreter, avoid taking on an advocacy role. However, sometimes, *not* to take action is morally unacceptable. Perhaps someone is at risk of having surgery on the wrong part of the body. If the risk to a patient's safety, health, well-being or human dignity is serious enough, you may think that you have no other moral choice but to take action or speak up. It might simply be inhumane to stand by and do nothing.

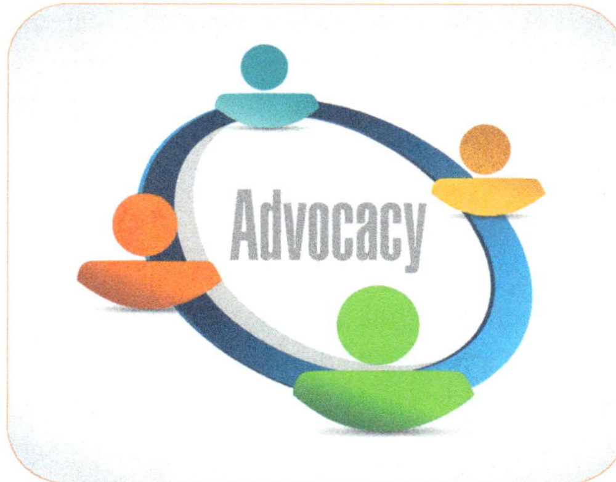

For example, you would not allow a bleeding patient to be ignored. After all, you have a simple, moral duty to help someone in extreme circumstances. No professional code of any profession has the right to ban anyone from acting morally. When we advocate, we are acting not so much as professional interpreters but rather as human beings.

Ethical dilemmas and advocacy

Whenever you advocate, you breach your ethical requirements such as impartiality and professional boundaries. If you face competing ethical or moral demands, you face an ethical dilemma. Whatever action you take, you will violate an ethical or moral requirement. Situations for interpreters that call for advocacy are, by definition, *ethical dilemmas*. The interpreter needs to choose between two options. None of the options is ideal. The interpreter needs to decide which is the "lesser evil," in other words, which one of the non-ideal options is the least harmful.

Weighing the pros and cons

Consider this example. The patient has an allergy to penicillin. You know that from a previous encounter. This time, the patient doesn't mention his allergy to the doctor, who prescribes a medication that you know contains penicillin. Should you look away and pretend it does not exist to respect interpreter role boundaries and remain impartial? Or should you set aside your professional ethics and act as you choose?

Neither of these two choices is appropriate because they show no effort to weigh the pros and cons. In a situation like this one, you need to engage in conscious decision-making before taking action. In fact, the first question to ask yourself here is: *should* I advocate?

Should I advocate?

The Advocacy Road Map

How to use the road map

Making decisions about advocacy is not easy. In García-Beyaert (2015), community interpreters were introduced to a simple "road map" to help them make decisions about advocacy–starting with whether or not to advocate at all. After all, only when the risk is important enough should you even consider advocating. Deciding whether a risk is serious enough to justify advocacy is your decision.

The road map discussed on the next pages will help by walking you through three simple steps to guide your decision-making process. The steps are presented in the form of questions. You decide the answer to each question before moving on to the next step.

Step 1: Decide why you want to advocate

The first step when you make a decision about advocacy as an interpreter is self-awareness. *Why* do you want to advocate? What causes you to feel or think the need to do so? If you are doing so for yourself, to feel better or because you are angry or upset—please do not advocate. Instead, ask yourself: *Is there a risk to someone's safety, health, well-being or human dignity?*

How Not to Advocate

Too often, interpreters advocate because they think they know better than others or because they have a great desire to help. These are not good or sufficient reasons to advocate. Advocacy is a decision to make based on the serious risk of harm to the patient.

Even when advocating is the right thing to do–it must be done in an appropriate and professional way. Here are examples of advocacy that were inappropriate.

I once interpreted for a poor family that had come to the U.S. for medical treatment. They had very little money and felt quite isolated due to the language barrier. So I went to church and told their story to my congregation. Soon, the family began to receive visits from church members. I know this helped them feel better during their stay in this country.

If I'm interpreting and I feel that the patient should get a second opinion, I probe the patient to see if this is what s/he wants. After I interpret the provider's diagnosis, I ask the patient (in the target language, of course), "Do you want to see another doctor?"

One provider was so rude to my patient, that at the end of the session, I offered to rebook the patient's appointment with a different provider. I never want any of my patients to be seen by that provider![4]

Step 2: Assess risk

The second step is to determine how serious the risk is. If you didn't advocate, would someone's safety, health, well-being or human dignity be at *serious* risk? If not, there is no need to take action. You can always monitor the situation to decide whether or not to advocate later. Your opinion might change if the risk changes.

If you think the risk is very serious, so serious that you are willing to step out of your professional role, consider advocacy. But remember: now you are acting as a human being. You have stepped out of your role as a professional interpreter. There might be consequences, even serious consequences. You could lose your job–or never be asked to interpret for the language service again. You might be stripped of your certification or even trigger a lawsuit or a court case. Be careful when you assess risk. Take this decision seriously.

4 Retrieved from https://embracingculture.com/wp-content/uploads/2014/12/ce_express_02_08.pdf

Step 3: Take action

The third step helps you decide *when* and *how* to take action–if it is truly needed. First, you will need to decide if the risk to the patient (or, in principle, anyone else) is *imminent* or not. Imminent means that something is about to happen. For example, if you know a domestic violence victim's bruises are from her husband because she told you so in the waiting room, but the patient doesn't tell the nurse, there is no *imminent* danger that you know of. The situation is serious and requires taking action soon, but it is not imminent. It would be imminent if the patient told you that she saw her husband following her before she came into the hospital and that she fears for her life right now.

If the risk is truly imminent, you would take action on the spot. You could disclose the situation to a health professional or call 911.

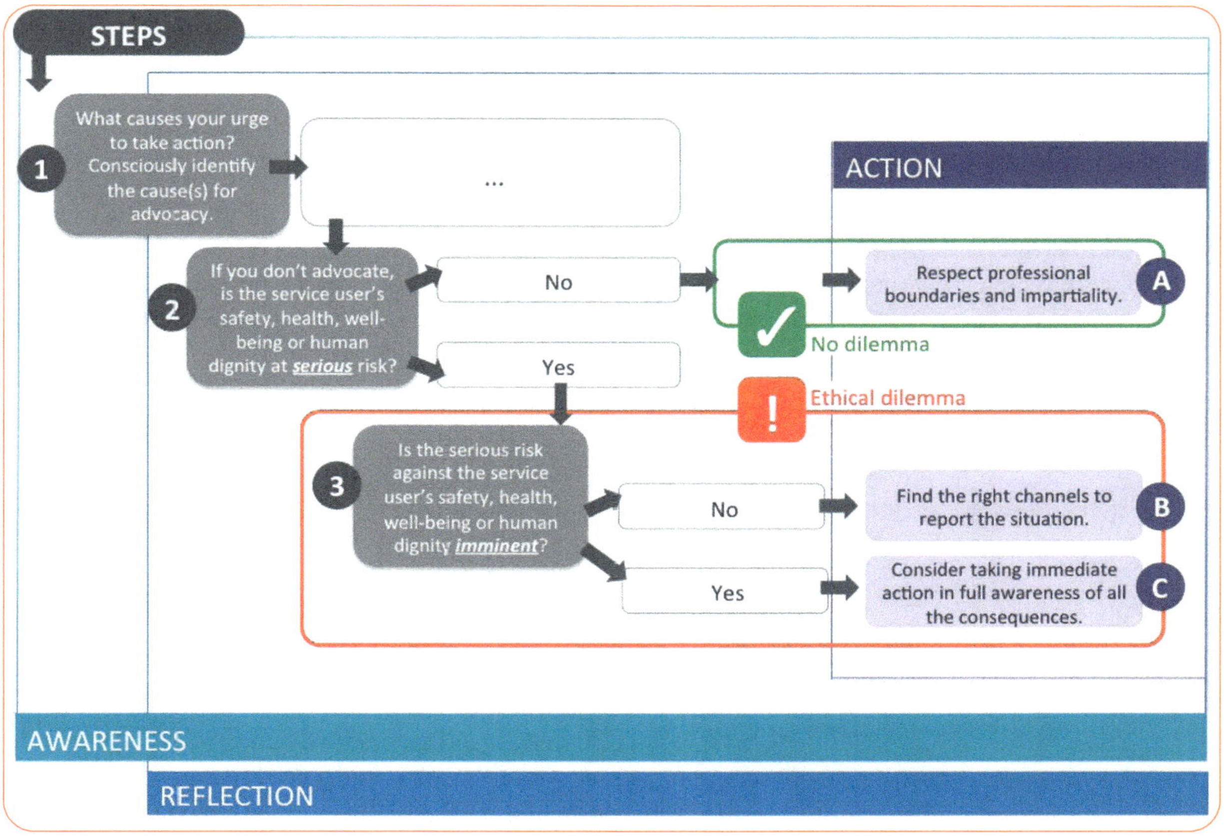

Figure 5-C: **A Road Map for Advocacy. Source: García-Beyaert (2015).**

How to advocate

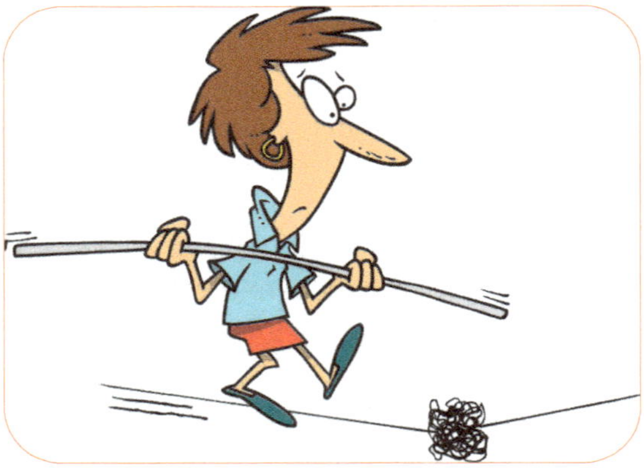

Action A: Continue interpreting

As you answer the questions in the Advocacy Road Map for steps 1, 2 and 3, you face different choices. If the risk of harm is not serious, simply act as a professional interpreter.

Actions B and C: Ethical dilemma zone!

If you do take action, it could be immediate, if the risk is imminent, or you could take action after the session. Whatever you decide to do, remember to always consider all your options carefully. You are in the ethical dilemma zone!

Action B: The risk is serious but not imminent

Use the system in place

If the risk of harm is serious, but not likely to happen very soon, consider taking action after the session, but try to work within the system in place. In other words, don't take a big burden on your shoulders or try to correct the situation alone. Taking action for nonurgent situations usually means reporting the problem to the appropriate person or office.

Reporting a problem

Let's say that a provider insulted a patient by making racist remarks that you interpreted. The patient was too timid to speak up. You think the provider might act the same way with other patients. After the session, you could find the right channels to report the situation. Depending on your employment status, what you decide to do could be quite different.

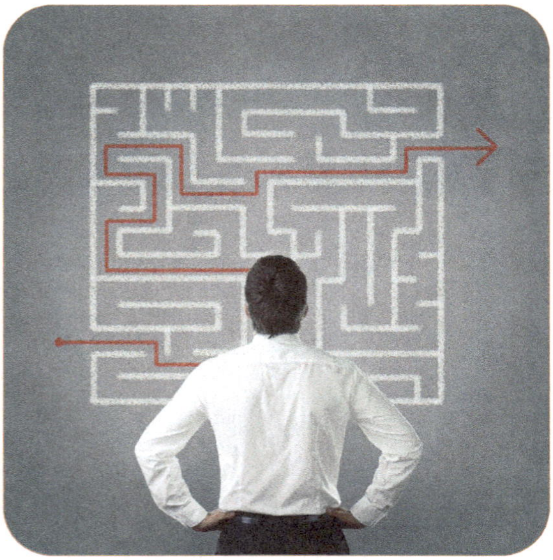

Employed interpreters

If you are a staff interpreter employed by the institution, or a bilingual employee who interprets as an extra duty, you could speak to the provider directly. If you don't think you can do so, instead you could report the situation to someone within the institution. When you make that report, you would try to follow established rules for reporting critical incidents. If you don't know the rules, you could report the incident to your supervisor. You might be asked to write a report. Respect patient confidentiality.

Self-employed and agency interpreters

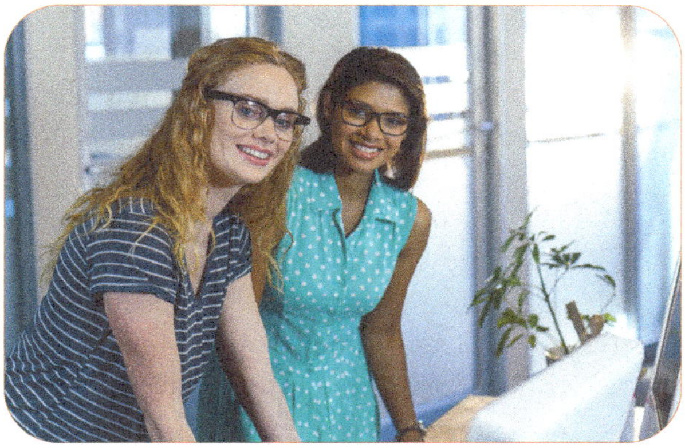

If you are a self-employed interpreter (a freelance interpreter or a contract interpreter) or an agency interpreter (an interpreter who works for a language service as an employee), you usually should not report to the institution where you interpreted (e.g., a health department). Instead, report to the agency that hired or contracted you. That agency assumes legal liability for your conduct. The agency will need to decide what to do about the situation you report. As a contract or agency interpreter, be especially careful before you reveal any details. Which information is confidential? Which is not? Think carefully.

Action C: The risk is serious and imminent

Liability

If the risk for the patient is not only serious but also imminent, then and only then consider taking action on the spot. Keep in mind that you are now acting not as an interpreter but as a human being. The consequences are your responsibility. Yet the legal liability for your actions could affect many parties–including the agency you work for (if you are an employee) or the agency that hired you (if you are self-employed). Think hard about the potential consequences of your advocacy–good and bad–because they could affect many other people and also organizations.

The penicillin example

Let's go back to the penicillin story. Imagine that a nurse is about to administer a drug to which you know the patient is allergic because it contains penicillin. What would you do? You might suggest that the provider ask, again, if the patient is allergic to any medication. If that doesn't work, you could step out of role to suggest that the nurse ask about allergies to penicillin. If at all possible, you would want that information to come from the patient, but if all else fails you could consider disclosing the allergy to prevent harm. Note that in its code of ethics, NCIHC specifically states that advocacy should be engaged in *only* after trying other options: "Advocacy must only be undertaken after careful and thoughtful analysis of the situation and if other less intrusive actions have not resolved the problem" (NCIHC, 2004, p. 3).

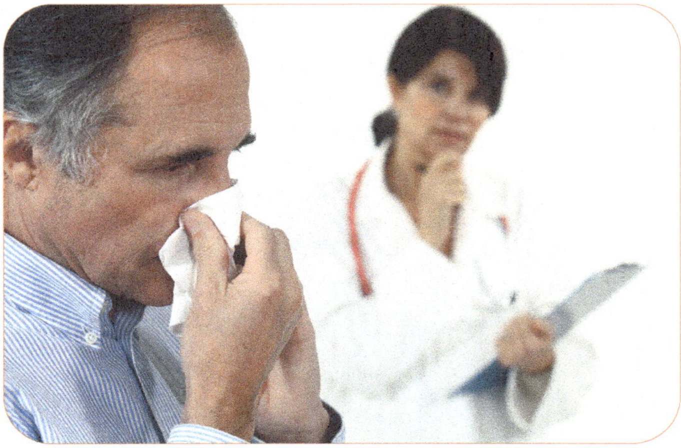

Review

Human situations in medical interpreting can be extreme. If you see an individual at risk of harm, especially a risk to a patient's safety, health, well-being or human dignity, you might want to advocate for that person. Yet each time you do, you are stepping out of your role as a professional interpreter. Situations that call for advocacy create an ethical dilemma. Two or more ethical or moral demands compete with each other.

The Advocacy Road Map included in this section offers a visual tool to guide your decision-making about advocacy. It includes a simple three-step process. The main criteria for decision-making are: 1. Decide why you want to advocate. 2. Assess the seriousness of the risk. 3. Determine how imminent a serious risk is. By walking yourself through these steps, you can decide whether or not to take action outside your role as a professional interpreter. Always remember that if you do, you are acting as a human being with a conscience. Sometimes advocacy is the right thing to do. Sometimes it is the *only* right thing to do.

Anesthesia 1

Advisory

This chapter involves a visit to a medical office and preparation for anesthesia prior to surgery.

Notes for acting out role plays

1. If you are acting out this role play for practice or in class, you might wish to read the role play first before acting it out.
2. This is a long role play. Consider switching the person who plays the interpreter at the beginning of each new section.
3. The English-only version that follows the English-Spanish version should be used for role players who do not interpret Spanish. If you are working with other individuals who speak your (non-Spanish) working languages, the person who plays the patient should sight translate that text into the other working language while acting out the role play. (The sight translation doesn't need to be exact. Just provide the general meaning.)
4. Remember, keep the role play real! Use your best acting skills. Don't interrupt. Don't help the interpreter or speak too slowly. Don't stop to discuss anything. Keep discussions for the end!

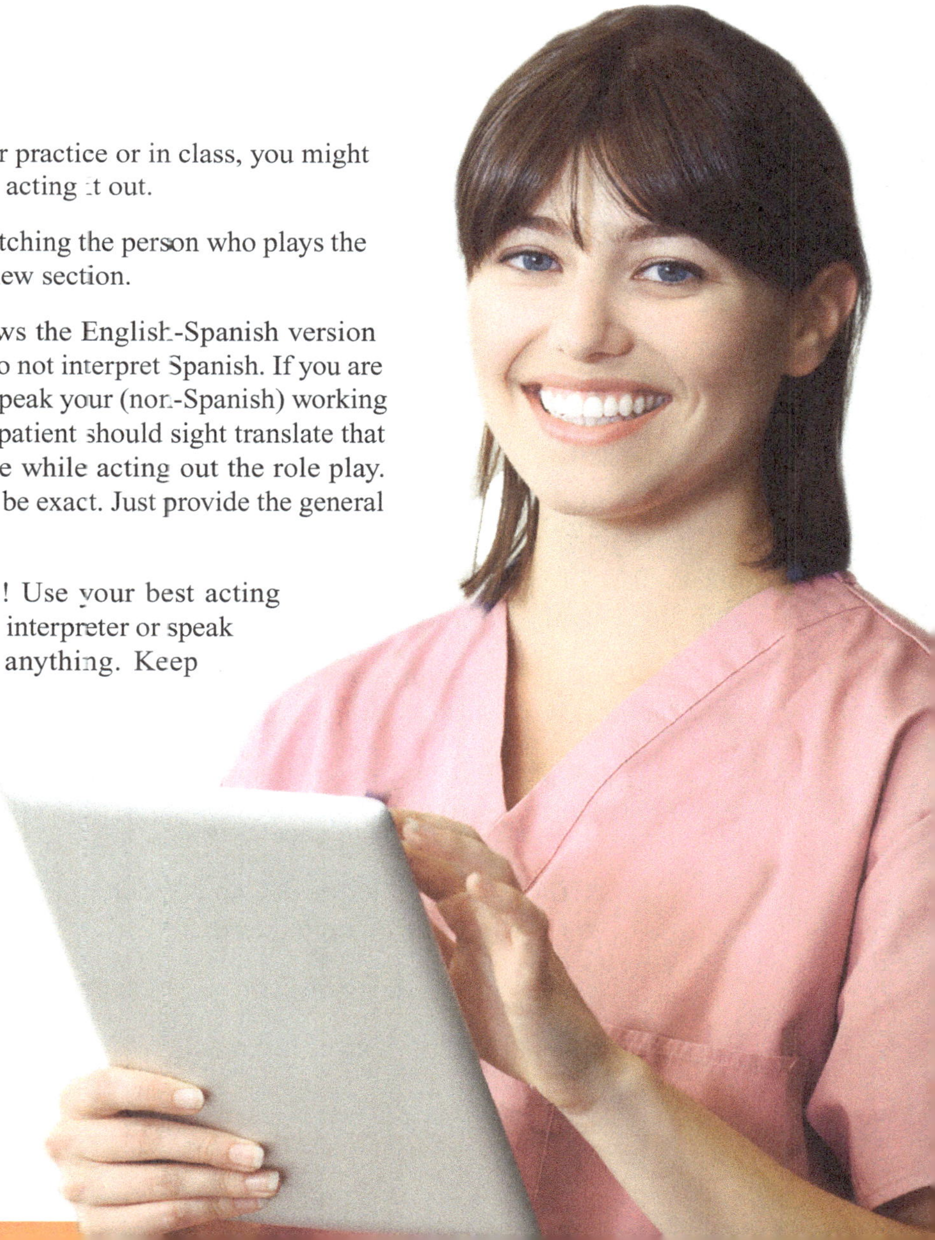

Note: *This patient is a 68-year-old woman, originally from Cuba (in the English-Spanish version of the role play). She has come for a presurgical checkup to clear her for anesthesia. The interpreter walks into the room where the nurse practitioner and patient are already seated.*

Preparation for anesthesia role play (English-Spanish)

PART 1

INTERPRETER: Good morning. My name is ______________. I'm your interpreter. I'd like to let you know that everything you say will be interpreted, and everything will be kept confidential. Please speak directly to each other, not to me, and pause when I make this signal *(raises hand)* so I can interpret.	**INTERPRETER:** Buenos días. Me llamo ______________. Soy su intérprete. Quisiera informarle que yo interpretaré todo lo que usted dice y que todo será confidencial. Por favor dirijánse directamente el uno al otro. Cuando yo le hago esta señal *(raises hand)*, por favor haga una pausa y permítame interpretar.

NURSE PRACTITIONER: Good morning, please have a seat.

PATIENT: Buenos días.

NURSE PRACTITIONER: Hello, Asteria Ruiz? Buenas tardes, my name is Jill.

PATIENT: ¿Buenas tardes?

NURSE PRACTITIONER: Oh, well, that's the only Spanish I know, so I have a translator here to help.

PATIENT: Muy bien, doctora, muy bien.

NURSE PRACTITIONER: Please have a seat, Mrs. Ruiz. So, as I was saying, I'm a nurse practitioner here in the anesthesia department and my job is to make sure everything is safe to go ahead and give you anesthesia for your surgery.

PATIENT: Muy bien, muy bien, pero llámeme Asteria. Cuando me dice "Sra. Ruiz," me hace sentir muy vieja.

NURSE PRACTITIONER: Very good, Asteria. Oh, I'm sorry. Can you wait just one minute, I left part of your file at another desk, I'll be right back.

PATIENT: ¡Por supuesto, doctora! *(Nurse practitioner leaves the room; patient turns to interpreter.)* Good morning. ¡Oh! ¿Usted habla español, ¿verdad? Y usted es enfermera?

INTERPRETER: No, yo soy intérprete.

PATIENT: ¿Y qué trabajo hace usted?

INTERPRETER: Yo interpreto. Como la enfermera no habla español y usted no habla inglés, yo les voy a servir como intérprete.

PATIENT: ¿Y es lo único que hace en todo el día? ¿Trabaja aquí todo el día, así?

INTERPRETER: Sí. Éste es mi trabajo. *(Nurse practitioner enters the room.)*

PATIENT: *(to the nurse practitioner)* ¿Puedo hacer una pregunta?

NURSE PRACTITIONER: Sure, go ahead.

PATIENT: ¿Me van a dormir completamente o me van a poner un sedante o cómo es eso? Es que la última vez que—

NURSE PRACTITIONER: Actually, we'll get to all of that, but I have some questions I wanted to ask about your health history first. Then I'll do a brief physical exam, listen to your heart and lungs and then we'll talk about anesthesia options. Will that be all right?

PATIENT: Claro que sí, doctora. Usted es la que manda. Aunque para serle franca, estoy un poco ansiosa.

NURSE PRACTITIONER: That's normal. Let's see if we can get through these questions first. Maybe that will help set you at ease. OK?

PATIENT: Vaya doctora.

NURSE PRACTITIONER: OK, so to start, how are you feeling, and how would you say your health is in general?

PATIENT: Muy bien doctora. ¡Más sana que una pera!

NURSE PRACTITIONER: All right, now, Mrs. Ruiz, can you tell me what they will be doing in this surgery?

PATIENT: Sí. A mí lo que va a hacer el doctor es quitármelo todo, de un tajo. Me va a quitar la matriz. Todo el equipo entero.

NURSE PRACTITIONER: OK, that's also what I have in your chart. I just wanted to make sure we were all on the same page. It says here that you're going to have a radical hysterectomy and lymphectomy. Is that what you understand?

PATIENT: Sí, doctora. Así es. Me van a quitar todo lo malo y espero que, si Dios quiere, lo vamos a resolver.

NURSE PRACTITIONER: Very good, Mrs. Ruiz. Now can you tell me if you are taking any medicines regularly?

PATIENT: Bueno, de vez en cuando me tomo mi Motrín si me duele la cabeza, y a veces me tomo algo para dormir porque me pongo muy nerviosa.

NURSE PRACTITIONER: And do you know the name of that medicine you take for sleeping?

PATIENT: Es algo así como Lorazam.

NURSE PRACTITIONER: Lorazepam or Ativan?

PATIENT: Sí, esa es la talla.

NURSE PRACTITIONER: That's often used for anxiety. Do you suffer from anxiety?

PATIENT: Pues, usted sabe doctora, con tantas cosas en la vida, los hijos, los nietos, uno se pone nerviosa. Y luego con esto. Como le dije, doctora, me fui para hacerme un simple Papanicolau, pensé que iba a ser salchicha. Y mire no más. No es cosa fácil dormir.

NURSE PRACTITIONER: And is that every night?

PATIENT: Pues antes...cada muerte de obispo. Ahora, usted sabe, es con más frecuencia.

NURSE PRACTITIONER: How often would you say you take that medicine?

PATIENT: Bueno, la tomé anoche, es que estaba nerviosa por este *apoingmen*, y la cirugía. Y creo que la tomé hace tres noches también.

NURSE PRACTITIONER: So, on average, would you say you take it twice a week, three times a week, five times a week?

PATIENT: Oh no, doctora, nada de eso.

NURSE PRACTITIONER: So how often would you say you take it?

PATIENT: Vaya, como una o dos veces a la semana. Quizás tres.

NURSE PRACTITIONER: All right. And when was the last time you took Motrin?

PATIENT: Oh eso, muy retirado.

NURSE PRACTITIONER: And when was the last time you took it?

PATIENT: Bueno, como a mi me dijeron que no debo tomarlo durante dos semanas antes de la operación y yo siempre sigo lo me dicen los doctores al pie de la letra, es que ustedes son los que mandan, no lo he tomado desde el comienzo del mes, el dos, creo. Tampoco he tomado aspirina, ni ibuprofén ni nada que lo contenga. ¿No está bien así, doctora?

NURSE PRACTITIONER: Excellent, Mrs. Ruiz. That's to protect you from bleeding unnecessarily.

PATIENT: Eso es lo que le dije a mi vecina. Le dije, "Estos doctores son todo poderosos benditos sean, y voy a hacer exactamente lo que me dicen". Algunas personas no quieren escuchar y yo digo—*(Nurse practitioner interrupts.)*

NURSE PRACTITIONER: Very good, Mrs. Ruiz.

PATIENT: Pues sí, yo siempre trato de cumplir con lo que me digan y gracias a Dios aquí estoy hasta ahora.

NURSE PRACTITIONER: All right, can you tell me if you have any allergies to medicines or anything else?

PATIENT: Pues, ahora mismo estoy con una coriza, no sé si es por el polen, pero no es mucho. Lo que me preocupa es que la última vez que me pusieron anestesia, tuve un problema grave. ¡Ave María! ¡Muchacha, casi me muero! Es que no podía respirar, fue una emergencia, casi me ahogo, no podía respirar.

NURSE PRACTITIONER: Oh yes, I see here in your chart that you were given some epinephrine at the dentist with a local anesthesia and you had a reaction. OK. Let me get that into your chart here, your workup for this anesthesia. I'll make sure the doctors see this, so they are prepared. Can you tell me what happened?

PART 2

PATIENT: Bueno, me pusieron la inyección esa, ¡y el corazón me latía como que se me quería salir del pecho! ¡Ave María Santísima!

NURSE PRACTITIONER: And what happened after that? What did you do?

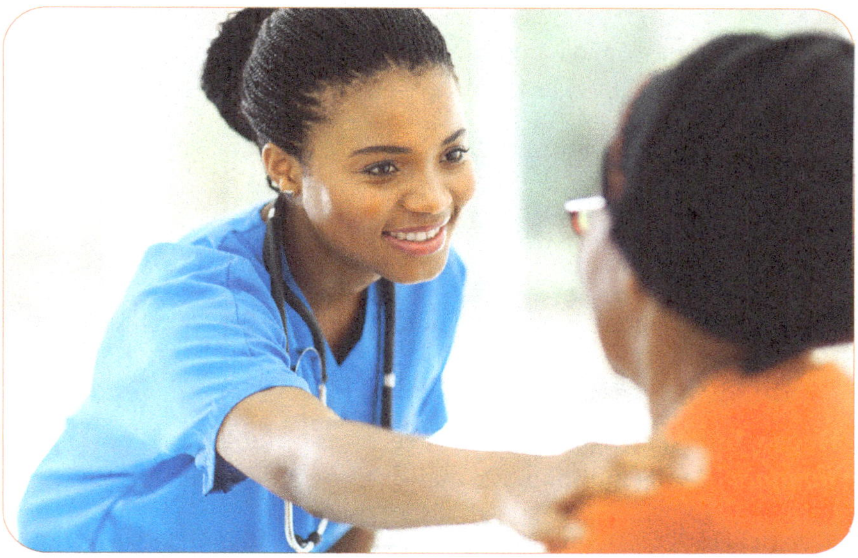

PATIENT: Después de un tiempo, se me fue calmando y ya. ¡Pero, como usted sabe, sentí que se me iba el caballo!

NURSE PRACTITIONER: And have you had anesthesia since then?

PATIENT: No, no, doctora.

NURSE PRACTITIONER: So you just had local anesthesia that one time?

PATIENT: No, no, no. La tuve con las niñas.

NURSE PRACTITIONER: What happened then? Did you have an epidural?

PATIENT: ¡Qué va, chica! ¡En mi tiempo no tenían esas cosas! Pero nacieron por cesárea. Pero eso fue en La Habana.

NURSE PRACTITIONER: Is that where you're from originally, Asteria?

PATIENT: Sí. Yo soy cubana, gracias a Dios.

NURSE PRACTITIONER: Oh? And why were your girls born by C-section?

PATIENT: Pues, con la primera, yo no era muy ancha de la cadera y no se me salía. Entonces me hicieron una cesárea. Con la segunda, pues ya sabe, tuvo que ser igual con la matriz, toda partida así.

NURSE PRACTITIONER: So you had general anesthesia those two times?

PATIENT: ¡Claro que sí! Y después me quedé arrullada como bebé en la cuna.

NURSE PRACTITIONER: Let's see then. That was two C-sections? Did you ever have anesthesia for anything else? Any kind of a study?

PATIENT: Sí. La segunda vez, después de la cesárea, se infectó la herida y viera. ¡Ave María Santísima! ¡Qué clase de peste! Me tuvieron que abrir de nuevo, limpiarlo todo.

NURSE PRACTITIONER: OK. And everything went well, with the anesthesia?

PATIENT: Sí, sí.

NURSE PRACTITIONER: And was that the only other time you had anesthesia?

PATIENT: Después también, cuando me hicieron un *tamitac*, después de mis cesáreas.

NURSE PRACTITIONER: Oh, so you had some cosmetic surgery?

PATIENT: Bueno, usted sabe, después de todas estas cirugías y los dos embarazos, luego me hicieron un *tamitac*. Menos mal. No hay mal que por bien no venga, ¿no?

NURSE PRACTITIONER: I guess so. And did you have a reaction to the anesthesia those times after that first reaction?

PATIENT: No, solamente un dolor de cabeza. ¡Pero tremendo dolor de cabeza, chica!

NURSE PRACTITIONER: OK. It seems like we can assume that the one time when you had the respiratory reaction, it was probably due to the epinephrine, and that isn't usually part of getting general anesthesia, but I'm going to note all this in your chart and leave it up to the anesthesiologist. You'll meet him or her the day of the procedure, and you can discuss it. I'll also let them know about the headaches. Maybe they can try to prevent that this time.

PATIENT: Bueno, pero espero que sea un doctor. Yo quiero que me vigile un doctor hombre. No quiero que sea una doctora. Las mujeres, para este trabajo, pues no son para eso.

NURSE PRACTITIONER: Well, I'm not sure who it will be, but I can assure you they'll take good care of you, and whoever it is will be qualified. In fact, it's usually a team of at least two doctors and a nurse for the anesthesia part of the surgery.

PATIENT: *Oká.*

NURSE PRACTITIONER: Mrs. Ruiz, you said you have a little bit of a runny nose, can you tell me what color it is? Is it clear, yellow or green?

PATIENT: Es clara, es un tincito nada más, desde hace poco. Es la temporada.

NURSE PRACTITIONER: And you sound pretty sure that it's just a little bit of hay fever. Did you have a temperature with that?

PATIENT: No, doctora, nada de temperatura ni na'.

NURSE PRACTITIONER: And have you had a cold or a cough or fever during the last two weeks?

PATIENT: No, doctora.

NURSE PRACTITIONER: Ms. Ruiz, how would you say your health is in general?

PATIENT: Vaya, yo digo que no está tan mal como algunas personas, diría que bastante bien. Como dije, más sana que una pera.

NURSE PRACTITIONER: Do you get any regular exercise?

PATIENT: Vivo en un quinto piso, y no uso el ascensor. Tengo un mes de visita aquí con mi hijo, pero cuando estoy en casa, la verdad es que camino mucho, camino por lo menos una hora todos los días. Ahorita voy a caminar.

NURSE PRACTITIONER: Oh, that's wonderful. Do you walk every afternoon?

PATIENT: No, no. Dije que voy a caminar *ahorita*.

NURSE PRACTITIONER: Well, it's beautiful outside, but be careful not to get overheated.

PATIENT: No, no. Voy a caminar *ahorita*. Durante el día, especialmente en Miami, hace mucho calor, así que acostumbro caminar en la noche.

NURSE PRACTITIONER: How about walking uphill? Do you get out of breath? Do you have any trouble with stairs? Can you go up two flights of stairs without any trouble?

PATIENT: Bueno, lo normal. Me agito[5] un poco como cualquiera.

NURSE PRACTITIONER: Does it make you stop because you're short of breath or need to rest?

PATIENT: No, no, no, no, no. Nada así. No, yo siempre he cuidado la cintura, siempre he hecho mi ejercicio.

NURSE PRACTITIONER: Good, that's great. Uh...do you have any problems with your heart?

PATIENT: A veces pienso que...que quizá, a veces siento piquetillos aquí...

NURSE PRACTITIONER: Have you ever seen a doctor about it?

5 What meaning does "agitarse" have in Spanish? Why do we call this a false cognate or "false friend"?

PATIENT: Bueno, hablé con mi doctora, pero ella me dijo que no era nada.

NURSE PRACTITIONER: Have you ever had an electrocardiogram? Any other kind of a heart exam?

PATIENT: Sí, sí, sí. Me hicieron todo antes de hacerme el *tamitac.*

NURSE PRACTITIONER: And was everything OK? Did they tell you there was any kind of a heart problem?

PATIENT: Oh, eso, no. Me dijeron que todo estaba normal, todo bien, fuerte como una yegua.

NURSE PRACTITIONER: OK, it sounds like you don't have any kind of a heart problem. But that was, let's see, in 1992. I think I'm going to recommend another EKG before this surgery just to make sure everything is fine, since this will be a longer surgery.

PATIENT: Como usted diga, doctora.

NURSE PRACTITIONER: Do you have any problems with your lungs, Mrs. Ruiz?

PATIENT: Pues, no sé. Como le digo, a veces me agito cuando subo unos tres o cuatro pisos, y una vez cuando cogí frialdad,[6] me puse muy mal, pasé seis semanas con una tos. Mi doctora me dijo que era algo así como una reacción en las vías áreas o bronquitis o algo así.

NURSE PRACTITIONER: Reactive airway disease?

PATIENT: Sí, sí, eso es lo que fue.

NURSE PRACTITIONER: And do you use any medicines for that, inhalers or nasal sprays?

PATIENT: Bueno, ya no.

NURSE PRACTITIONER: But you were prescribed something for that?

PATIENT: Me dió un aparato de esos, una bombita. Aluero, floruto o algo así para asma, pero yo no soy asmática.

NURSE PRACTITIONER: Was it Albuterol?

PATIENT: ¡Esa es la talla! ¡Albuterol! Pero lo usé esa vez, nada más.

NURSE PRACTITIONER: All right. Have you ever had bronchitis, bronchilitis or pneumonia?

PATIENT: No, que yo sepa, no.

NURSE PRACTITIONER: Have you ever tested positive for tuberculosis?

PATIENT: Bueno, en eso sí. Una vez salí como usted dice y tuve que tomar medicina durante unos seis meses. Pero no vieron nada. Me dijeron que no tenía la enfermedad pero que tenía que tomar las medicinas, una cápsula para prevenir.

NURSE PRACTITIONER: And when was that?

---

6 What is "coger frialdad" in Venezuela? In Nicaragua? In México? In the United States?

PART 3

PATIENT: ¡Uuh! Hace mucho tiempo, hace como unos 15 o 17 años, cuando llegué a Miami.

NURSE PRACTITIONER: OK. Let's see, do you have any problems with your liver?

PATIENT: No, nunca me han diagnosticado con nada así.

NURSE PRACTITIONER: Have you ever had hepatitis?

PATIENT: No, doctora, gracias a Dios.

NURSE PRACTITIONER: Have you ever had problems with your gallbladder, gallstones, for example?

PATIENT: No, doctora.

NURSE PRACTITIONER: How about your stomach or intestine?

PATIENT: A veces me pongo muy *elaste*.

PATIENT: *(to interpreter) Jani*, de dónde tú eres?

INTERPRETER: Soy de aquí.

PATIENT: ¡Ah, por eso, *Jani*, *elaste* quiere decir muy grande así, muy llena, inflada.

NURSE PRACTITIONER: And do you have heartburn or acid reflux?

PATIENT: Eso sí.

NURSE PRACTITIONER: And do you take anything for that?

PATIENT: Tums, me como unos Tums.

NURSE PRACTITIONER: How about your kidneys?

PATIENT: No, doctora.

NURSE PRACTITIONER: Have you ever had bladder infections or urinary tract infections or problems with your bladder?

PATIENT: No, tampoco doctora. Gracias a Dios.

NURSE PRACTITIONER: Do you have any problems with your thyroid?

PATIENT: No. Gracias a la Virgin Santísima.

NURSE PRACTITIONER: Do you have chronic headaches or migraines?

PATIENT: A veces me dan dolores de cabeza, pero dolor así fuerte, inaguantable, solamente esa vez después del *tamitac*.

NURSE PRACTITIONER: OK. Do you have diabetes?

PATIENT: No. Yo no soy diabética.

NURSE PRACTITIONER: High blood pressure?

PATIENT: La doctora me dice que estoy a punto de, pero no tomo nada todavía. Me dice que por el momento estoy bien, pero que me va a vigilar.

NURSE PRACTITIONER: Do you have any problems with your blood? Do you have trouble clotting or do you have any kind of blood disorder?

PATIENT: ¿La anemia se considera como una condición de la sangre?

NURSE PRACTITIONER: Well, not exactly a disorder, but why? Have you been told that you're anemic?

PATIENT: Pues hace años, pero me dieron medicina. Ferros algo.

NURSE PRACTITIONER: Ferrous sulfate? Iron?

PATIENT: Sí, sí, sí. Eso es, doctora.

NURSE PRACTITIONER: And did that help?

PATIENT: Sí, sí. Tomé esa medicina y no tuve ese problema más nunca.

NURSE PRACTITIONER: Good. Do you ever have trouble healing, for example, if you cut yourself in the kitchen, do you stop bleeding quickly?

PATIENT: Yo creo que en eso soy normal.

NURSE PRACTITIONER: How about your vaccines? Are you up to date on all your vaccines? Let's see if your doctor sent us any of that information. *(looks through file and computer)* Ah, yes, even your tetanus, which you had in April. Very good. Now, does anyone in your family have a problem with their blood, or has anyone had a bad experience with anesthesia?

PATIENT: No, doctora. Pero a la mayoría jamás les han puesto anestesia, solamente a mí, y gracias a Dios todo ha salido bien. Pero eso de coágulos, ¿va a ser un problema? ¿Es un riesgo muy grande? Porque no recuerdo que me hayan mencionado algo así.

NURSE PRACTITIONER: No, it's not really a problem, but they'll give you some special stockings to put on when you get there. The stockings help with circulation and help reduce the risk of blood clots.

PATIENT: Vaya usted, doctora.

NURSE PRACTITIONER: Well, Mrs. Ruiz, I mean Asteria, I think you are going to do well. Now, I need to tell you about the possible risks of anesthesia.

PATIENT: Vaya, doctora.

NURSE PRACTITIONER: Now, anytime you have anesthesia there is always a risk, but people who are pretty healthy, as you are, really don't have much trouble. There is a small risk of a stroke or even death, but actually, you're safer getting anesthesia than you are every time you get in your car on the highway. You're actually safer getting anesthesia, according to the statistics. There will be a team of people taking care of you and checking your breathing, your blood pressure, your heartbeat and your pulse the entire time. You'll be in good hands. Do you have any questions about that so far?

PATIENT: No doctora, usted me explicó todo, bien clarito.

NURSE PRACTITIONER: Well, good. You're probably going to do just fine. Now, here are some instructions in English, which I'm going to explain to you. I'll give you the same document in Spanish as well, but let me just talk you through this. It says that you're scheduled for a 10:30 procedure on Wednesday and that you'll need to be in the surgical waiting room by 8:30 in the morning. Is that what they told you?

PATIENT: Sí. Así es.

NURSE PRACTITIONER: All right. Now, here are some specific eating and drinking instructions. You can have a normal dinner or evening meal, but nothing too heavy. But after 12:00 midnight on Tuesday, you cannot eat anything or drink any milk or nonclear liquids. You can have clear apple juice or 7 Up or water up until four hours before your scheduled arrival.

PATIENT: Bien. Nomás tomaré mi tincito de café antes de salir de la casa.

NURSE PRACTITIONER: Asteria, you really should not drink anything for six hours before the procedure, for your own safety. The doctors don't want you to have anything in your stomach, just in case you vomit. If you do vomit and there's anything in your stomach, it can go to your lungs and cause pneumonia. It's very important that you follow these instructions. If you don't, the doctors will cancel the surgery. So not even a little bit of coffee or even water, all right?

PATIENT: ¿Y si no puedo dormir, o tengo un dolor de cabeza?

NURSE PRACTITIONER: You can take your sleeping medicine with a little water during the night. But if you're going to take it, try to do it before midnight so you aren't still feeling the effects in the morning. If your head is really hurting in the morning, you can take Tylenol with a little sip of water, just enough to get it down. All right? It's really for your own safety.

PATIENT: Bueno, doctora, entiendo.

NURSE PRACTITIONER: OK. It looks like you have an appointment with Dr. Redding at 2:00 this afternoon. If you have any questions about the surgery itself, you can ask her about it. But if everything is clear about the anesthesia, then I'm going to ask you to sign here, which is just indicating that I went over the instructions with you and that you agree to follow them. And here is your copy of the same thing in Spanish. All right?

PATIENT: Sí, doctora.

NURSE PRACTITIONER: Well, then, I guess that's it. Don't worry, Mrs. Ruiz, they're very good here and they'll take good care of you.

PATIENT: Bueno, muchas gracias doctora, que Dios le bendiga.

Preparation for anesthesia role play (English only)

Note: Feel free to change the name of the patient to fit the language you interpret to from English.

PART 1

INTERPRETER: Good morning. My name is ___________. I'm your interpreter. I'd like to let you know that everything you say will be interpreted, and everything will be kept confidential. Please speak directly to each other, not to me, and pause when I make this signal (*raises hand*) so I can interpret.

NURSE PRACTITIONER: Good morning, please have a seat.

PATIENT: Good morning.

NURSE PRACTITIONER: Hello, Asteria Ruiz? (*Substitute any name that you choose for the patient's name.*) Good afternoon, my name is Jill. I don't speak your language, so I have a translator here to help.

PATIENT: Very good, doctor, that's very good.

NURSE PRACTITIONER: Please have a seat, Mrs. ________. So, as I was saying, I'm a nurse practitioner here in the anesthesia department and my job is to make sure everything is safe to go ahead and give you anesthesia for your surgery.

PATIENT: Very good, very good, but call me Asteria. (*Substitute the patient name that you decided on.*) When you call me Mrs. _________, it makes me feel so old!

NURSE PRACTITIONER: Very good, Asteria. Oh, I'm sorry. Can you wait just one minute, I left part of your file at another desk, I'll be right back.

PATIENT: Of course, doctor! (*Nurse practitioner leaves the room; patient turns to interpreter.*) Good morning. Oh! You speak __________, right? Are you a nurse?

INTERPRETER: I'm an interpreter.

PATIENT: And what's your job? What do you do?

INTERPRETER: I interpret. Since the nurse doesn't speak ________, and you don't speak English, I'll interpret for you.

PATIENT: And is that all you do all day? You work here the whole day doing that?

INTERPRETER: Yes, this is my job. (*Nurse practitioner enters the room.*)

PATIENT: (*to the nurse practitioner*) Can I ask a question?

NURSE PRACTITIONER: Sure, go ahead.

PATIENT: Are you going to put me completely asleep, or give me a sedative or what's gonna happen? It's just that the last time that—

NURSE PRACTITIONER: Actually, we'll get to all of that, but I have some questions I wanted to ask about your health history first. Then I'll do a brief physical exam, listen to your heart and lungs and then we'll talk about anesthesia options. Will that be all right?

PATIENT: Of course, doctor! You're the boss. Even though, to be honest, I'm a wee bit anxious.

NURSE PRACTITIONER: That's normal. Let's see if we can get through these questions first. Maybe that will help set you at ease. OK?

PATIENT: Go ahead, doctor.

NURSE PRACTITIONER: OK, so to start, how are you feeling; how would you say your health is in general?

PATIENT: Very good, doctor. I'm fit as a fiddle!

NURSE PRACTITIONER: Well that's great. All right, now, can you tell me what they will be doing in this surgery?

PATIENT: Yes. What the doctor is gonna do to me is take it all out, the whole kit and kaboodle, in one fell swoop. He's gonna take out my uterus. Everything, the whole works.

NURSE PRACTITIONER: OK, that's also what I have in your chart. I just wanted to make sure we were all on the same page. It says here that you're going to have a radical hysterectomy and lymphectomy. Is that what you understand?

PATIENT: Yes, doctor. That's right. They're gonna take out all the bad stuff, and I hope that if God wills, we'll find a solution.

NURSE PRACTITIONER: Very good, Mrs. _______________. Now can you tell me if you are taking any medicines regularly?

PATIENT: Well, once in a while I take a Motrin if my head hurts, and sometimes I take something to sleep because I get anxious a lot.

NURSE PRACTITIONER: And do you know the name of that medicine you take for sleeping?

PATIENT: It's something like Lorazam.

NURSE PRACTITIONER: Lorazepam or Ativan?

PATIENT: Yes! You hit the nail on the head!

NURSE PRACTITIONER: That's often used for anxiety. Do you suffer from anxiety?

PATIENT: Well, you know, doctor, with all the things in life, the kids, the grandchildren, it makes you anxious. And then all this. As I said, doctor, I went to have a simple Pap smear. I thought it was gonna be a piece of cake. And look. It's not an easy thing to fall asleep at night.

NURSE PRACTITIONER: And is that every night?

> **PATIENT:** Well...once in a blue moon. Now, you know, it's more often.

NURSE PRACTITIONER: How often would you say you take that medicine?

> **PATIENT:** Well, I took it last night. It's just that I was nervous about this appointment and the surgery. And I think I took it three nights ago too.

NURSE PRACTITIONER: So, on average, would you say you take it twice a week, three times a week, five times a week?

> **PATIENT:** Oh no, doctor, nothing like that.

NURSE PRACTITIONER: So how often would you say you take it?

> **PATIENT:** Well, you know, like once or twice a week. Maybe three.

NURSE PRACTITIONER: All right. And when was the last time you took Motrin?

> **PATIENT:** Oh, well. A long time back.

NURSE PRACTITIONER: And when was the last time you took it?

> **PATIENT:** Well, since they told me that I shouldn't take anything for two weeks before the operation, and I always do exactly what the doctors tell me, to the letter of the law, it's that you guys are the boss, so I haven't taken it since the beginning of the month, since the second, I think. I haven't taken aspirin either, not ibuprofen or anything that has aspirin in it. Did I do it like I was supposed to, doctor?

NURSE PRACTITIONER: Excellent, Mrs. _________. That's to protect you from bleeding unnecessarily.

> **PATIENT:** That's what I told my neighbor. I said, "Those doctors are all-powerful, bless them, and I'm gonna do exactly what they say." Now, you know some people don't want to listen—(*Nurse practitioner interrupts.*)

NURSE PRACTITIONER: Very good, Mrs. ______________.

> **PATIENT:** Well, yes, I always try to do what they tell me, and, thank God, I'm still here so far.

NURSE PRACTITIONER: All right, can you tell me if you have any allergies to medicines or anything else?

> **PATIENT:** Well, right now I have a runny nose.[7] I don't know if it's pollen, but it's not running a lot. What worries me is the last time I had anesthesia, I had a really serious problem. Saints alive! Girl, I almost died! I couldn't breathe, it was an emergency. I almost suffocated.

NURSE PRACTITIONER: Oh yes, I see here in your chart that you were given some epinephrine at the dentist with a local anesthesia and you had a reaction. OK. Let me get that into your chart here, your workup for this anesthesia. I'll make sure the doctors see this so they are prepared. Can you tell me what happened?

7 What are some regionalisms for "runny nose" or "cold" in your other language?

PART 2

PATIENT: Well, they gave me that injection and my heart was beating like it was gonna burst outta my chest. My lord!

NURSE PRACTITIONER: And what happened after that? What did you do?

PATIENT: After a while, it started getting better, and that was it. But you know, I felt like I was gonna kick the bucket!

NURSE PRACTITIONER: And have you had anesthesia since then?

PATIENT: No, no, doctor.

NURSE PRACTITIONER: So you just had local anesthesia that one time?

PATIENT: No, no, no. I had it when I had the girls.

NURSE PRACTITIONER: What happened then? Did you have an epidural?

PATIENT: What are you thinking, girl! In my time, we didn't have those things. But they were born by Caesarean. Only that was in the capital of my country.

NURSE PRACTITIONER: Where are you from originally?

PATIENT: I'm _____________(*insert any nationality that makes sense*), thank God.

NURSE PRACTITIONER: Oh? And why were your girls born by C-section?

PATIENT: Well, with the first girl, I wasn't very wide-hipped and she wouldn't come out. So they did a Caesarian. With the second one, well, you know, they had to do the same thing, me having a womb like that, all cut up like that.

NURSE PRACTITIONER: So you had general anesthesia those two times?

PATIENT: Of course! And after that, I slept like a baby in a cradle.

NURSE PRACTITIONER: Let's see then. That was two C-sections? Did you ever have anesthesia for anything else? Any kind of a study?

PATIENT: Yes, the second time, after the Caesarian the wound got infected, and you should have seen it. Oh my God. What a stink! They had to open me up again, clean it all out.

NURSE PRACTITIONER: OK. And everything went well, with the anesthesia?

PATIENT: Yes, yes.

NURSE PRACTITIONER: And was that the only other time you had anesthesia?

PATIENT: I had it again after that, when they did a *tamitác*, after my Caesarians.

NURSE PRACTITIONER: Oh, so you had some cosmetic surgery?

PATIENT: Well, you know, after all those surgeries and the two pregnancies, after that they gave me a *tamitac*. Thank goodness. Every cloud has a silver lining, no?

NURSE PRACTITIONER: I guess so. And did you have a reaction to the anesthesia those times after that first reaction?

PATIENT: No, just a headache. But what a headache, girl!

NURSE PRACTITIONER: OK. It seems like we can assume that the one time when you had the respiratory reaction, it was probably due to the epinephrine, and that isn't usually part of getting general anesthesia, but I'm going to note all this in your chart and leave it up to the anesthesiologist. You'll meet him or her the day of the procedure, and you can discuss it. I'll also let them know about the headaches. Maybe they can try to prevent that this time.

PATIENT: OK, but I hope it'll be a male doctor. I want a male doctor to take care of me; I don't want it to be a lady doctor. Women, for this work, well, they weren't cut out for this.

NURSE PRACTITIONER: Well, I'm not sure who it will be, but I can assure you they'll take good care of you, and whoever it is will be qualified. In fact, it's usually a team of at least two doctors and a nurse for the anesthesia part of the surgery.

PATIENT: Okey-dokey.

NURSE PRACTITIONER: You said you have a little bit of a runny nose, can you tell me what color it is? Is it clear, yellow or green?

PATIENT: It's clear, it's just a tiny little bit, it just started. It's the season.

NURSE PRACTITIONER: And you sound pretty sure that it's just a little bit of hay fever. Did you have a temperature with that?

PATIENT: No, doctor, no temperature, no nothing.

NURSE PRACTITIONER: And have you had a cold or a cough or fever during the last two weeks?

PATIENT: No, doctor.

NURSE PRACTITIONER: How would you say your health is in general?

PATIENT: Well, I'd say it's not as bad as some other folks, I'd say it's good. Like I said, I'm fit as a fiddle.

NURSE PRACTITIONER: Do you get any regular exercise?

PATIENT: I live on the fifth floor, and I don't use the elevator. I've been visiting here for a month with my son, but when I'm home, the truth is I walk a lot. I walk at least an hour every day. I'm gonna go walking in a little while.

NURSE PRACTITIONER: Oh, that's wonderful. Do you walk every afternoon?

PATIENT: No, no. But today, yes, I'm gonna go walking in a while.

NURSE PRACTITIONER: Well, it's beautiful outside, but be careful not to get overheated.

PATIENT: No, no. I usually walk in the evening.

NURSE PRACTITIONER: How about walking uphill? Do you get out of breath? Do you have any trouble with stairs? Can you go up two flights of stairs without any trouble?

PATIENT: Well, the usual. I get a little out of breath, like anybody.

NURSE PRACTITIONER: Does it make you stop because you're short of breath or need to rest?

PATIENT: No, no, no, no. Nothing like that. No, I've always taken care of my figure; I've always done my exercise.

NURSE PRACTITIONER: Good, that's great. Uh...do you have any problems with your heart?

PATIENT: Sometimes I think that...maybe, sometimes I feel little needle sticks here...

NURSE PRACTITIONER: Have you ever seen a doctor about it?

PATIENT: I asked my doctor, but she said it was nothing.

NURSE PRACTITIONER: Have you ever had an electrocardiogram? Any other kind of a heart exam?

PATIENT: Yes, yes. They did all that before the *tamitac*.

NURSE PRACTITIONER: And was everything OK? Did they tell you there was any kind of a heart problem?

PATIENT: Oh, none of that. They told me everything was normal, fine. I'm strong as a mare.

NURSE PRACTITIONER: OK, it sounds like you don't have any kind of a heart problem. But that was, let's see, in 1992. I think I'm going to recommend another EKG before this surgery just to make sure everything is fine, since this will be a longer surgery.

PATIENT: Whatever you say, doctor.

NURSE PRACTITIONER: Do you have any problems with your lungs?

PATIENT: I don't know. Like I said, sometimes I get a little out of breath, when I climb up three or four floors, and once when I caught a chill[8] I got really sick. I had a cough for six weeks. My doctor told me that it was something like a reaction in the airways or bronchitis or something like that.

NURSE PRACTITIONER: Reactive airway disease?

PATIENT: Yes, yes. That's what it was.

NURSE PRACTITIONER: And do you use any medicines for that, inhalers or nasal sprays?

PATIENT: Well, not anymore.

---

8 What is "to catch a chill" in your other language? Is there more than one way to say it?

NURSE PRACTITIONER: But you were prescribed something for that?

PATIENT: She gave me one of those devices, a little puffer. *Aluero, floruto* or something like that for asthma, but I don't have asthma.

NURSE PRACTITIONER: Was it Albuterol?

PATIENT: You got it! Albuterol! But I just used it that one time, that's it.

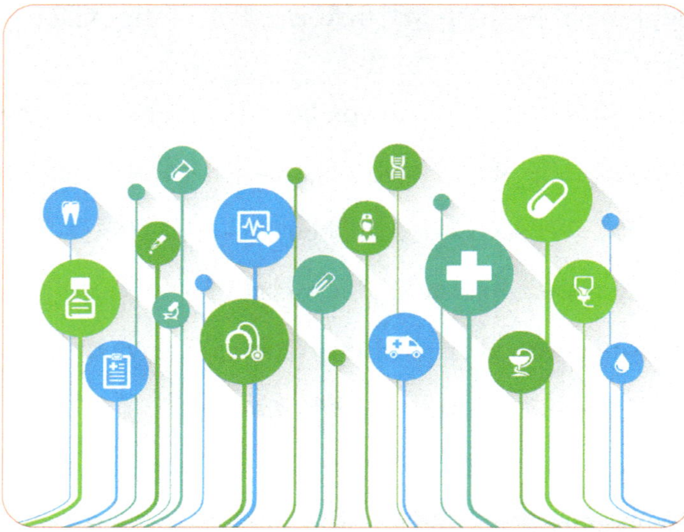

NURSE PRACTITIONER: All right. Have you ever had bronchitis, bronchilitis or pneumonia?

PATIENT: No, not that I know of, no.

NURSE PRACTITIONER: Have you ever tested positive for tuberculosis?

PATIENT: Well, that, yes. Once it came back like you say, and I had to take medicine, for about six months. But they didn't see anything. They told me I didn't have the disease but I had to take the medicines, a capsule for prevention.

NURSE PRACTITIONER: And when was that?

PATIENT: Hmm. It was a long time ago, about 15 or 17 years ago, when I first came to this country.

PART 3

NURSE PRACTITIONER: OK. Let's see, do you have any problems with your liver?

PATIENT: No, I've never been diagnosed with anything like that.

NURSE PRACTITIONER: Have you ever had hepatitis?

PATIENT: No, doctor, thank God.

NURSE PRACTITIONER: Have you ever had problems with your gallbladder, gallstones, for example?

PATIENT: No, doctor.

NURSE PRACTITIONER: How about your stomach or intestine?

PATIENT: Sometimes I get really *elaste*.

PATIENT: (*to interpreter*) Honey, where are you from?

INTERPRETER: I'm from here.

PATIENT: ¡Ah, that's why you don't get it. Honey, *elaste* means really big, like this, very full, bloated.

NURSE PRACTITIONER: And do you have heartburn[9] or acid reflux?

PATIENT: That, yes.

NURSE PRACTITIONER: And do you take anything for that?

PATIENT: Tums, I take some Tums.

NURSE PRACTITIONER: How about your kidneys?

PATIENT: No, doctor.

NURSE PRACTITIONER: Have you ever had bladder infections or urinary tract infections or problems with your bladder?

PATIENT: No, not that either, doctor. Thank God.

NURSE PRACTITIONER: Do you have any problems with your thyroid?

PATIENT: No. Thanks to the blessed one.

NURSE PRACTITIONER: Do you have chronic headaches or migraines?

PATIENT: Sometimes I get headaches, but really bad pain like that, intolerable, just that time after the *tamitac*.

NURSE PRACTITIONER: OK. Do you have diabetes?

PATIENT: No. I'm not a diabetic.

NURSE PRACTITIONER: High blood pressure?

9 What is "heartburn" in your other language? What are some other terms?

PATIENT: The doctor told me that I'm right on the borderline, but I still don't take anything. She said that for the time being I'm fine, but she's gonna watch over me.

NURSE PRACTITIONER: Do you have any problems with your blood? Do you have trouble clotting, or do you have any kind of blood disorder?

PATIENT: Is anemia supposed to be a blood disorder?

NURSE PRACTITIONER: Well, not exactly a disorder, but why? Have you been told that you're anemic?

PATIENT: Well, years ago, but they gave me medicine. Ferris something.

NURSE PRACTITIONER: Ferrous sulfate? Iron?

PATIENT: Yes, yes, yes, that was it, doctor.

NURSE PRACTITIONER: And did that help?

PATIENT: Yes, yes. I took that medicine and I never had that problem ever again.

NURSE PRACTITIONER: Good. Do you ever have trouble healing, for example, if you cut yourself in the kitchen, do you stop bleeding quickly?

PATIENT: I don't think so, for that I think I'm normal.

NURSE PRACTITIONER: How about your vaccines? Are you up to date on all your vaccines? Let's see if your doctor sent us any of that information. (*looks through file and computer*) Ah, yes, even your tetanus, which you had in April. Very good. Now, does anyone in your family have a problem with their blood, or has anyone had a bad experience with anesthesia?

PATIENT: No, doctor. But most of them have never had anesthesia, just me, and thank God, everything turned out fine. But what you said about clots, is that gonna be a problem? Is it a big risk? Because I don't remember if they ever mentioned anything like that to me.

NURSE PRACTITIONER: No, it's not really a problem, but they'll give you some special stockings to put on when you get there. The stockings help with circulation and help reduce the risk of blood clots.

PATIENT: Of course, doctor.

NURSE PRACTITIONER: Well, I think you are going to do well. Now, I need to tell you about the possible risks of anesthesia.

PATIENT: Go ahead, doctor.

NURSE PRACTITIONER: Now, anytime you have anesthesia there is always a risk, but people who are pretty healthy, as you are, really don't have much trouble. There is a small risk of a stroke or even death, but actually, you're safer getting anesthesia than you are every time you get in your car on the highway. You're actually safer getting anesthesia, according to the statistics. There will be a team of people taking care of you and checking your breathing, your blood pressure, your heartbeat and your pulse the entire time. You'll be in good hands. Do you have any questions about that so far?

PATIENT: No doctor, you explained everything to me, perfectly clearly.

NURSE PRACTITIONER: Well, good. You're probably going to do just fine. Now, here are some instructions in English, which I'm going to explain to you. I'll give you the same document in your language as well, but let me just talk you through this. It says that you're scheduled for a 10:30 procedure on Wednesday, and that you'll need to be in the surgical waiting room by 8:30 in the morning. Is that what they told you?

PATIENT: Yes. That's right.

NURSE PRACTITIONER: All right. Now, here are some specific eating and drinking instructions. You can have a normal dinner or evening meal, but nothing too heavy. But after 12:00 midnight on Tuesday, you cannot eat anything or drink any milk or nonclear liquids. You can have clear apple juice or 7 Up or water up until four hours before your scheduled arrival.

PATIENT: OK, I'll just have my little itty bitty coffee before leaving the house.

NURSE PRACTITIONER: You really should not drink anything for six hours before the procedure, for your own safety. The doctors don't want you to have anything in your stomach, just in case you vomit. If you do vomit and there's anything in your stomach, it can go to your lungs and cause pneumonia. It's very important that you follow these instructions. If you don't, the doctors will cancel the surgery. So not even a little bit of coffee or even water, all right?

PATIENT: And if I can't sleep or if I have a headache?

NURSE PRACTITIONER: You can take your sleeping medicine with a little water during the night. But if you're going to take it, try to do it before midnight so you aren't still feeling the effects in the morning. If your head is really hurting in the morning, you can take Tylenol with a little sip of water, just enough to get it down. All right? It's really for your own safety.

PATIENT: Well, all right, doctor, I understand.

NURSE PRACTITIONER: OK. It looks like you have an appointment with Dr. Redding at 2:00 this afternoon. If you have any questions about the surgery itself, you can ask her about it. But if everything is clear about the anesthesia, then I'm going to ask you to sign here, which is just indicating that I went over the instructions with you, and that you agree to follow them. And here is your copy of the same thing in your language. All right?

PATIENT: Yes, doctor.

NURSE PRACTITIONER: Well, then, I guess that's it. Don't worry, they're very good here and they'll take good care of you.

PATIENT: Well, thank you very much, doctor. May God bless you.

What's important to know about this chapter?

Overview

This is an appointment in preparation for anesthesia, and the practitioner will conduct a health history, from head to toe. The interpreter will need to know the corresponding vocabulary, including the major body parts and organs.

Terminology

See the illustration at the end of this chapter and the terminology that accompanies this dialogue. As you go through the chapter, note any new or useful terms and learn them in both or all your working languages. Add them to the illustration, the glossary in the back of this book (Appendix 3) or in the margins of the dialogue. Here are some basic vocabulary words and concepts that may be useful:

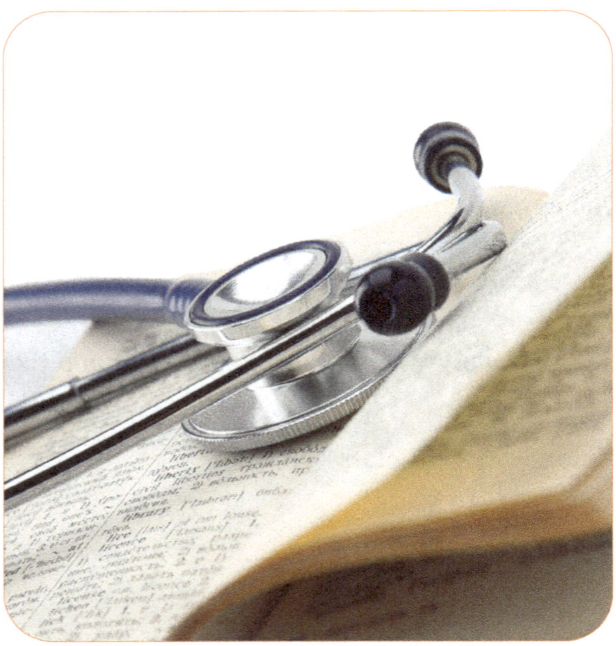

Health practitioner: This dialogue features a nurse practitioner. In the United States, you may work with nurse practitioners, registered nurses, licensed vocational nurses, clinical nurse specialists, physician's assistants, medical assistants, attending physicians, resident physicians, physician fellows, interns and medical students. Each of these titles might or might not have an equivalent in your other working language(s), and the titles may also vary from one health organization to another.

Interpreter titles: The health providers and healthcare staff you work with might or might not understand the difference between an interpreter and a translator, as in this dialogue. Sometimes it may be appropriate to clarify the difference, and at other times not.

Health history: In preparation for a patient who will have a procedure under anesthesia, it is typical to go through a health history and talk about the health or problems associated with all major systems and organs. Some patients might also be asked additional questions about pediatric diseases, pregnancies or prostate cancer.

"Just an interpreter"

It's not unusual for interpreters to hear questions or comments similar to the one from this patient, who wants to know what the interpreter's "real job" is and is surprised to learn that interpreting *is* a job—and that the interpreter does it all day long. It might be interesting to check in with yourself from time to time to learn how *you* feel about the amazing job you do and what a skilled and demanding profession healthcare interpreting is.

Idiomatic expression and more

The patient in this dialogue has a bubbly personality and uses many idiomatic expressions. These are one of the harder aspects of a language to command—and to interpret. It will also be impossible to come up with one "correct" interpretation because there are so many variations from region to region, depending on the location and social group where a language is spoken. Talk with colleagues; then discuss some of the expressions used here and collect translations for them. For example, try to find good translations for these phrases: *to be on the same page; once in a blue moon; to hit the nail on the head; to the letter of the law; a runny nose; to catch a chill; hysterectomy; lymphectomy; to kick the bucket; the whole kit and caboodle; if God wills; every cloud has a silver lining; to be cut out for something.*

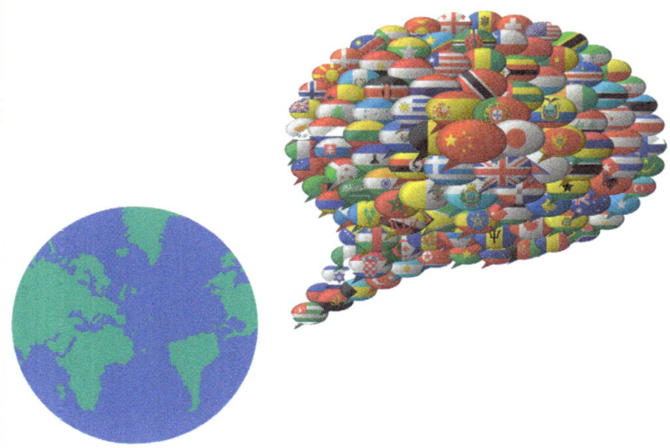

Pidgin

In addition to more traditional idiomatic expressions, this patient has some of her own, often a mix of her first language and the one spoken in the new country: for example, *tamitac* (tummy tuck), *Jani* (honey, used to address a person) and *elaste* (elastic or stretched out, bloated). Sometimes, as here, what the patient says might not even be a true word but a term that is unique to the patient, to a small group or to a city or region.

Birth by Caesarian-section (C-section)

In the United States, for many years, after a woman had a C-section, she was usually scheduled for C-sections for all subsequent births. That situation has changed. But what is the expectation in the patient's country or other places in the world, rural and urban?

Gender and practitioner

People from different parts of the world have varying opinions about gender appropriateness for certain jobs. They might prefer male doctors or female nurses, for example. In this case, the patient has opinions that are probably considered somewhat prejudicial, even in her own culture; she is from a generation when there were few women physicians or scientists. You might have patients whose religious or cultural norms prohibit receiving healthcare from a different gender practitioner. If this is significant in the encounter you are interpreting for, you might want to alert the practitioner to ask about the patient's preference. Otherwise, interpret everything as it is uttered and remember *you are not responsible for the consequences—only the accuracy of the interpreting.*

Gender and the interpreter

Of course, there will be situations in which individual or cultural norms will make it uncomfortable, difficult or even impossible to interpret for a certain patient depending on gender. For cultural and/or religious reasons, a patient might request or insist on having an interpreter of a particular gender.

Then there is the question of personal comfort. Think about males interpreting for females at gynecological appointments, or females interpreting for male patients at urology appointments in an erectile dysfunction clinic. How comfortable is the patient,

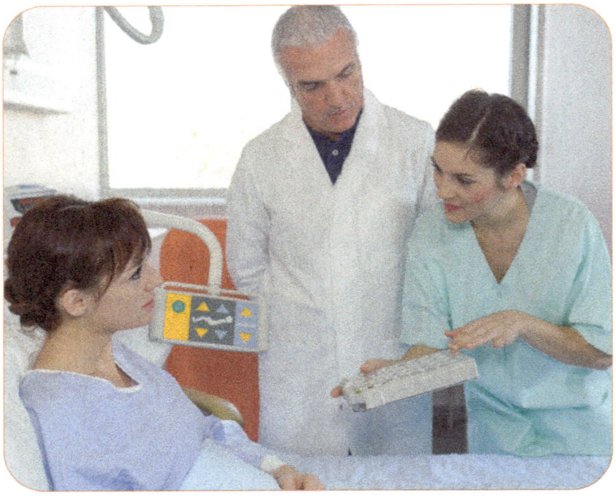

and how comfortable is the interpreter? It is most convenient in such cases if this decision is made in advance. If the situation is unforeseen, particularly if the patient does not mention it but you sense discomfort or distress, you might need to bring it to the attention of the provider by suggesting that the provider ask about the patient's preferences.

In a while

What is "a while"? A bit, a time, a spell, a few minutes, a few hours, a few days? There are so many ways to say "a while" and so many meanings for such a term. Does it mean right away, in an hour, in the evening? Check in on your patient's place of origin and the variety of the language you are interpreting, in case terms that refer to periods of time mean different things in different places. They often do, even within the same language.

Open-ended questions

Sometimes practitioners ask questions that leave the answers open to many kinds of narratives, including personal or anecdotal histories of symptoms and experiences. This nurse practitioner wants to know if the patient has any liver conditions that might put her at risk when receiving anesthesia and she may have limited time to get that information. She can ask, "Do you have any problem or condition of the liver?" or "Have you ever been diagnosed with a liver problem?" As the interpreter, it's important to be as accurate in the interpreting of the question as possible and allow the practitioner to formulate the question as she sees fit, however tempting it might to be to change it in order to get a short answer.

Lengthy passages

If the interpreter is in consecutive mode and finds a passage too long to comfortably manage, what strategies can she use to break up the message or handle it more smoothly while still being accurate?

Nothing to eat or drink

Perhaps surprisingly, "nothing to eat or drink" can be interpreted in different ways. In this case, it means that literally nothing can pass between someone's lips (or nasogastric or other feeding tube) into the stomach, including water or any amount of food, unless specifically stated. If you sense this might not be the actual case (someone drank a little juice, some coffee, ate a hamburger) as the interpreter, advise the practitioner to inquire about it for clarity. If you do so, *be transparent and report to the patient exactly what you said to the provider.*

Being left alone with the patient

Should you be alone with the patient? Why or why not? What could you do instead? Some hospitals have instituted policies requiring the interpreter to leave the room if the provider does so in order to avoid leaving interpreters alone with patients. Do you agree with such policies? Why or why not?

Ethics and standards: Reflect and practice

For each of the exercises on the NCIHC national ethics and standards in this book, you will need to access the NCIHC *National Code of Ethics for Interpreters in Health Care* and *National Standards of Practice for Interpreters in Health Care* (NCIHC 2004 and 2005, respectively).

These documents are available at www.ncihc.org (currently under the heading "Resources"). You might find it easier to print them or save both documents on the desktop of your computer or device. For this exercise, you will need to look at the *National Standards of Practice for Interpreters in Health Care*, p. 5.

Goal 1: Accuracy

Translation and paraphrasing

1. Look at the first six NCIHC standards of practice related to accuracy (Standards 1 to 6, NCIHC, 2005, p. 5). Working individually, *paraphrase* the objective, its related ethical principle and the six standards (in other words, all the text in bold on p. 5).

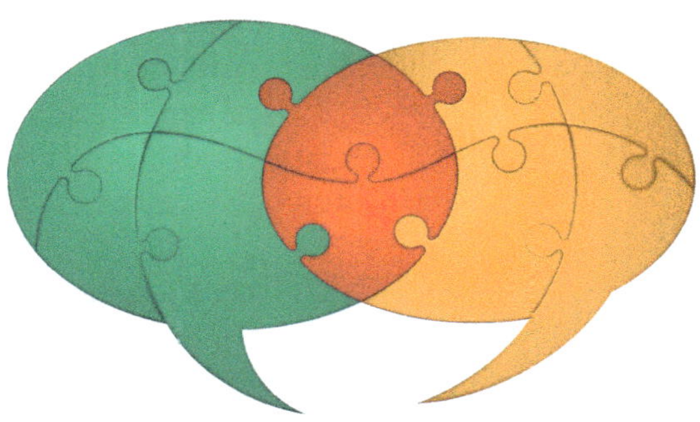

2. Working individually, *translate* the original text of these standards into your other working language(s) or interpret it into sign language.
3. Find a partner or partners. Compare, discuss and modify your translations and paraphrasing until you are satisfied with your final products as a group.
4. If you can, pick a group representative and discuss your final versions with any other groups that share your working languages. Compare and discuss your differences.

Suggested reading

Roat, C. E. (2010). *Healthcare Interpreting in Small Bites: 50 Nourishing Selections from the "Pacific Interpreters Newsletter," 2002-2010*. Victoria, British Columbia: Trafford, pp. 21-24.

Consider and discuss

1. **Standard 1** Four health providers come into a clinical appointment one after another to speak with a patient: a doctor, a nurse, a social worker and a speech therapist. Each provider asks the parent the same questions about the child, including which therapies the child is receiving (physical, occupational, speech), for how long and how often. After the fourth provider asks these same questions, the parent turns to the interpreter, exasperated and says, "Es como que una no sabe lo que hace la otra. ¿Cuántas veces me van a hacer estas mismas preguntas? ¿Se las tengo que contesta otra vez?/It's as if one of them has no idea what the other one is doing. How many times are they going to ask me the same questions? Do I have to answer them again?" With *accuracy* and transparency in mind, how should the interpreter respond, and to whom?

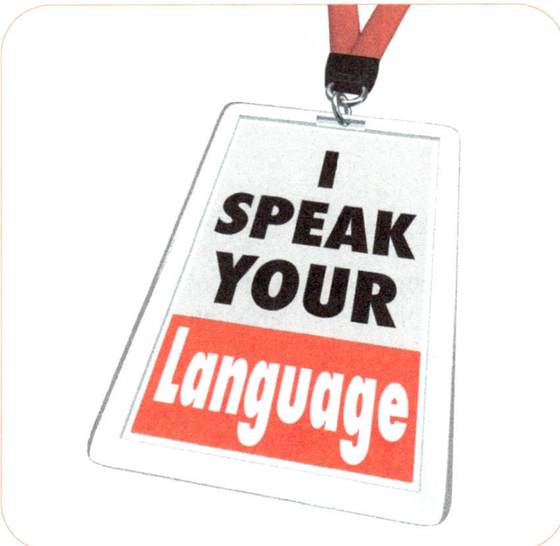

What might be challenging for the interpreter who faces a decision like this in real life?

Standard 2 A healthcare provider gives a child's father a detailed explanation of chromosomal mitosis and specific translocation of genes on a chromosome as a way of explaining a genetic syndrome. You interpret accurately, maintaining the practitioner's register. You can tell the father is in a fog, not understanding the provider. From earlier conversation, you know the father is a field worker who has finished no more than third grade in his country. He listens intently and respectfully, giving no verbal indication of a lack of understanding, but to you, his facial expression suggests profound confusion. Should you indicate to the provider that you suspect a problem of understanding, even if the patient isn't saying anything? How might one phrase it to instill confidence in the accuracy and transparency of the interpreting? Is doing so advocacy? How does intervening in this way affect interpreter neutrality?

Pick which approach from the five below you think might work best:

1. Just interpret.
2. Tell the provider you don't think the parent understands and that this might be due to low education (third grade) and his background as an agricultural worker.
3. Interpret, then ask the father if he understands the provider.
4. Interpret, then ask the provider's permission to check for understanding.
5. Interpret, then intervene to tell the provider something like, "The interpreter is concerned there might be a break in communication about the genetic syndrome," or, "As the interpreter, I'm afraid that what I just interpreted isn't clear—you might want to check for understanding," and report what you have just said to the patient.

What are the possible consequences of each of these five scenarios? *After* choosing an answer, you may consult the answer provided upside down, below.

2. **Standard 2** A patient uses many idiomatic and colorful expressions. Should the interpreter try to interpret these as faithfully as possible, replace them with simple equivalents that the practitioner will understand, or follow each expression (faithfully rendered) with a brief paraphrase? Is there another strategy? How might changing the speech patterns, faithfully interpreting them or using another strategy impact communication?
3. **Standard 3** An interpreter walks into a gynecology oncology room where a patient and six family members are waiting for the doctor. Upon entry, the English-speaking grown children of the patient rush to the interpreter and tell her that they don't want anything said to their mother about the diagnosis. They insist she would get too upset and shouldn't be told. What should the interpreter say or do? How is this decision related to the principle of accuracy? How might the interpreter prevent such ethical challenges from arising in the first place?
4. **Standard 4** An interpreter is in a family meeting with many participants (foster parent, godparent and wife, two oncologists, child-life specialist, social worker, child protective services worker,

Scenario 1) does not solve the problem.
Scenario 2) sounds condescending and inappropriate.
Scenarios 3) and 4) involve the interpreter taking over the provider's job. These actions are not recommended.
Scenario 5) could be acceptable.
For Scenario 6), ideally the interpreter would request the patient to clarify the terms.

nurse). The interpreter has been working in simultaneous mode for most of the meeting, but suddenly two separate side conversations erupt, in addition to two conversations directed at the patient. (The impact on the interpreter's concentration is like hearing classical, reggae, hip-hop and bluegrass music from multiple speakers at once, and then needing to reproduce or remember all the different tunes.) How do such side conversations affect the interpreter's accuracy? What can the interpreter say or do to manage the flow of communication and be accurate?

5. **Standard 4** Upon answering each and every question asked by a physician, the patient enters into a nonstop, three-minute monologue. Some of the information is relevant and important; some is irrelevant, irritating and confusing. The doctor begins to ignore the interpreter's rendition. Sometimes the doctor talks over the interpreter to the assistant in the room or interrupts the interpreter. Some important health information might be lost or ignored. What is the impact on accuracy? Whose responsibility is it to manage patient participation? What could the interpreter do to improve the quality of communication without stepping out of his or her role?
6. **Standard 6** An elderly Spanish-speaking LEP patient who has resided in the United States for 20 years narrates her history and describes her gastrointestinal health symptoms to the doctor, repeatedly using terms like *elaste* and *mosa* and a home remedy called *anemia*. The interpreter believes the patient means she is bloated and has used enemas for constipation (rather than that she has anemia or has used anemia) but isn't sure. How should the interpreter clarify the confusion?

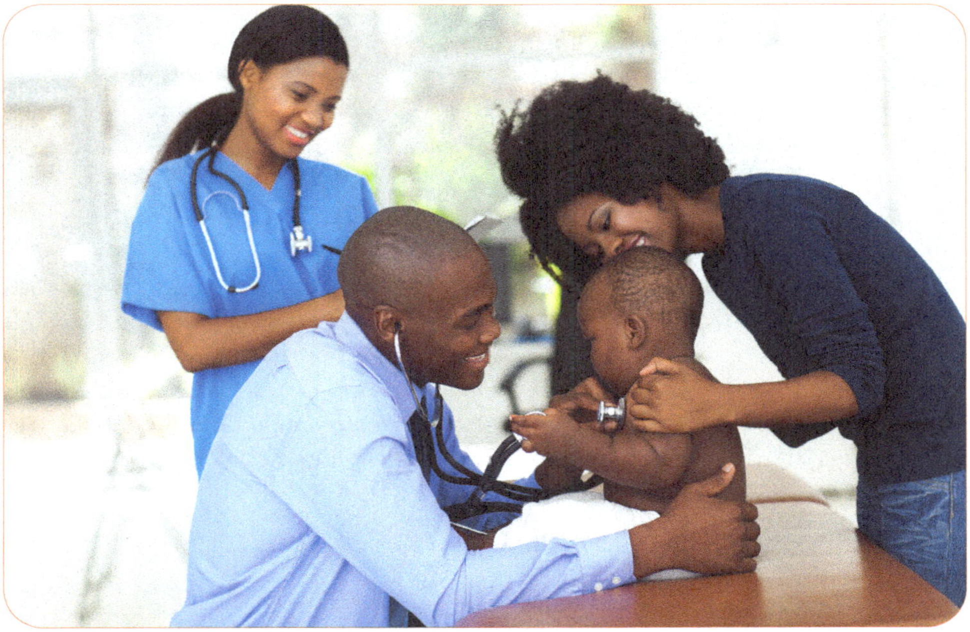

Occupational therapy for interpreters

EXERCISES FOR THE TONGUE, HEART AND MIND

Suggested reading for Spanish speakers, until the book is available in your language[10]

Martín del Campo, M. (1999). *Amor y Conquista: La novela de Malinalli mal llamada la Malinche.*

Read the following excerpts from del Campo's book and consider any parallels you find to medical interpreting. For those who do not read Spanish, the following excerpts from the book above are helpful. They are taken from the masterfully told story of one of the first interpreters between Europeans and nations of the Americas. This powerful novel recounts a 16th-century interpreter's pain and joy and her intelligent survival through a turbulent period of history. This book is a fascinating work for interpreters and history lovers. Here are some excerpts: see if you can find out what is relevant in them for interpreters in healthcare.

Malinalli, upon hearing the language of her childhood, discovers that she can interpret:

> "In the evening I realized that the Totonacas hidden in the brush were spying on us...We said hello, it was the only thing that we had learned from the prisoners. They talked to us but we didn't understand them. We responded in Maya, one of them understood. He tried to talk to us, but his pronunciation was so bad we couldn't understand him. Then one of them started to talk in another language. I was dumbstruck when I understood him. Something moved from the depths of my memory and, without realizing it, I answered him with fluidity, without doubts or tripping over myself. I talked and talked in that language and felt happy" (p. 71)[11]
>
> *"En la tarde me di cuenta de que nos espiaban los totonacas ocultos en la maleza...Los saludamos, era lo único que habíamos aprendido de los prisioneros, nos hablaron, no les entendíamos. Les respondimos en maya, uno nos comprendió, intentó hablarnos, pronunciaba tan mal que no le comprendimos. Entonces, uno de ellos, comenzó a hablar en otro idioma, quedé atónita al entenderlo, algo se me removió del fondo de la memoria y, sin darme cuenta, le contesté con fluidez, sin dudas o tropiezos, hablé y hablé en ese idioma sintiéndome feliz" (p. 71).*

10 Publisher's note: The book by Martîn del Campo is the only Spanish-language "suggested reading" in this book. It is a valuable work, and the author has included in this section English translations of relevant excerpts for non-Spanish readers of this textbook.

11 Translated by the author.

Jerónimo informs Malinalli that she will be the official interpreter:

"You'll be the interpreter of Don Hernando." Jerónimo's voice was hoarse with emotion. "If you serve him well, great will be your rewards. Praise God who put you in our path!" (p. 72).

"-Serás la intérprete de don Hernando - la voz de Jerónimo estaba ronco de emoción- , si lo sirves bien, grandes serán tus recompensas. ¡Alabado sea Dios que te puso en nuestro camino!" (p. 72).

Malinalli thinks about her role as interpreter:

"For the first time in my life I was escorted by a soldier, as if I were someone important. My friends were surprised upon seeing me" (p. 72).

"Por primera vez en mi vida fui escoltada por un soldado, como si fuera principal, mis amigas se sorprendieron al verme" (p. 72).

* * *

"My new work was more arduous than all my previous work put together" (p. 126).

"Mi nuevo trabajo es más arduo que todos los anteriores juntos" (p. 126).

* * *

"I grew up as a slave among many, now I am 'Marina,' indispensable for communication between the captain and the Totonaca nobles and all the other chiefs whose lands we crossed" (p. 126).

"Crecí siendo esclava entre muchas, ahora soy 'Marina', indispensable para la comunicación entre el capitán, los señores Totonacas, y los demás principales por cuyas tierras atravesamos" (p. 126).

Malinalli talks to herself about her doubts and the personal and historical implications of her role:

"At each stage on the route toward Tenochtitlan, with every step I take, my soul molts like a caterpillar transforming into a butterfly, and now I don't know what I am changing into" (p. 115).

"En cada etapa de la ruta hacia Tenochtitlan, con cada paso que avanzo, se me muda el alma como gusano al transformarme en mariposa y ahora no sé en que me estoy convirtiendo" (p. 115).

* * *

"At the beginning I swore a false oath to the captain. After Tlazcallan the change began, but I didn't realize it until after what happened at Chollolan. Now I don't know who I am. You should have seen it, only vultures remained, the sweet acid smell...the fallen temples of the Gods and dead priests. I'm cold...they call me, 'wretched,' 'damned,' 'traitor'" (p. 116).

"Al inicio juré en falso ayudar al capitán, después de Tlazcallan empezó el cambio, pero no me di cuenta sino hasta lo ocurrido en Chollolan. Ya no sé quién soy. Vieras, sólo quedaron zopilotes, un olor ácido-dulzón...los templos de dioses caídos y sacerdotes muertos. Tengo frio...me dicen 'desgraciada,' 'maldita,' 'traidora'" (p. 116).

* * *

"I had to translate. I hoped he would talk without needing to be tortured. I couldn't breathe" (p. 118).

"Tuve que traducir. Esperé que hablese sin necesidad de tortura. Me faltó el aire" (p. 118).

And Malinalli also thinks about what they say to her:

"Damn you...may your death be violent, may you never know peace, may your children be born under an evil star and may they bring you only suffering" (p. 118).

"Maldita seas...que tu muerte sea violenta, que nunca encuentres paz, que tus hijos nazcan con mala estrella y sólo te provoquen sufrimientos" (p. 118).

"Just an interpreter"

Malinalli's story and her time in history were pivotal. In the book, like many girls from poor families in her world, she was sold, bought, given away, used to pay off debt, trafficked and forced to switch languages, religions, national identities and allegiances many times, before falling into the hands of the Spanish invaders. Yet, just as Europeans invaded the Americas, Malinalli found herself in a unique position as an interpreter with some opportunities, power and influence. She was also in a precarious position where how she performed her work could affect whether she and others lived or died.

In popular culture, Malinalli is often blamed for the next five hundred years of the suffering of Indigenous Peoples at the hands of European invaders. Her role was far more complex than this simplification suggests. She was able, sometimes, to make a difference. Who knows? Perhaps she influenced the following standards for interpreting first published by Spain during the Spanish conquest of the Americas. Note how incredibly modern these standards sound:

> *"Interpreters had to be duly sworn to perform their task 'well and faithfully,' expressing the matter before them 'clearly and frankly,' 'without hiding or adding anything,' 'without acting in favor of any of the parties,' and 'without deriving any profit from their task other than the pay due to them'" (Pöchhacker, 2007, p. 13).*

About this time, legislation by Spain included 14 laws regarding interpreter conduct in the Spanish colonies. These laws include the following:

- *"that the interpreters for the Indian language(s) shall have the necessary capacities and qualities...*
- *that the interpreters shall not accept or ask for presents or gifts...*
- *that the interpreters shall not hold private meetings with Indian clients;*
- *that the interpreters shall not act as advocates for the Indians" (Pöchhacker, 2007, p. 13).*

Given her real-life story, talents and skills, this interpreter must have thought quite a bit about her place and role as an interpreter and whether she should be an impartial facilitator, someone who sided with those in power or an advocate of her own people and other Indigenous groups. She almost certainly thought about the importance, limitations, pleasures and frustrations of her role. As a medical interpreter, you may find many parallels with her experience.

Now list as many such parallels as you can find.

Medical terminology: The human body

On the next pages you will find two anatomical drawings, the first drawing with labels in English and Spanish (Figure 1-A) and the second drawing with only blank lines (Figure 1-B).

Study Figure 1-A. If you interpret in any other spoken language(s) than Spanish and English, then go to Figure 1-B, which has blank labels. Write in the appropriate translations of each English term on the blank line. To do so, use a reliable medical glossary, consult fellow interpreters, research the information on the Internet and/or use any other resource that you trust in order to find the correct terms to insert on the blank lines.

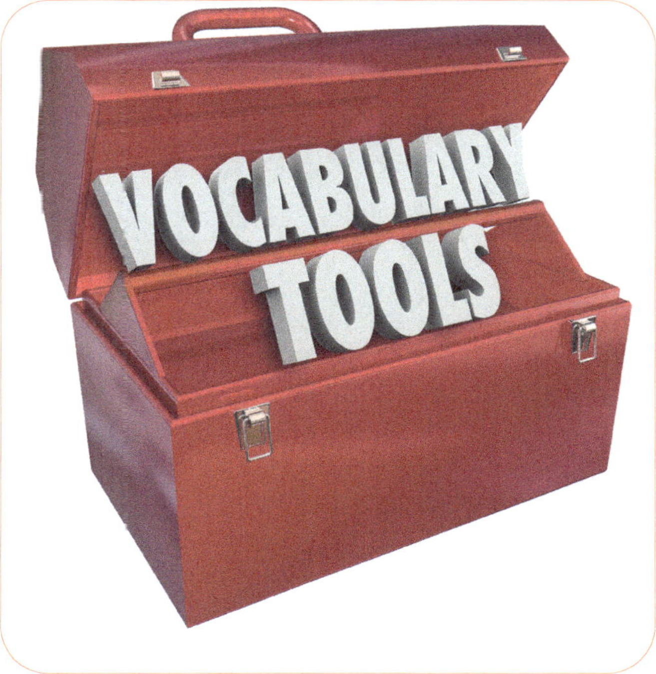

Now, test yourself. Turn to Figure 1-B. If you are an English-Spanish interpreter, or a sign language interpreter, see if you can say or sign the correct terms for each part of the human body in both or all your working languages. If you have a different language pair and have already filled in the blank, cover the blanks to test yourself.

Now turn to Figure 1-C. Write all the terms you can think of in both or all your working languages for human genitalia.

Keep studying these terms until you can interpret all of them into your working languages.

Medical terminology: The human body

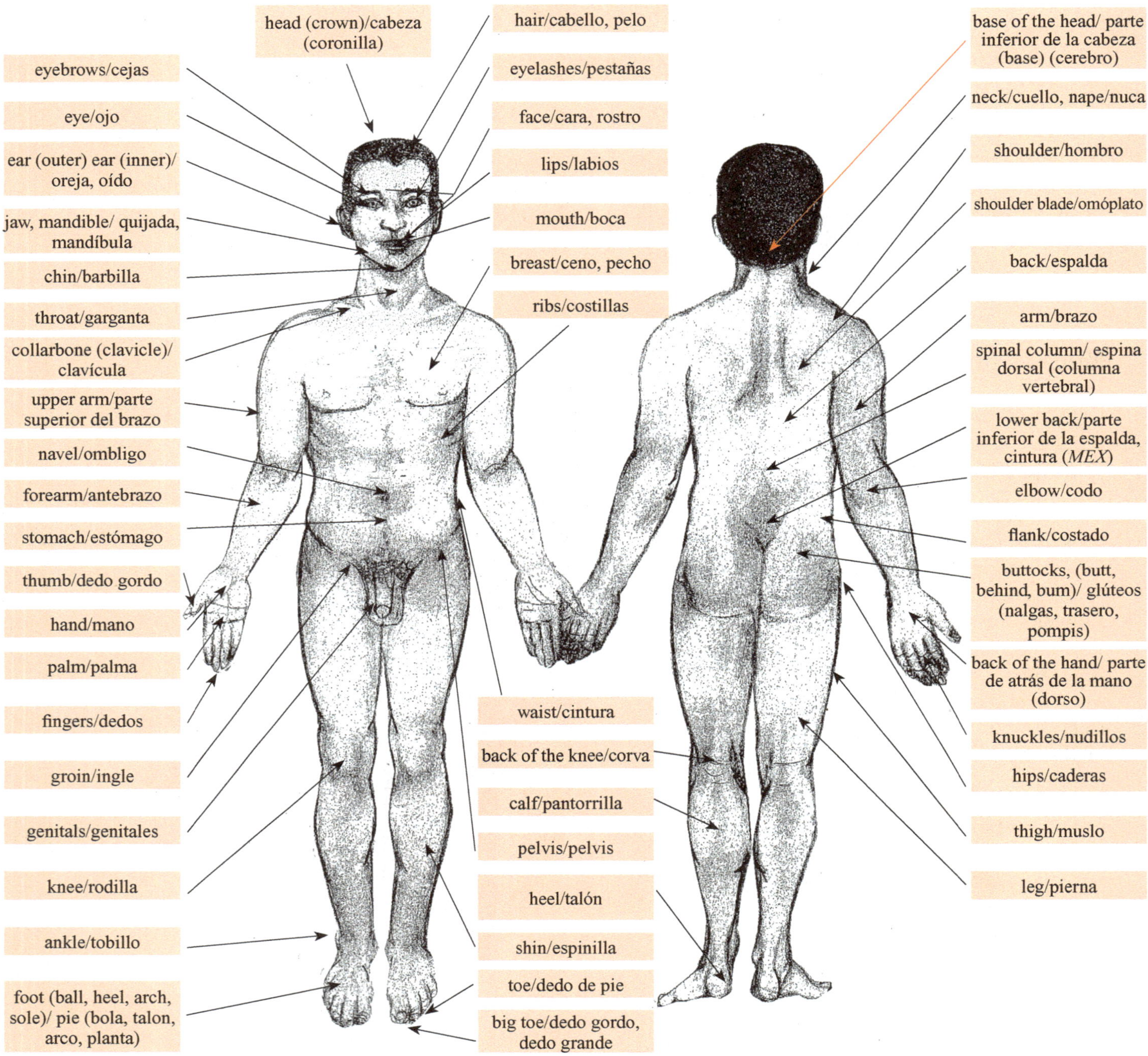

Figure 1-A: The human body (English and Spanish)

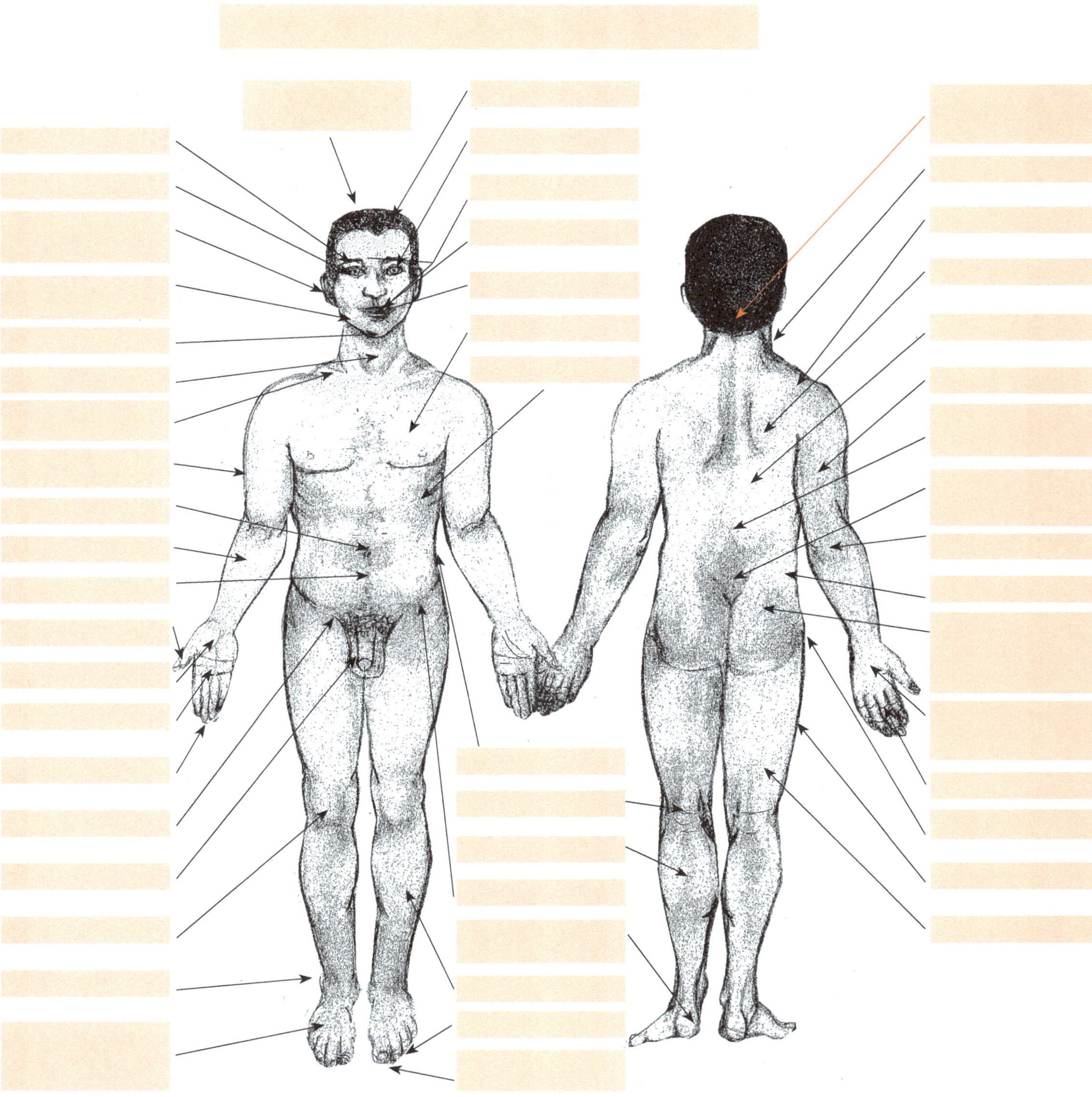

Figure 1-B: The human body (blank labels)

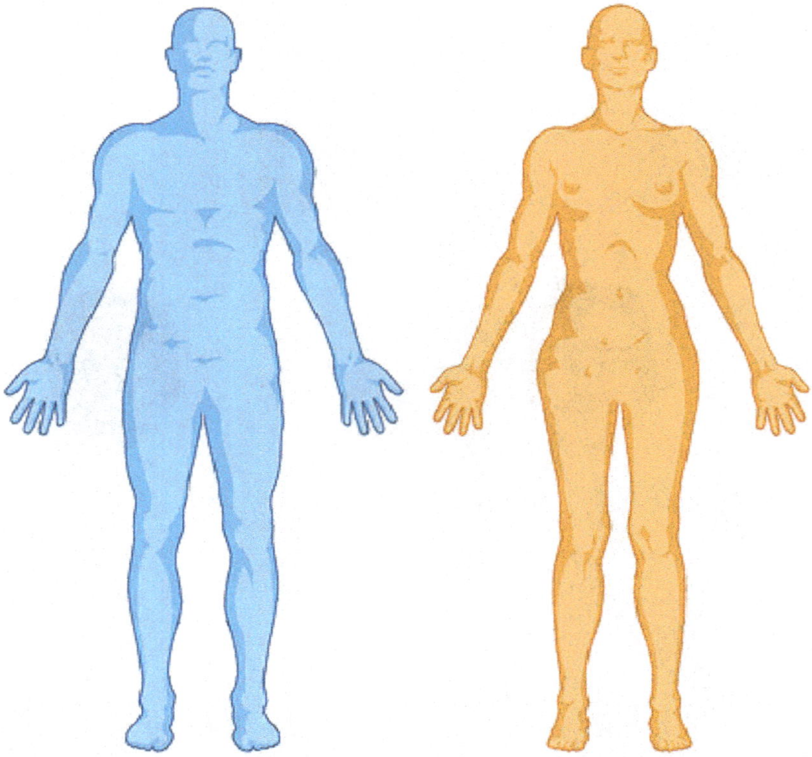

Figure 1-C: Human Genitalia

In the blanks below, for both (or all) your working languages write down as many terms as you can find for external male and female genitalia.

Male

Female

Medical terminology list

The Human Body

VOCABULARY FOR GRAPHIC–IN ENGLISH	VOCABULARY FOR GRAPHIC–IN SPANISH	ANY OTHER LANGUAGE
ENGLISH	SPANISH	
abdomen	abdomen	
ankle	tobillo	
arm	brazo	
back	espalda	
back of the hand	parte de atrás de la mano (dorso)	
back of the knee	corva	
ball, heel, arch of foot	bola, talon, arco del pie	
base of the head	parte inferior de la cabeza (base) (cerebro)	
big toe	dedo gordo, dedo grande	
breast	seno, pecho	
buttocks, (butt, behind, bum)	glúteos (nalgas, tresero, pompis)	
calf	pantorrilla	
chest	pecho	
chin	barbilla	
collarbone (clavicle)	clavícula	
ear (outer) ear (inner)	oreja, oído	
elbow	codo	
eye	ojo	
eyebrows	cejas	
eyelashes	pestañas	
face	cara, rostro	
fingers	dedos	
flank	costado	
foot (ball, heel, arch, sole)	pie (bola, talon, arco, planta)	
forearm	antebrazo	
genitals	genitales	
groin	ingle	

VOCABULARY FOR GRAPHIC—IN ENGLISH	VOCABULARY FOR GRAPHIC—IN SPANISH	ANY OTHER LANGUAGE
hair	cabello, pelo	
hand	mano	
head (base, crown)	cabeza (base, coronilla)	
hell	talón	
hips	caderas	
jaw, mandible	quijada, mandíbula	
knee	rodilla	
knuckles	nudillos	
leg	pierna	
lips	labios	
lower back	parte inferior de la espalda, cintura	
mouth	boca	
nape	nuca	
navel	ombligo	
neck	cuello, nuca	
palm	palma	
pelvis	pelvis	
ribs	costillas	
shin	espinilla	
shoulder	hombro	
shoulder blade	omóplato	
spinal column	espina dorsal (columna vertebral)	
stomach	estómago	
thigh	muslo	
throat	garganta	
thumb	dedo gordo	
toe	dedo de pie	
upper arm	parte superior del brazo	
waist	cintura	

Endocrinology—Pediatric 2

Advisory

This dialogue takes place during a visit to a medical office and discusses pediatric health problems, such as pituitary and neurological conditions, impaired vision and raising a child with birth defects and serious health conditions.

This appointment involves a family with little formal education. In the Spanish version below, the family comes from El Salvador. The family includes the mother, father, the three-year-old female patient, an energetic toddler sibling and a newborn.

One of the challenges for the interpreter might be the difference in communication styles between the provider and the family. The provider would probably prefer getting simple answers to straightforward questions. This provider would also likely want to hear a sequential narration of the medical history (beginning to end) rather than the family's non-chronological answers (jumping around).

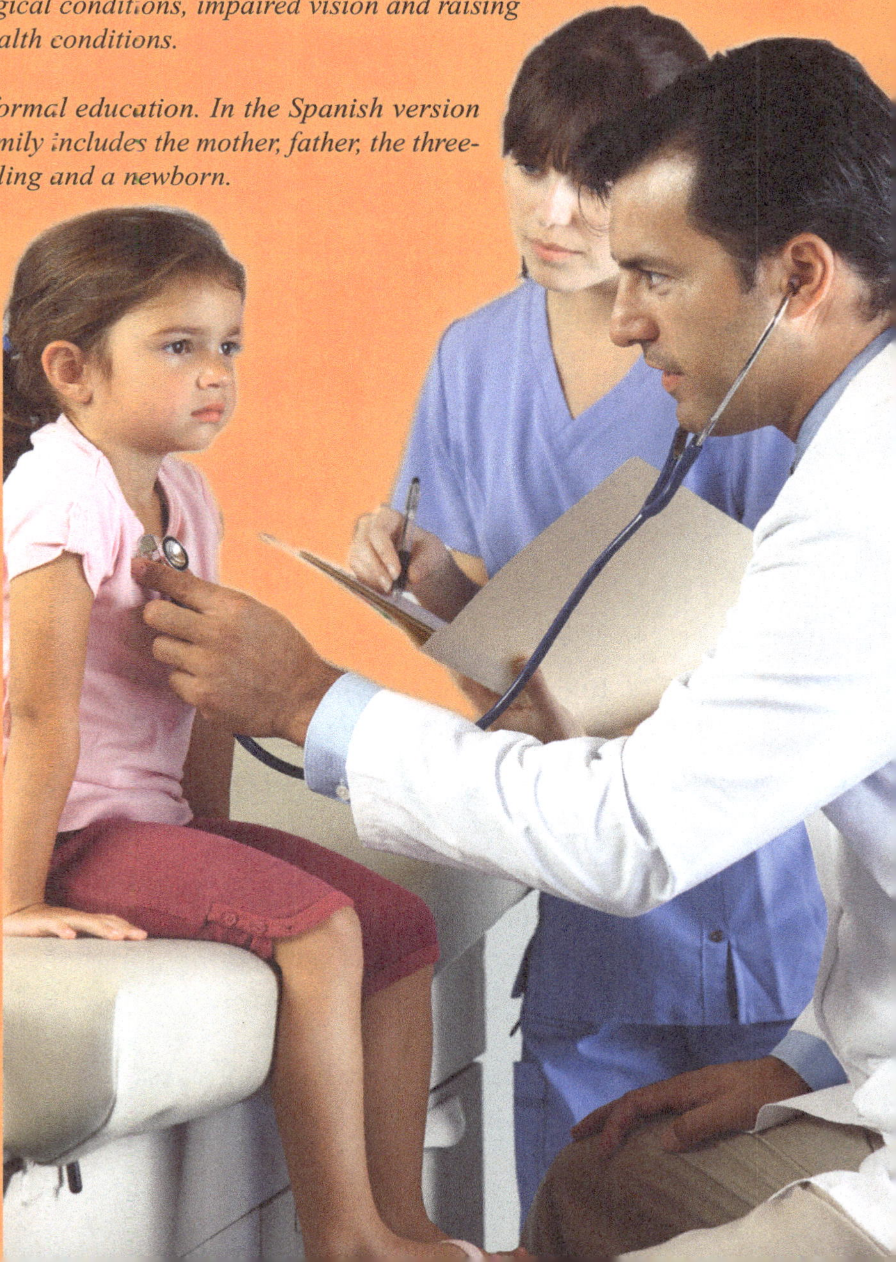

Note for both dialogues

The interpreter arrived on time, contrary to what the doctor suggests.

Pediatric endocrinology role play (English-Spanish)

Note about the English-Spanish dialogue: *In El Salvador and other parts of Latin America, there is frequent use of "voseo," or the pronoun "vos," instead of "tú," which changes the verb conjugation.*

PART 1

INTERPRETER: Good afternoon. My name is ___________. I'm your interpreter. I'd like to let you know that everything you say will be interpreted, and everything will be kept confidential. Please speak directly to each other, not to me, and pause when I make this signal *(raises hand)* so I can interpret.	**INTERPRETER:** Buenas tardes. Me llamo _____________. Soy su intérprete. Quisiera informarle que yo interpretaré todo lo que usted dice y que todo será confidencial. Por favor dirijánse directamente el uno al otro. Cuando yo le hago esta señal (*raises hand*), por favor haga una pausa y permítame interpretar.

DOCTOR: Good afternoon, *buenos tardes. (Doctor tries to say a greeting in the patient's language but makes mistakes with grammatical errors.)* Mrs. Duarte, Mr. Duarte. The interpreter is finally here. Now we can talk.

MOM AND DAD: Buenas tardes.

DOCTOR: So, what's the name of the doctor who referred you to us from the clinic?

DAD: Es la Dra. Quiñónez.

DOCTOR: OK. Did she explain to you why you're here today?

MOM: Es por el crecimiento. Y el ojo. Dicen que no está creciendo bien. Pero dejamos la cita para el ojo hasta el 15 de diciembre.

DOCTOR: Right, well, that's good. But we need to talk about—*(turns to kids)* Shh! We need to talk about why you are here today in *this* clinic. Did she explain that to you?

MOM: Nos dijo que es por el crecimiento. ¿Veá? Y de sus piernas, ella está aguadita de aquí en sus piernitas y su ojo.

DOCTOR: OK. Well, that's true. *(turns to kids again)* Shh! Be quiet! *(to parents)* But it seems that Clara has several problems, and we need to talk about all these things today. You know she had a study done a couple of weeks ago, right?

DAD: Sí.

MOM: Fue aquí que lo hicieron, sí, esa cosa en el tubo, *emarrái.*

DOCTOR: Did anyone talk to you about the results of the MRI? Did anyone tell you anything about the result?

MOM: No, nadie nos ha dicho.

DOCTOR: All right, well, we're going to talk about all that. But first I need to talk to you a little bit about her medical history. Now, where was Clara born?

DAD: En El Salvador.

DOCTOR: Salvador. And when did you come to this country?

MOM: El 14 de sectiembre del año pasado. Hace un año ya.

DAD: Todo estaba bien cuando nació, estaba bonita, gordita, rosadita, todo. Todo bien hasta que se enfermó y su ojo se puso así. Y pue' también sufre porque no puede hacer del baño muy bien. Popó.

DOCTOR: Wait a minute, wait a minute, let's back up here. Now, Mrs. Duarte, can you tell me if there were any problems or complications during the pregnancy?

MOM: *(distracted from the conversation, to child)* Clarita, vení, dale el juguete a tu hermano. No, no...

DAD: *(to Mom)* Te está preguntando algo, contestá vos.

MOM: *(to Dad)* ¿Qué me preguntó?

DAD: Sobre cuando estabas preñada—si tuviste problemas.

MOM: Sí. Es que ella quiso venir antes de tiempo.

DOCTOR: *(Kids are making lots of noise.)* Mr. Duarte, I think that if you want to go back out to the waiting room with the children until I can finish this part, then I can invite you back in when I'm ready to talk to you about the information that I have. I think I can talk to Mom about this other part of her early history. I do want you to come back in after because it will be very important for you to hear what I need to explain to you. All right?

DAD: Está bien. *(Dad leaves with the children.)*

DOCTOR: So she was a preemie?

MOM: Es que se me iba a caer.

DOCTOR: All right, so she was born early. At how many weeks was she born?

MOM: No, no. Ella nació bien, completó los nueve meses.

DOCTOR: *(irritated)* I thought you said she came early.

MOM: Sí, tuve que ir al hospital y me dieron medicina. Luego estuve bien hasta los nueve meses completos.

DOCTOR: And how did she do when she was born? Did she have any problems?

> **MOM:** Ella estaba muy bien.

DOCTOR: So you never saw anyone for any of her problems until you came here?

> **MOM:** No.

DOCTOR: Did she ever have any convulsions or seizures?

> **MOM:** No, nunca.

DOCTOR: And who was the first person to notice she had a problem?

> **MOM:** Fue la Dra. Quiñónez. Es ella que es su doctora, que siempre la ve.

DOCTOR: So, Dr. Quiñónez was the first one to notice her eye?

> **MOM:** No, fue cuando se enfermó. Primero se puso chelita, pues ella es chelita, pero se puso más chelita. Luego fue cuando los ojos se le pusieron así y la lengua le colgaba pa' fuera así y se puso aguadita de las piernas.

DOCTOR: Wait, wait, wait. So she got sick? When was that? You said she was fine until you came to this country.

> **MOM:** A los seis meses.

DOCTOR: And what happened?

> **MOM:** Es que se enfermó y se veía muy mal. Los ojos se le fueron así y hacía muecas con su cara y su lengua le colgaba así, y de aquí para abajo se puso aguadita.

PART 2

DOCTOR: And did that last a long time?

> **MOM:** Pue' unos dos o tres meses de la lengua. Pero los ojos se le quedaron así y las piernas, pues están aguaditas hasta ahora.

DOCTOR: Did they tell you anything about what happened? Did they tell you what kind of a problem they thought she had?

> **MOM:** Nomás lo de su ojo.

DOCTOR: Right, the hypo-septo-optic dysplasia. Did they tell you anything else?

> **MOM:** Bueno, no sé de ese nombre que usted dice, ¿veá? Pero esa cosa con el ojo, que dijeron que tuvo un problema con el ojo.

DOCTOR: Did they tell you anything else?

MOM: No, nada.

DOCTOR: All right. Did they give her any medicine?

MOM: No, no le dieron medicina. Nomás le frotaron. Así se mejoró, con frotaciones.

DOCTOR: Wow. I can't believe this. And they just said it was her eye?

MOM: Sí.

DOCTOR: Tell me about her legs. When did she sit up? When did she start to walk?

MOM: Pues, desde que se enfermó se quedó aguadita. Yo la sentaba y se caía. Tuve que ponerle almohadas para que se sentara bien.

DOCTOR: And walking?

MOM: Pues ella camina, pero está aguadita, se cae enseguida. La chineo cuando se pone de pie, se cae en seguida.

DOCTOR: And how about her vision? Do you think she sees well? I mean, does she run into walls or anything?

MOM: Sí, creo que ve bien, se cae pero es por las piernas, no por la vista.

DOCTOR: Well, I wonder. Anyway, so Dr. Quiñónez was the first person to notice something?

MOM: No, fue allí en el otro hospital, el general. Aquí tengo sus papeles, ¿los quiere ver?

DOCTOR: Yes, yes! *(Examines chart.)* Oh, I'm so glad you brought the chart. This really helps me a lot. Make sure you bring this with you any time you see any kind of doctor. It will really help. Otherwise they won't be able to help you. This tells me everything I wanted to know.

MOM: Sí, siempre tengo mis copias. La doctora me dijo que le diera estas copias, son para usted.

DOCTOR: *(to the interpreter, referring to the mother, sounding upset)* So *why* didn't she give them to me before?

DOCTOR: *(to mother)* And nobody's ever talked to you about what they think the problem might be?

MOM: No.

DOCTOR: OK. I think if your husband wants to come back in the room, he could come now. I want him to hear this too.

DAD: *(Father comes back into the room.)*

DOCTOR: All right, Mr. and Mrs. Duarte. I'm glad you're here, Mr. Duarte. I need to tell you about some very important information that will impact Clara for the rest of her life, and your lives too. Now, first of all, I need to explain to you several things. Clara has various problems, but the underlying problem she has is in her brain.

DAD: Entonces, ¿no va a ocupar cirugía?

DOCTOR: No, she doesn't need surgery.

MOM AND DAD: ¡Qué bien! No ocupa cirugía.

DOCTOR: Now, I mean she doesn't need surgery for the problem she has in the brain. She may need surgery to fix her eye. It's just the right eye, right?

DAD: Sí, es que estas cosas al lado aquí. *(Gestures showing outside corners of eyes and temples.)* Es que tiene una corta y la otra larga.

DOCTOR: Right, the hypo-septo-optic dysplasia. Just one eye is affected, the right eye. Now, I want to talk to you about the problem she has with her brain. I believe the problem she has with her eye is caused by the problem she has in her brain. The eye is only a symptom that something else is wrong. Clara has *several* problems, and I believe most of them are caused by the problems in her brain. *¿Comprende*?

MOM AND DAD: Sí.

DOCTOR: Now, I'm a brain specialist. Clara has a problem with something in the brain called the hypothalamus. It's very small and it's right in the center of the brain, on the midline.

DAD: Sí, la doctora nos dijo algo de una glándula.

DOCTOR: Ah! *(to the interpreter, sarcastically)* So there is some information after all! *(to parents)* Right, we're getting to that. The hypothalamus is very important. It sits just on top of something else called the pituitary gland. The pituitary gland is only the size of your thumbnail, this big, but it's responsible for hormone production and controls six very important systems in your body.

DAD: Me acuerdo de algo así.

DOCTOR: It's sometimes called "the master gland." It affects her thyroid gland, which produces the hormone that gives you energy, and it affects the production of cortisol, which is the hormone that helps your body in times of stress. When you're ill, for example, it affects the production of growth hormone, which is responsible for your growth and bones, and it affects the production of the hormones responsible for sexual development and the regulation of water and urine production. Clara's problem is that this part of the brain didn't develop correctly, and so it affects all these other systems in her body.

DAD: Entonces, ¿sucedió después de que nació?

PART 3

DOCTOR: No, it happened in utero, during development.

(There is a long pause. The mother and father appear upset by this news and get tears in their eyes.)

DOCTOR: So this is what I believe Clara's problem is. She suffers from what I believe is called hypopituitarism. It may be the reason she got sick at six months. If her cortisol production were affected, then she wouldn't have had sufficient cortisol to help her through the illness, and perhaps this is how she ended up with the eye and tongue problem and the weakness problem. Is this making sense to you?

MOM: Sí.

DAD: Pero yo no entiendo, ella platica, hace todo. Cuando usted empezó a hablar por teléfono aquí en la oficina, ella agarró su juguete y empieza a hablar, agarra el periódico. ¿Veá? Agarra creyones y cuando usted escribe ella empieza a rayar, juega con su hermanito.

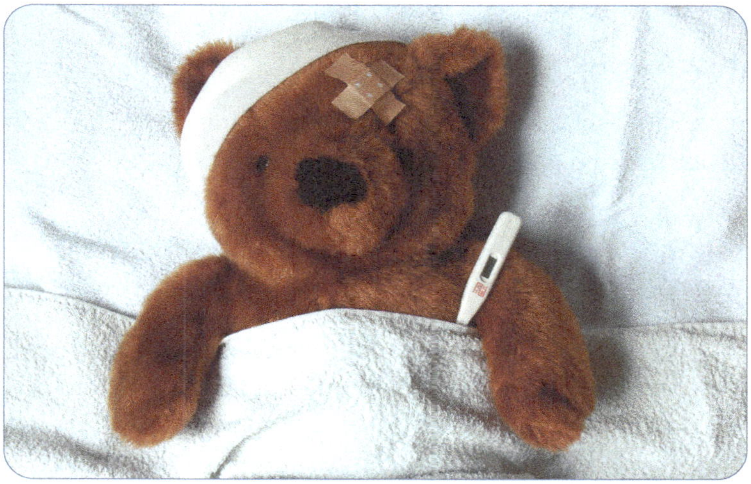

DOCTOR: *(sarcastically)* Well, she does have *some* brain function *(shaking his head)*. We're talking about a small, very specific part of her brain. Before I forget, I want to write down the name of this disease for you. It's very important that you have this somewhere. I'm going to write it on the back of my card. Here. Now, if she ever ends up in the emergency room for any reason, it's very important that you show them this card and the name of the problem she has, hypopituitarism. Whoever sees her will need to know this right away. You'll need to get her immediate help. If you show them this card, they should treat her right away and not let you sit there for hours. It's very important. It could be life-threatening. You need to remember that, do you understand?

MOM AND DAD: Sí.

DOCTOR: I'll see if I can find one of those pamphlets for medical alert bracelets out front. You can get her a bracelet or a necklace with the name of the condition on the back. That way if she's ever in trouble and you're not around, then she'll have the bracelet on to identify the condition.

MOM: Sí, yo tengo una tía diabética y ella anda uno de esos.

DOCTOR: Now, this is all the bad news I'm going to give you today, but there is some good news. All right?

MOM AND DAD: Sí.

DOCTOR: Now, for all these problems I've talked about, there are medicines we can give Clara to replace the hormones her body isn't making. Now you understand, we can't do anything about the damage that may have already occurred to the brain, but we can do a lot to prevent any damage in the future. What we have to do is determine which systems are affected and go from there. I don't think that it's affecting the water or urine production. If that were the case, we'd see her urinating all the time, and she doesn't do that, so I think we're OK there. As far as the sex hormones and sexual development, we'll have to wait until she's a little older, about the time she should be menstruating. For the time being, I don't think we can do anything about that except to wait and see. I do suspect she may have problems with her other systems, including her growth.

DAD: Pero ella hace muchas cosas.

DOCTOR: Yes, but she doesn't do what other children her age are doing and she's a little small. The main thing is, I don't want to start her on any medicines until we know exactly what we're dealing with.

DAD: Entonces, ¿no hay qué hacer nada por ahora?

DOCTOR: Well, there are some studies I'd like to do. I'd like for her to have some blood tests that will look for levels of certain substances in her blood and that may tell us about which hormones are lacking and causing her problems. I'd also like for her to get some x-rays of her hands. This is going to tell us what stage of development her body is at in terms of her growth and if it corresponds to her age. In addition, and this is the last thing, I'd like her to get some scans of her brain so we can take a look at brain structure and see if we can learn anything about what's going on from that. All right?

MOM AND DAD: Sí

DOCTOR: Now, I also want you to come back in about a month, after we have the results of all these studies, all right? So, take these papers up front and they'll help you schedule all of these appointments. Do either of you have any questions?

MOM AND DAD: No, doctor. Muchas gracias. Que Dios le bendiga doctor, *(turns to interpreter)* y a usted también, señorita.

DOCTOR: You're very welcome. So we'll see you in about a month.

MOM AND DAD: Muchas gracias.

Pediatric endocrinology role play—hypopituitarism (English only)

Note: Feel free to change the name of the patient to fit the language you interpret to from English.

PART 1

DOCTOR: Good afternoon, Mrs. (__________), Mr. (_________). *(Insert an appropriate family name.)* The interpreter is finally here. Now we can talk. *(Doctor tries to say a greeting in the patient's language but makes mistakes with grammatical errors.)*

MOM AND DAD: Good afternoon.

INTERPRETER: Good afternoon. My name is ___________. I'm your interpreter. I'd like to let you know that everything you say will be interpreted, and everything will be kept confidential. Please speak directly to each other, not to me, and pause when I make this signal *(raises hand)* so I can interpret. *(Interpreter repeats this passage in the patient's language.)*

DOCTOR: So, what's the name of the doctor who referred you to us from the clinic?

DAD: It's Dr. Quiñónez.

DOCTOR: OK. Did she explain to you why you're here today?

MOM: It's because of her growth. And her eye. They say she isn't growing well. But the eye appointment isn't until December 15.

DOCTOR: Right, well, that's good. But we need to talk about—*(turns to kids)* Shh! We need to talk about why you are here today in *this* clinic. Did she explain that to you?

MOM: They say it's because of her growth. Right? And her legs, she's wobbly here in her legs. And her eye.

DOCTOR: OK. Well, that's true. *(turns to kids again)* Shh! Be quiet! *(to parents)* But it seems that Clara has several problems, and we need to talk about all these things today. You know she had a study done a couple of weeks ago, right?

DAD: Yes.

MOM: They did it here, yes, that thing in the tube, *emarrái.*

DOCTOR: Did anyone talk to you about the results of the MRI? Did anyone tell you anything about the result?

MOM: No, nobody's talked to us.

DOCTOR: All right, well, we're going to talk about all that. But first I need to talk to you a little bit about her medical history. Now, where was Clara born?

DAD: In _______ *(Choose an appropriate country.)*

DOCTOR: I see. And when did you come to this country?

MOM: The 14th of September, last year. It's been quite a year already.

DAD: Everything was fine when she was born, she was pretty, nice and chubby and pink and everything. Everything was OK until she got sick and her eye got like that. And she also suffers because she can't go to the bathroom very well. To poop.

DOCTOR: Wait a minute, wait a minute, let's back up here. Now, Mrs. (________), can you tell me if there were any problems or complications during the pregnancy?

MOM: *(distracted from the conversation, to child)* Clara, come here. Give the toy to your brother. No, no...

DAD: *(to mother)* Hey, answer, he's asking you something.

MOM: *(to father)* What did he ask me?

DAD: About when you had your little bun in the oven[12]—if you had any problems.

MOM: Yes. She wanted to come out before it was time.

DOCTOR: *(Kids are making lots of noise.)* Mr. Duarte. *(Substitute the other family name you chose, if you did so.)* I think that if you want to go back out to the waiting room with the children until I can finish this part, then I can invite you back in when I'm ready to talk to you about the information that I have. I think I can talk to Mom about this other part of her early history. I do want you to come back in after because it will be very important for you to hear what I need to explain to you. All right?

DAD: All right. *(Dad leaves with the children.)*

DOCTOR: So she was a preemie?

MOM: Well, she was going to come out.

DOCTOR: All right, so she was born early. At how many weeks was she born?

MOM: No, no. She was on time, she made it through nine months.

DOCTOR: *(irritated)* I thought you said she came early.

MOM: Yes, I had to go to the hospital and they gave me medicine. Then I was fine until the end of nine months.

DOCTOR: And how did she do when she was born? Did she have any problems?

12 To have a "bun in the oven" means to be pregnant.

MOM: She was just fine.

DOCTOR: So you never saw anyone for any of her problems until you came here?

MOM: No.

DOCTOR: Did she ever have any convulsions or seizures?

MOM: No, never.

DOCTOR: And who was the first person to notice she had a problem?

MOM: It was Dr. Quiñónez. That's her regular doctor; she always sees her.

DOCTOR: So, Dr. Quiñónez was the first one to notice her eye?

MOM: No, it was when she got sick. First she got pale, well, she is really light-skinned, but she got even lighter. After that is when her eyes got like that, and her tongue was hanging out like this, and she got all floppy in her legs.

DOCTOR: Wait, wait, wait. So she got sick? When was that? You said she was fine until you came to this country.

MOM: At six months of age.

DOCTOR: And what happened?

PART 2

MOM: Well, she got sick and looked really bad. Her eyes went like this and she made strange faces, and her tongue hung out like this, and from here down she was really, really floppy.

DOCTOR: And did that last a long time?

MOM: Well, the tongue thing lasted two or three months. But her eyes stayed like that, and her legs, well, they're still wobbly today.

DOCTOR: Did they tell you anything about what happened? Did they tell you what kind of a problem they thought she had?

MOM: No. Just about her eye.

DOCTOR: Right, the hypo-septo-optic dysplasia. Did they tell you anything else?

MOM: Well, I don't know anything about that thing you just said, you know? But that thing with the eye, they said she had a problem with her eye.

DOCTOR: Did they tell you anything else?

MOM: No, nothing.

DOCTOR: All right. Did they give her any medicine?

MOM: No, they didn't give her any medicine. They just massaged her. She got better with that, with massages.

DOCTOR: Wow. I can't believe this. And they just said it was her eye?

MOM: Yep.

DOCTOR: Tell me about her legs. When did she sit up? When did she start to walk?

MOM: Well, since she got sick she stayed floppy. I would sit her up and she would fall. I had to put pillows around her so she could sit up right.

DOCTOR: And walking?

MOM: Well, she walks, but she's wobbly, she falls right away. I hold on to her when she gets up, but she falls right away.

DOCTOR: And how about her vision? Do you think she sees well? I mean, does she run into walls or anything?

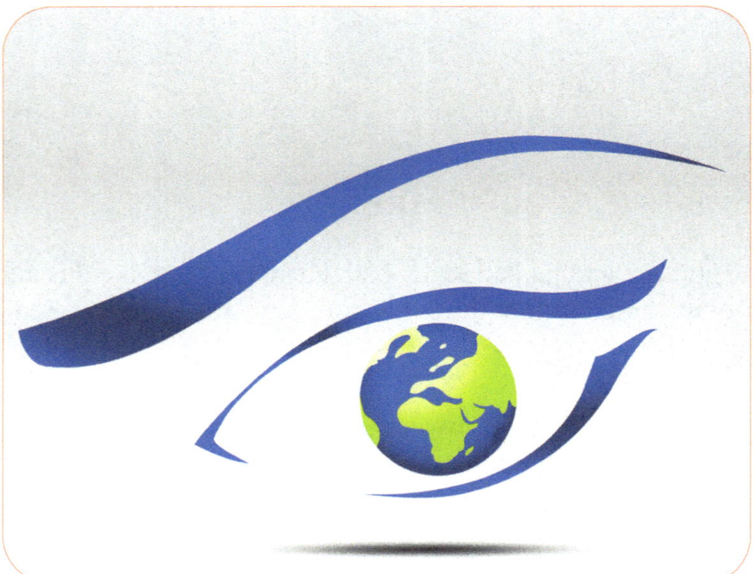

MOM: Yes, I think she sees OK, she falls; but it's her legs, not her seeing.

DOCTOR: Well, I wonder. Anyway, so Dr. Quiñónez was the first person to notice something?

MOM: No, it was at that other hospital, the county hospital. I have the papers here, do you want to see them?

DOCTOR: Yes, yes! *(examines chart)* Oh, I'm so glad you brought the chart. This really helps me a lot. Make sure you bring this with you any time you see any kind of doctor. It will really help. Otherwise they won't be able to help you. This tells me everything I wanted to know.

MOM: Yes, I always have my copies. The doctor told me to give you these copies; they're for you.

DOCTOR: *(to the interpreter, referring to the mother, sounding upset)* So *why* didn't she give them to me before?

DOCTOR: *(to mother)* And nobody's ever talked to you about what they think the problem might be?

MOM: No.

DOCTOR: OK. I think if your husband wants to come back in the room, he could come now. I want him to hear this too.

DAD: *(Father comes back into the room.)*

DOCTOR: All right, Mr. and Mrs. Duarte. I'm glad you're here, Mr. Duarte. I need to tell you about some very important information that will impact Clara for the rest of her life, and your lives too. Now, first of all, I need to explain to you several things. Clara has various problems, but the underlying problem she has is in her brain.

DAD: So then she doesn't need a surgery?

DOCTOR: No, she doesn't need surgery.

MOM AND DAD: Oh that's great! She won't need a surgery!

DOCTOR: Now, I mean she doesn't need surgery for the problem she has in the brain. She may need surgery to fix her eye. It's just the right eye, right?

DAD: Yes, it's these things on the side here. *(Gestures showing outside corners of eyes and temples.)* One of 'em is short and the other's long.

DOCTOR: Right, the hypo-septo-optic dysplasia. Just one eye is affected, the right eye. Now, I want to talk to you about the problem she has with her brain. I believe the problem she has with her eye is caused by the problem she has in her brain. The eye is only a symptom that something else is wrong. Clara has *several* problems, and I believe most of them are caused by the problems in her brain. Understand?

MOM AND DAD: Yes.

DOCTOR: Now, I'm a brain specialist. Clara has a problem with something in the brain called the hypothalamus. It's very small, and it's right in the center of the brain, on the midline.

DAD: Yes, the doctor said something to us about a gland.

DOCTOR: Ah! *(to the interpreter, sarcastically)* So there is some information after all! *(to parents)* Right, we're getting to that. The hypothalamus is very important. It sits just on top of something else called the pituitary gland. The pituitary gland is only the size of your thumbnail, this big, but it's responsible for hormone production and controls six very important systems in your body.

DAD: I remember something about that.

DOCTOR: It's sometimes called "the master gland." It affects her thyroid gland, which produces the hormone that gives you energy, and it affects the production of cortisol, which is the hormone that helps your body in times of stress. When you're ill, for example, it affects the production of growth hormone, which is responsible for your growth and bones, and it affects the production of the hormones responsible for sexual development and the regulation of water and urine production. Clara's problem is that this part of the brain didn't develop correctly, and so it affects all these other systems in her body.

DAD: So then it happened after she was born?

PART 3

DOCTOR: No, it happened in utero, during development.

(There is a long pause. The mother and father appear upset by this news and get tears in their eyes.)

DOCTOR: So this is what I believe Clara's problem is. She suffers from what I believe is called hypopituitarism. It may be the reason she got sick at six months. If her cortisol production were affected, then she wouldn't have had sufficient cortisol to help her through the illness, and perhaps this is how she ended up with the eye and tongue problem, and the weakness problem. Is this making sense to you?

MOM: Yes.

DAD: But I don't understand, she talks, she does everything. When you started talking on the telephone just now here in the office, she grabbed her toy telephone. She starts talking; she grabs the newspaper. Right? She grabs crayons, and when you write, she starts to scribble, she plays with her little brother.

DOCTOR: *(sarcastically)* Well, she does have *some* brain function (*shaking his head*). We're talking about a small, very specific part of her brain. Before I forget, I want to write down the name of this disease for you. It's very important that you have this somewhere. I'm going to write it on the back of my card. Here. Now, if she ever ends up in the emergency room for any reason, it's very important that you show them this card and the name of the problem she has, hypopituitarism. Whoever sees her will need to know this right away. You'll need to get her immediate help. If you show them this card, they should treat her right away and not let you sit there for hours. It's very important. It could be life-threatening. You need to remember that, do you understand?

MOM AND DAD: Yes.

DOCTOR: I'll see if I can find one of those pamphlets for medical alert bracelets out front. You can get her a bracelet or a necklace with the name of the condition on the back. That way if she's ever in trouble and you're not around, then she'll have the bracelet on to identify the condition.

MOM: Yes, I have an aunt with diabetes, and she goes around with one of those.

DOCTOR: Now, this is all the bad news I'm going to give you today, but there is some good news. All right?

MOM AND DAD: Yes.

DOCTOR: Now, for all these problems I've talked about, there are medicines we can give Clara to replace the hormones her body isn't making. Now you understand, we can't do anything about the damage that may have already occurred to the brain, but we can do a lot to prevent any damage in the future. What we have to do is determine which systems are affected, and go from there. I don't think that it's affecting the water or urine production. If that were the case, we'd see her urinating all the time, and she doesn't do that, so I think we're OK there. As far as the sex hormones and sexual development, we'll have to wait until she's a little older, about the time she should be menstruating. For the time being I don't think we can do anything about that except to wait and see. I do suspect she may have problems with her other systems, including her growth.

DAD: But she does a lot of things.

DOCTOR: Yes, but she doesn't do what other children her age are doing and she's a little small. The main thing is, I don't want to start her on any medicines until we know exactly what we're dealing with.

DAD: Then we don't need to do anything for now?

DOCTOR: Well, there are some studies I'd like to do. I'd like for her to have some blood tests that will look for levels of certain substances in her blood, and that may tell us about which hormones are lacking and causing her problems. I'd also like for her to get some x-rays of her hands. This is going to tell us what stage of development her body is at in terms of her growth, and if it corresponds to her age. In addition, and this is the last thing, I'd like her to get some scans of her brain so we can take a look at brain structure and see if we can learn anything about what's going on from that. All right?

MOM AND DAD: Yes.

DOCTOR: Now, I also want you to come back in about a month, after we have the results of all these studies, all right? So, take these papers up front, and they'll help you schedule all of these appointments. Do either of you have any questions?

MOM AND DAD: No, doctor. Thank you very much. God bless you, and you too, Miss Interpreter.

DOCTOR: You're very welcome. So we'll see you in about a month.

MOM AND DAD: Thank you so much.

What's important to know about this chapter?

Terminology

See the illustration at the end of this chapter and the terminology that accompanies this dialogue. As you go through the chapter, note any new or useful terms and learn them in both or all your working languages. You can find a general introduction to endocrinology and much of the related vocabulary online, for example:

> "Endocrinology is a complex study of the various hormones and their actions and disorders in the body. Glands are organs that make hormones. These are substances that help to control activities in the body and have several effects on the metabolism, reproduction, food absorption and utilization, growth and development etc.
>
> Hormones also control the way an organism responds to their surroundings and help by providing adequate energy for various functions.
>
> The glands that make up the endocrine system include the pineal, hypothalamus, pituitary, thyroid, parathyroid, thymus, adrenals, pancreas, ovaries and testes."[13]

Formal education and health literacy

The family in this dialogue has little formal education. They depend on the knowledge and expertise of health practitioners and face many challenges navigating the healthcare system. They may tell their health history in a non-chronological or nonlinear style. If the provider is irritated by this style of speech, the interpreter might find the situation awkward and difficult.

Dialect or regional variety

As often happens, this family speaks a major world language (in this case, Spanish) but speaks a regional variety (Salvadoran). In addition to some other unique vocabulary that might challenge the interpreter, this family uses a form of the second person informal pronoun *you* (vos) along with its verb conjugation. (In Spanish, this is sometimes referred to as the "*voseo,*" when "*vos*" is used instead of "*tú*" and can be found in other countries, such as Spain, Argentina and Uruguay.)

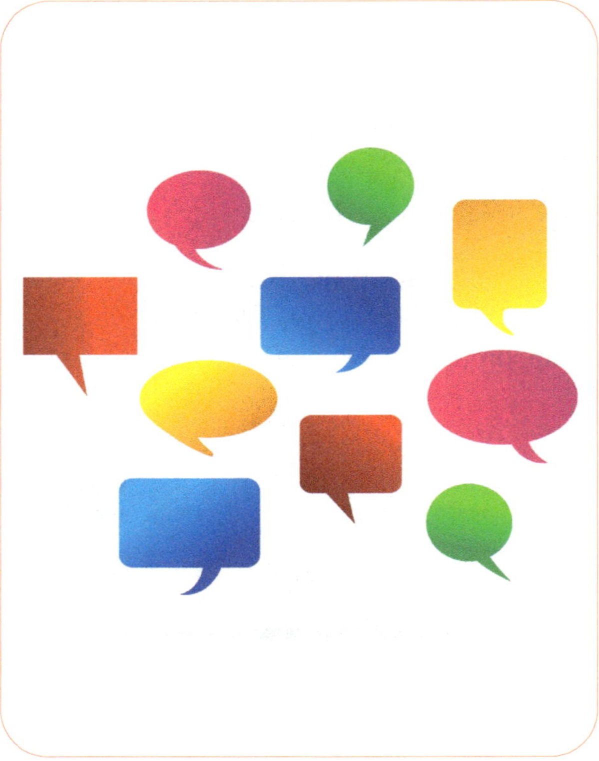

13 Retrieved from: www.news-medical.net/health/What-is-an-Endocrinologist.aspx

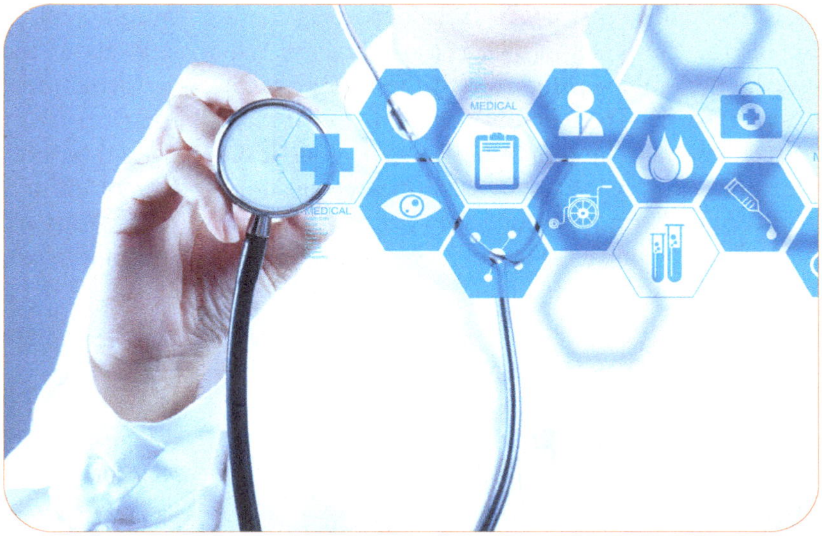

If you meet a person using a regional variety or dialect of a language you interpret for and you do not know it well, you can state up front that you are less familiar with it and make sure to ask for clarifications or repetition when you need to. Do your best and be transparent about your misgivings or doubts. If communication gets awkward, you can excuse yourself. If you know ahead of time, it could be easier to make the right decision. Still, there may be difficulty in getting another interpreter who is both fluent in the relevant regional variety and qualified to interpret. An experienced, qualified interpreter who declines the assignment might be replaced by someone less skilled. Use your best judgment when making such decisions.

Health concepts

Do an Internet search for the following terms and concepts:

1. patient-centered care
2. health literacy
3. informed consent

Write a brief description or definition of each one.

Practitioner language dilemma

In this dialogue, the practitioner begins by greeting the patient's family in their language, even though that greeting has errors. Should the interpreter relay the greeting as is, for example, by repeating *"Goods afternoon,"* or interpret it as it was intended, *"Good afternoon"*? If the interpreter politely corrects the practitioner, "*Good* afternoon," it might heighten the doctor's awareness of the importance of speaking through the interpreter.

Blame the interpreter

The physician's comment about the interpreter "finally" arriving strongly implied that the interpreter was late. Sometimes interpreters who run from assignment to assignment with no scheduled transportation time *are* late. Other times, clinicians are behind on their schedules and lose an interpreter (who has been called somewhere else), then have to wait for a new interpreter and blame the replacement. Such blame may be inappropriate. The interpreter might be misscheduled. Almost anything can happen.

In this case, the interpreter was punctual, but the doctor seems to comment on the interpreter's tardiness. Is it important for the interpreter to correct this misstatement? It might seem insignificant and not worth addressing, or it might indicate a problem. Be sure to consider how the interpreter is being portrayed, his or her professional integrity, the impact of the inappropriate clinician's commentary on the patient's trust in and regard for the interpreter and the interpreter's confidence in the clinician.

Blame the patient

From experience, the interpreter can become aware during a session like this that the parents may be blaming themselves for what has happened. The interpreter might want the doctor to address the fact that this condition is not in fact the parents' fault. Should the interpreter in such a case intervene? Why or why not? What is the role of the interpreter in such a case? Does the family's emotional state merit interpreter intervention? Could harm be done if the interpreter intervenes with a clarifying question? How is the interpreter's concentration or absorption of information impacted by emotional dilemmas like this?

Indirect conversation

At one point, in mid-sentence, the doctor turns to the children and says, "shh!" It is obvious to the interpreter that the parents have noticed the children's noise and attempted to get them to be quiet. They may be slightly stressed about it, or embarrassed. Should you interpret the doctor's "shh!"?

Private side conversations

Parents have a semi-private exchange in which basically one of them tells the other to pay attention to the doctor's question. How much of this exchange between the spouses should you interpret? Protocols regarding accuracy require the interpreter to interpret everything stated in the encounter. This couple makes private remarks in front of the interpreter. If the private remarks are not interpreted, the practitioner might feel excluded from the conversation and ask about it in case it includes important health information. If this were a conversation with a marriage and family counselor, behavioral specialist, social worker, psychologist, etc., it might reveal important information too. If the pace of the side conversation is too rapid for you to interpret, even in simultaneous mode, what could you do instead?

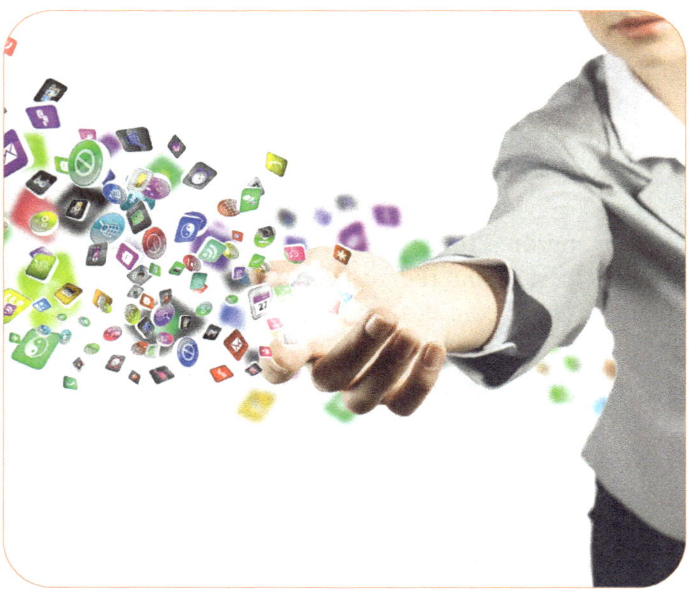

Gestational age and pregnancy dating

In different parts of the world, people calculate pregnancy differently. In this case, how are the patient and provider calculating pregnancy? In months or weeks? Health professionals and lay people (first-time mothers, those without access to clinical prenatal care, experienced unregulated midwives in the countryside and people in small villages without access to regulated professionals) might all think about date, measurements and describe pregnancies in different ways without realizing it.

For example, in some countries pregnancies might not be counted in weeks but in months. Others might date pregnancies from the date of conception (just after ovulation, days or weeks after a menstrual period); the first day or last day of the last menstrual period; the first day of the first missed period; or another date. In some cultures, pregnancies are dated from the moment the mother first feels movement; in others, pregnancies are not spoken of until three months' gestation.

Providers often ask pregnant women about birth histories and whether the baby was born "full term" or "to term." In the United States, health professionals usually date pregnancies in terms of weeks starting with the first day of the last menstrual period. Sometimes this calculation can be misleading or lead to inaccuracies. According to most recent definitions from the American College of Obstetricians and Gynecologists and the Society for Maternal-Fetal Medicine[14], it is preferable to use more specific labels than "term pregnancy," such as early term (37 weeks 0 days to 38 weeks 6 days), full

14 Definitions retrieved from www.smfm.org/publications/148-definition-of-term-pregnancy

term (39 weeks 0 days to 40 weeks 6 days), late term (41 weeks 0 days to 41 weeks 6 days) or postterm (42 weeks 0 days and longer). How professionals speak about this issue and what these terms mean may be different from how the question is being understood and answered by patients.

Interpreters may have to navigate this type of confusion by thinking quickly and deciding if cultural influences suggest a misunderstanding. If so, try to make your request for clarification transparent (interpret or report everything you say to one party for the other party).

Order of time and event

The doctor wants information in chronological order. He is obviously becoming irritated with the patient. The interpreter might feel that his bedside manner is unpleasant. Aware of the doctor's desire for a chronological narration of specific medical information, the interpreter could offer to clarify and obtain information. She could also restructure the solicited information. But is doing so part of the interpreter's job?

In fact, is doing so proper, improper or impractical? How? For example, the patient says, "It was Dr. Quiñónez. That's her regular doctor; she always sees her." The interpreter could render the message in a shorter English phrase, such as, "She's her regular doctor." Another interpretation, "She's her pediatrician," would give the doctor his short, straight answer, but it would be less complete, less accurate and also bring a change in register. It might lead the doctor to assume that the patient has a higher level of education and health literacy than he or she really has (including the patient's ability to understand basic health information and navigate the health system).

If a complex treatment plan follows this visit, *it is important for the doctor to have an accurate picture of the family's educational level and communication style*. They could all affect the parents' follow through and adherence to the treatment plan—and even the ability to understand it.

Comments made privately to the interpreter

In this dialogue, sometimes the doctor's frustration is clear. He makes a few private and even sarcastic remarks to the interpreter, such as the rhetorical question, "So, *why* didn't she give them to me before?" He is not expecting an answer: he is just venting to the interpreter.

Should this type of message be interpreted if it is not directed to the patient? Asking this question could have different results. If asked in a normal tone, the parents might simply give an explanation. If asked in a tone that accurately reflects the doctor's irritation, it could make the parents feel uncomfortable. They might feel demeaned, hurt or offended. (Having a limited ability to speak English does not make people less sensitive.)

Feeling offended or hurt could, in turn, prevent patients from communicating freely. As a result, everyone might get less out of the appointment, including the child. But then again—if you had a provider who was sarcastic, insulting and perhaps biased against people of your ethnicity, education and social class—wouldn't you want to know? Knowing could affect your decision about whether to stay with that doctor.

For all these reasons, the NCIHC national standards of practice (Standard 1) about accuracy specifically mentions "for example, an interpreter repeats all that is said, even if it seems redundant, irrelevant, or rude" (NCIHC, 2005, p. 5).

Sarcasm

How is sarcasm perceived cross-culturally? Does it vary among social classes? What can the interpreter do, if anything, when interpreting a negative remark or replicating a tone of voice that could be perceived by the patient as disrespectful or rude? Who is responsible for the remark? Might the patient think the tone comes from the interpreter? Does it matter? Interpreting in a

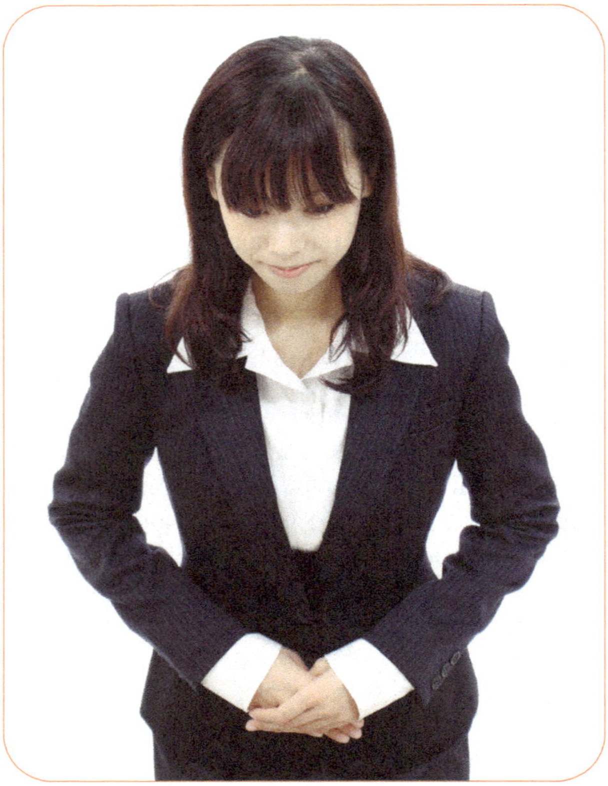

case like this one is complex. Interpreters are called on many times a day to use their sociocultural expertise to make decisions that can have serious consequences, some of them apparently subtle, and some that might affect health outcomes.

Interpreting tone

In this dialogue, the doctor comments, "Well, she does have *some* brain function." By emphasizing "*some*" this way, does the doctor mean, "The patient is very developmentally delayed and has very little brain function," or "Of course, she can do some things" or "Of course, she can do some things, you ignorant fools. Don't you know *anything*?" If the interpreter needs clarification, how can he or she ask for it? Is there a way to frame a request for clarification in a neutral way?

If the interpreter wants to raise consciousness (or is feeling feisty!), is there a way to ask for clarification that will alert the provider about the way he comes across? Sarcasm, irony and pointed tones can be understood differently in different cultures. It might be acceptable or considered offensive. However, in general, consciously intended put-downs (whether stated, implied or present only in the tone of voice of body language) are often more perceptible than providers realize. Simply because people do not speak a certain language does not make them blind to insults, but the provider might not be aware of that.

Simultaneous or consecutive?

The interpreter can interpret simultaneously or consecutively, as needed. In medical interpreting encounters, it's generally considered better to use consecutive, unless the situation veers out of control or when there is intense emotional content, for example, a patient recounting a rape or traumatizing event. In such cases, it might be better to switch to simultaneous rather than interrupt the speaker(s). Helping a patient or client share the story of a major trauma is often an essential part of therapy. In these situations too, it's often better not to interrupt, if possible.

But in many cases, the interpreter has to weigh other factors or constraints. Sometimes it just makes more sense for everyone to have a conversation at a normal flow without pauses. This is sometimes the case and then the interpreter might shift to simultaneous mode, including whispered interpreting (chuchotage). Some patients and providers are amazed and actually prefer it, "Wow! How do you do that? Just like at the United Nations!"

This question of when to switch modes in community (including medical) interpreting is now a national question that has no clear answers yet. The interpreter makes a decision, case by case.

Whichever mode you decide on, it's important to assess whether people are comfortable. It's also important to decide whether they can concentrate and take in information if you render it in simultaneous mode. If those present prefer consecutive interpreting, then you will need strong memory and note-taking skills to avoid interrupting too often, which can disrupt the flow. What are some nonintrusive ways you can get the provider or patient to pause if needed?

Clarification request—for the patient

In this dialogue, a point comes where the interpreter really wants to ask for clarification for a special purpose: to get the doctor to state the information in a different way, or to give further information. Sensing the parents' guilt and devastation after the doctor says, "No, it happened in utero, during development," the interpreter strongly senses that the parents feel guilt and shame. (Remember that at this point there was a long pause where *the mother and father appear upset by this news and get tears in their eyes.*)

Could the interpreter intervene to ask, "Excuse me, as the interpreter could I request you clarify whether this condition is the fault of the parents?" reporting what he or she said to the parents? In effect, the interpreter would be "asking" if the parents are responsible, through behaviors or actions, for the child's health issues. In reality, confident of the answer from previous experience, the interpreter would be *prompting* the physician with this question. Is this inappropriate intervention? Is it advocacy?

In this case, the interpreter has noticed something and asked herself: *Does the family's emotional state merit attention? Is there something that needs clarification? Could harm be done if nothing is acknowledged?* If the answer to any of these is "yes," then action may be needed. For example, if the parents are feeling emotionally impacted by the information (through guilt, sadness and fear for their child) they might not be able to concentrate or take in the information being presented to them. Is there another, less-intrusive way to ask the provider to address this concern?

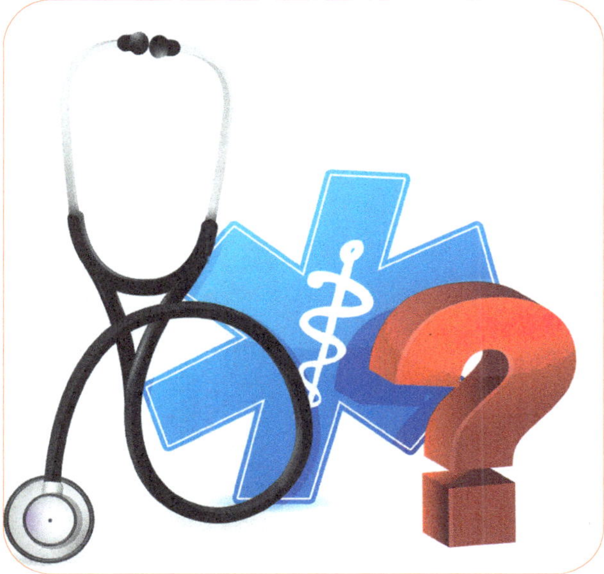

Important or inappropriate?

The interpreter is aware that the family will leave the consultation with little preparation for a possibly life-threatening emergency, which they might have difficulty communicating, especially with the language barrier. The doctor does not suggest a medic-alert bracelet, but the interpreter feels one is necessary for patient safety. Where does the "Do no harm" tenet of the national code of ethics fit in?[15]

Could a suggestion by the interpreter for the doctor to explore the possibility of a medic-alert bracelet end up being more harmful than failing to mention it, if the doctor does not do so? Does it mean crossing the line into advocacy?

How does interpreter intervention of this kind sit with the professional ethical requirement of accuracy versus the ethical requirement about advocacy? Would it be acceptable to suggest the bracelet in the presence of the doctor and the patient's family or better to raise the subject after the session in private with the doctor?

What about speaking to the parents alone to suggest looking into a medic-alert bracelet? Here the answer is clear: no. For the interpreter to make this suggestion to the parents might constitute, or be seen as, giving medical advice. Giving medical advice is not permitted for interpreters and in most states is probably not legal.

15 "Beneficence. A central value of the healthcare-interpreting profession is the health and well-being of the patient. This is a core value that is shared with other healthcare professions. It means that the members of these professions have as their essential obligation and duty to support the health and well-being of the patient and her/his family system of supports (e.g., family and community) and to do no harm (NCICH, 2004, p. 8).

Ethics and standards: Reflect and practice

Goal 2: Confidentiality

Translation and paraphrasing

1. Look at the two NCIHC standards of practice related to confidentiality (Standards 7 and 8, NCIHC, 2005, p. 6). Working individually, *paraphrase* the objective, its related ethical principle and the two standards.
2. Working individually, *translate* the original text of these standards into your other working language(s) or interpret it into sign language.
3. Find a partner or partners. Compare, discuss and modify your translations and paraphrasing until you are satisfied with your final products as a group.
4. If you can, pick a group representative and discuss your final versions with any other groups that share your working languages. Compare and discuss your differences.

Suggested reading

Roat, C. E. (2010). *Healthcare Interpreting in Small Bites: 50 Nourishing Selections from the "Pacific Interpreters Newsletter," 2002-2010.* Victoria, British Columbia: Trafford, pp. 31-34.

Consider and discuss

1. **Standard 7** An interpreter has been at an appointment with an elderly patient in a women's health clinic. During the course of the appointment, it is revealed that the woman is being abused by her husband, who has also been taking her pain medication, which she needs and suffers without. She and her son, present at the appointment, create a secure plan for storing her medication away from her husband. Three days later, the interpreter is in the emergency room (ER) with a patient in crisis with pain, anxiety and other psychiatric symptoms who reports no regular medication use. The interpreter discovers that this is the husband whose access to his wife's pain medication was probably cut off. Should the interpreter report this information to the attending ER physician? Why or why not?
2. **Standard 7** A few days later, the interpreter meets the same patient with a caregiver at a follow-up appointment. Should the interpreter fill the caregiver in on the problem of secure medication and the husband's access to it?
3. **Standard 7** A provider enters a hospital room with an interpreter to speak with an adult patient who has a lung infection. The patient's siblings are in the room. The provider mentions the patient's HIV-positive status. Should the interpreter proceed with the interpretation? Why or why not? What are the interpreter's options?
4. **Standard 8** If an interpreter takes notes or carries identifying patient information in writing, what personal consequences might there be for the patient? What personal measures might one take to prevent exposure or the loss of relevant information?

Occupational therapy for interpreters

EXERCISES FOR THE TONGUE, HEART AND MIND

"It is important, especially in emergency situations, not to have unnecessary delays... We really feel effective communication is fundamental to good quality care. It boils down to patient safety."

—Gayle Tang (Hua, 2006)

Suggested reading

Hua, V. (2006). Alameda County non-English speakers find ERs hard to reach: More than half of testers in study didn't get help. *San Francisco Chronicle*, February 17, 2006.

In the above-mentioned article, a writer for the *San Francisco Chronicle*, Vanessa Hua, described a study performed in Alameda County, California. The study examined the experience of limited or non-English speakers in getting emergency care. The goal was to provide research data to support claims of problematic access to care.

Background

According to U.S. Census Bureau data cited in the article, the number of people in this California county who do not speak English well is one in six. (More recent U.S. Census Bureau data suggest that one in five California residents is LEP—and one in three in some cities, such as San Francisco.)

Methodology and results

As part of the study, individuals speaking various languages who pretended to be patients made 551 calls to 12 different hospitals in the county. They called in complaining of symptoms that "were serious enough to warrant medical attention but not urgent enough to trigger an ambulance to be dispatched." The results were staggering, though perhaps not surprising. The following chart reflects some of the data found as a result of the study reported in the news article.

1. Describe how you felt when reading the data in this table.
2. Consider the following information: Federal law requires organizations that receive federal funding—including nearly all U.S. healthcare organizations—to take reasonable steps to prevent discrimination of the type documented in this article. The most important of these laws, often called language access laws, is Title VI of the U.S. Civil Rights Act of 1964. This law protects individuals from discrimination on the basis of race, color or national origin in any program or activity that receives federal financial assistance. How well do think the hospitals surveyed in the article comply with this law?
3. Consider the following scenario. A medical center operates a world-renowned organ transplant program. Intake appointments are four hours long. The first hour of orientation for patients, in English only, is followed by clinical appointments where interpreters are scheduled, if needed. In the United States, might the English-only orientation be considered a violation of an LEP and/or Deaf or Hard of Hearing person's civil rights? If so, how and why?
4. If you are familiar with language access laws in U.S. states or cities, or even other countries, that are similar to Title VI, list them.
5. Consider the following. An interpreter is concerned that patients at appointments in a county hospital who speak limited English are being told to go to another hospital or to come back with "someone who speaks English." She shares the following with management:

   Section 1557 of the Patient Protection and Affordable Care Act (42 U.S.C.

18116) provides that an individual shall not be excluded from participation in, be denied the benefits of, or be subjected to discrimination on the grounds prohibited under, among other laws, Title VI of the Civil Rights Act of 1964, under any health program or activity, any part of which is receiving federal financial assistance, or under any program or activity that is administered by an Executive Agency or any entity established under Title I of the Affordable Care Act or its amendments.[16]

The response the interpreter gets is, "I don't see how this applies. We are not a federal entity." What is incorrect in this answer?

6. In the article, Hua states, "Federal law requires hospitals receiving federal financial assistance to provide language services, including professional interpreters, at no cost to limited-English speakers. State law requires that hospitals have interpreters available, either on the premises or accessible by telephone, 24 hours a day" (Hua, 2006). What do you think are the reasons that interpreters (despite federal, state and city language access laws) are often not provided for LEP patients?
7. Access and read "The Department of Health and Human Services Language Access Plan 2013" at www.hhs.gov/sites/default/files/open/pres-actions/2013-hhs-language-access-plan.pdf. Describe the legal responsibility of healthcare organizations that need federal funds if a patient needs an interpreter. What exactly should the health organization do to comply with the law? Next, consider the most recent update to that plan, the HHS *Nondiscrimination in Health Programs and Activities,* a rule published in May 2016 and available at www.federalregister.gov/articles/2016/05/18/2016-11458/nondiscrimination-in-health-programs-and-activities#sec-92-201%20.
8. The Institute of Medicine (2000) estimated that as many as 98,000 people die each year because of preventable medical errors. Recent estimates are much higher: James (2013) in an evidence-based review suggests that between 210,000 and 400,000 patients suffer preventable harm that contributes to their deaths. This statistic means that medical errors are now *the third-leading cause of death in the United States after heart disease and cancer.* Robert Watcher, MD, chief of the division of Hospital Medicine at UCSF Medical Center states, "The most common causes of medical mistakes are communication lapses—the information didn't make it from place A to place B correctly, or from person A to person B correctly." The mistakes he refers to include "wrong diagnoses, wrong drugs, wrong doses, wrong patient and wrong body part" (UCSF, 2008, p. 4).
   Write a list of all the people and groups (the stakeholders) who might be affected by *one* patient death caused by communication barriers.
9. Briefly describe how LEP and Deaf or Hard of Hearing patients could become more aware of their legal rights to language assistance and interpreters. (See Appendix 1 and Appendix 2 for details.)

Language used by caller in alphabetical order	Percentage of callers hung up on or disconnected	Percentage connected to a speaker of his/her language	Percentage not connected to a speaker of his/her language	Never on hold longer than 10 minutes
Cantonese	63%	-	63% (inferred)	-
English	0%	-	-	100%
Spanish	-	62%	38% (inferred)	-
Tagalog	-	55%	45% (inferred)	-
Vietnamese	62%	50%	50% (inferred)	-

16 Retrieved from: www.hhs.gov/ocr/civilrights/understanding/race/index.html

10. Which of the following institutions, services or programs that receive federal finding would need to comply with Title VI requirements?
    - Alcohol and drug treatment centers
    - Day care centers
    - Domestic violence services
    - Senior centers
    - Community mental health services
    - Foster care and group homes
    - Healthcare professionals in private practice who have Medicaid patients
    - Homeless shelters
    - Hospitals
    - Skilled nursing facility
    - Nutrition programs
    - Sexual assault centers
    - State and county health departments
    - State and local income assistance programs
    - Government and nonprofit human service agencies

For more information about the law and regulations governing the provision of interpreter services, see Appendix 2.

Medical terminology: The pituitary gland

Locate the two anatomical drawings for the pituitary gland. The first drawing, as in Chapter 1, has labels in English and Spanish (Figure 2-A). The second drawing has the same graphic with blank lines instead of labels (Figure 2-B).

If you interpret in any other spoken language(s) than Spanish and English, then go to Figure 2-B, which has blank labels. Write in the appropriate translations of each English term on the blank lines, as you did in Chapter 1.

Now, test yourself, as you did in Chapter 1. Turn to Figure 2-B. If you are an English-Spanish interpreter, or a sign language interpreter, see if you can say or sign the correct terms for each part of the human body in both or all your working languages. If you have already filled in the blank, cover the blanks to test yourself.

Keep studying these terms until you can interpret all of them into your working languages.

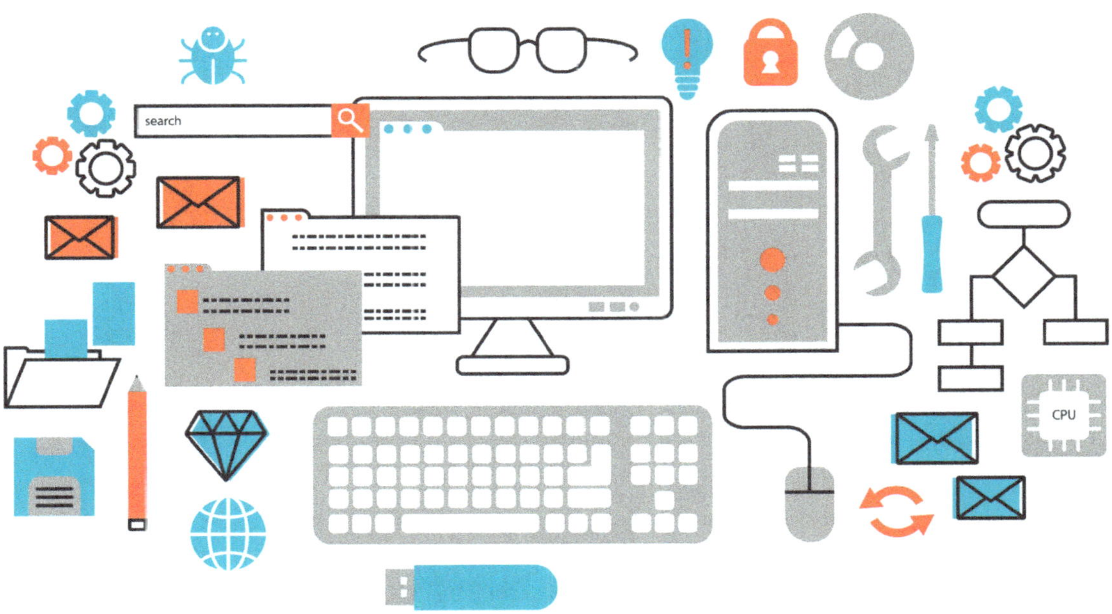

Medical terminology: The pituitary gland

Below you will find anatomical drawings relevant to the content of this chapter. Follow the instructions found at the end of Chapter 1 to study the terminology in this section.

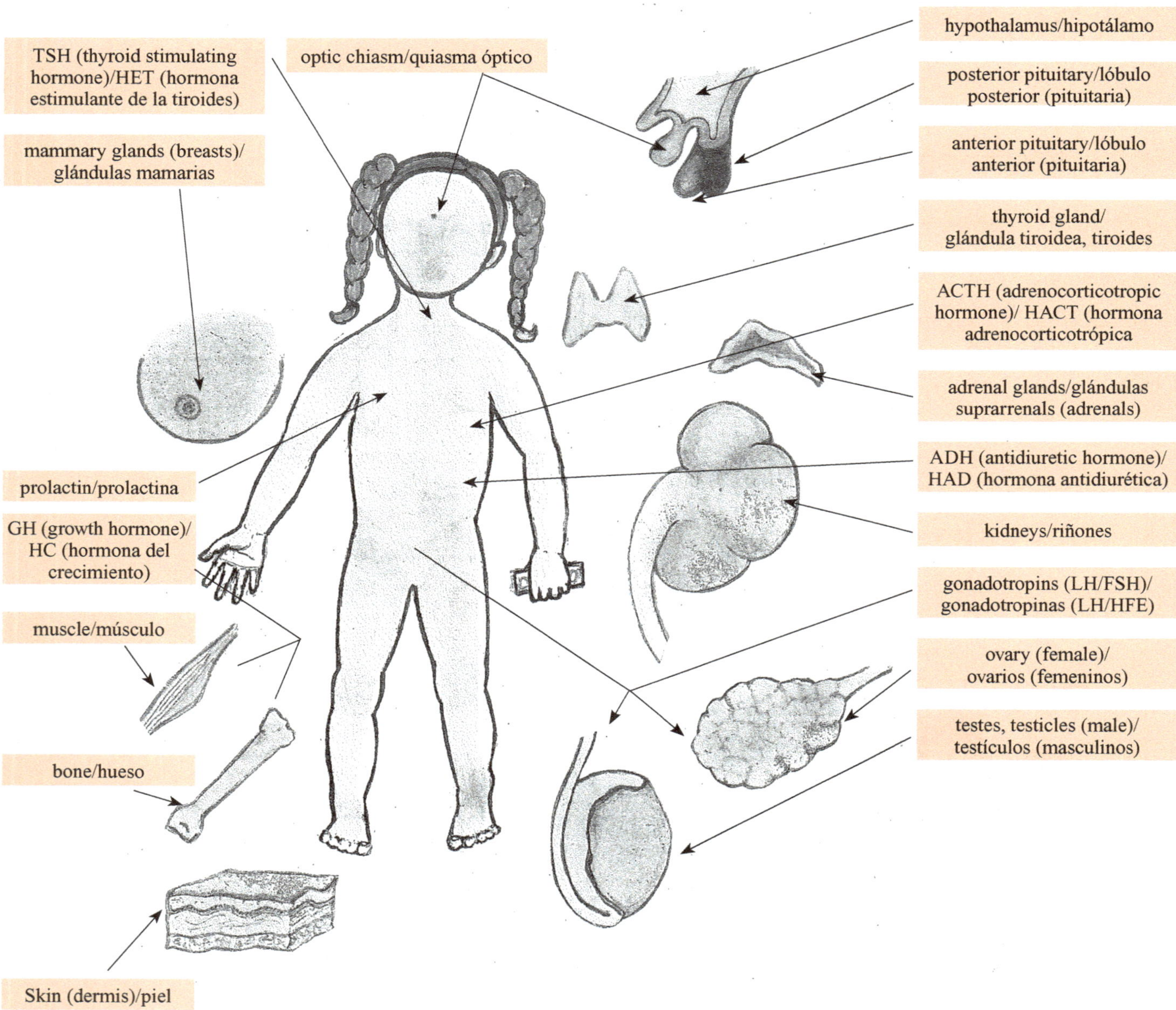

Figure 2-A: The pituitary gland (English and Spanish)

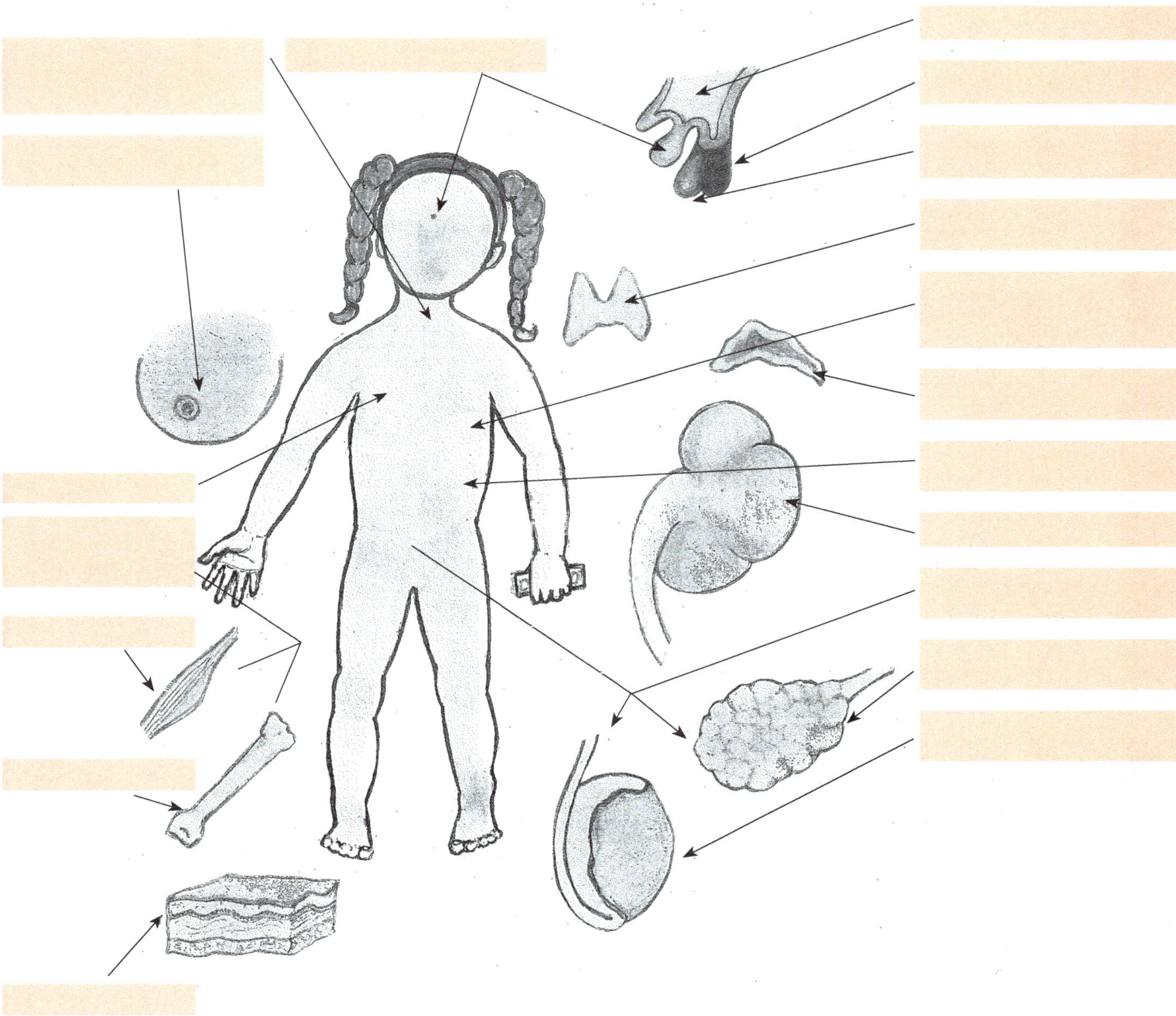

Figure 2-B: The pituitary gland (blank labels)

Medical terminology list

The pituitary gland

VOCABULARY FOR GRAPHIC–IN ENGLISH	VOCABULARY FOR GRAPHIC–IN SPANISH	ANY OTHER LANGUAGE
ACTH (adrenocorticotropic hormone)	HACT (hormona adrenocorticotrópica	
ADH (Antidiuretic Hormone)	HAD (hormona antidiurética)	
Adrenal glands	Glándulas suprarrenals (adrenals)	
Anterior pituitary	Lóbulo anterior (pituitaria)	
bone	hueso	
FSH (Follicle Stimulating Hormone)	HFE (hormona foliculoestimulante	
GH (Growth Hormone)	HC (hormona del crecimiento)	
Gonadotropins (LH/FSH)	Gonadotropinas (LH/HFE)	
Hypothalamus	Hipotálamo	
Kidneys	Riñones	
LH (Luteinizing Hormone)	HL (hormona luteinizante)	
Mammary glands (breasts)	Glándulas mamarias	
muscle	músculo	
Optic chiasm	Quiasma óptico	
Ovary (female)	Ovarios (femeninos)	
Oxytocin	oxitocina	
Pituitary gland (master gland)	Glándula pituitaria (hipófisis) (glándula de control maestro)	
Posterior pituitary	lóbulo posterior (pituitaria)	
prolactin	prolactina	
Skin (dermis)	piel	
Testes, testicles (male)	Testículos (masculinos)	
Thymus	Timo	
Thyroid gland	Glándula tiroidea, tiroides	
TSH (Thyroid Stimulating Hormone)	HET (hormona estimulante de la tiroides)	

HIV/AIDS 3

Advisory

This chapter includes content about sexual orientation, gender identity and intimate partner violence.

This appointment is a general medicine checkup for a patient with HIV. She has come to her regular checkup with the provider who has been her caregiver for several years.

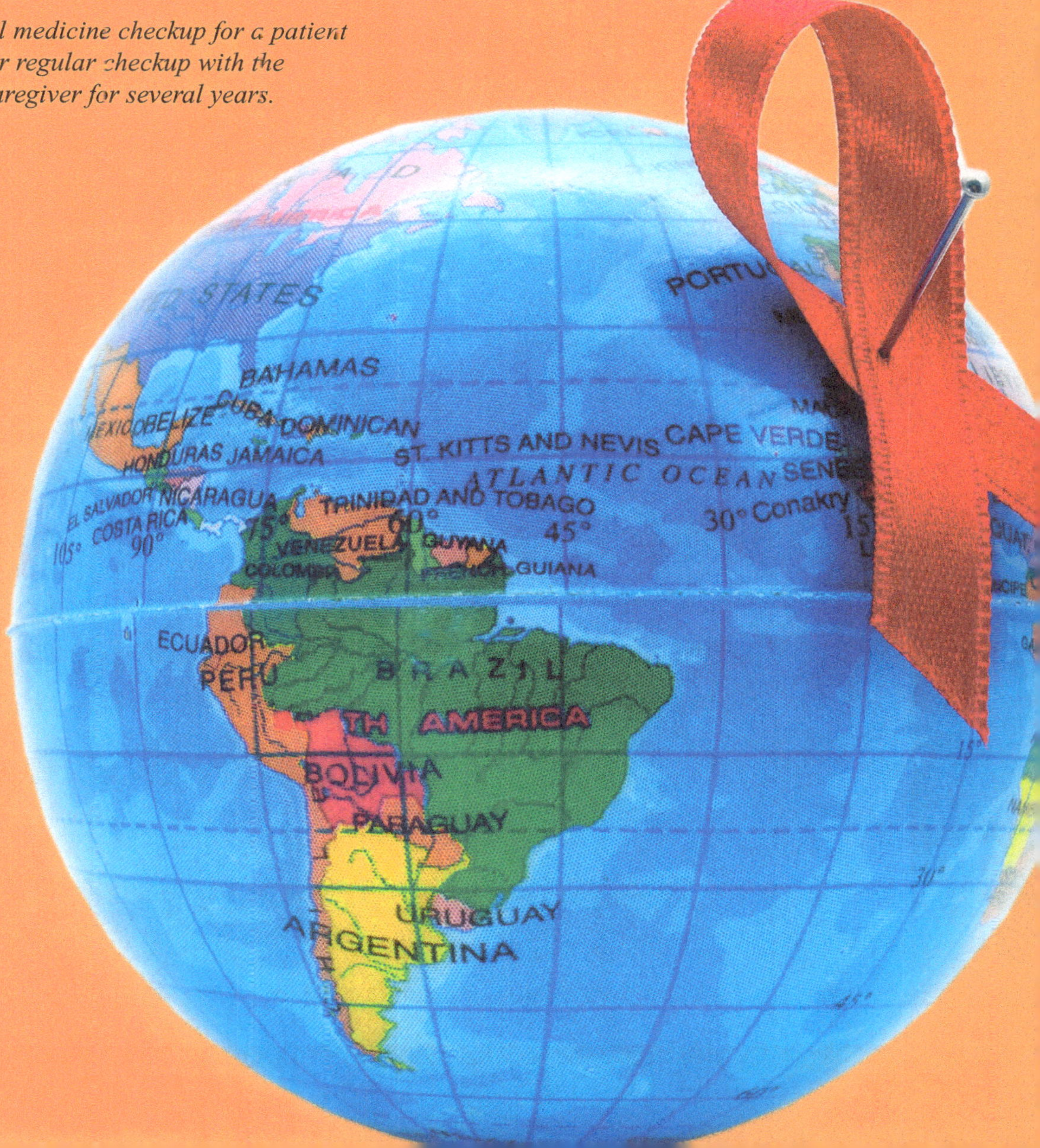

General medicine – HIV-positive and AIDS care role play (English-Spanish)

PART 1

INTERPRETER: Good afternoon. My name is _____________. I'm your interpreter. I'd like to let you know that everything you say will be interpreted, and everything will be kept confidential. Please speak directly to each other, not to me, and pause when I make this signal *(raises hand)* so I can interpret.	**INTERPRETER:** Buenas tardes. Me llamo _____________. Soy su intérprete. Quisiera informarle que yo interpretaré todo lo que usted dice y que todo será confidencial. Por favor dirijánse directamente el uno al otro. Cuando yo le hago esta señal *(raises hand)*, por favor haga una pausa y permitame interpretar.

DOCTOR: Hi, Olga. How are you? It's nice to see you. It seems like such a long time since you were here, but it was only three months ago. How are you?

PATIENT: ¡Buenas tardes, doctora! Estoy bien, muy bien. Gracias.

DOCTOR: Here Olga, have a seat over here. This is our interpreter today.

PATIENT: Hola.

DOCTOR: So, Olga. How are you? Tell me how you've been.

PATIENT: He estado bien, doctora. Todo bien.

DOCTOR: Well, that's good to hear. I'll just pull up your labs here *(checks computer)*. In the meantime, tell me, how are things at home?

PATIENT: Todo está bien.

DOCTOR: Good. I'm glad. How's your son doing?

PATIENT: Muy bien. Mucho mejor. El consejero y el grupo de apoyo le han ayudado mucho.

DOCTOR: Well, that's great. I'm so glad to hear that. He seems like a wonderful boy.

PATIENT: Sí. Gracias a Dios las cosas están mejor. De veras, es la luz de mi vida.

DOCTOR: OK. Here are your labs. Thank you for remembering to do the labs last week. That was very helpful.

PATIENT: Oh, doctora. Antes de que se me olvide, dijeron que se venció la orden y usted me tiene que dar otra.

DOCTOR: No problem. Let me do that right now. Here we go. It's all electronic now.

PATIENT: Gracias.

DOCTOR: This looks great, Olga. You know your T-cells look really good right now. Your viral load is really low.

PATIENT: ¡Qué bien! Es un milagro.

DOCTOR: Well, don't chalk it all up to miracles. You've been working really hard. How is that fungus?

PATIENT: Oh mira, doctora, desapareció. Mis uñas se miran normales ya.

DOCTOR: Yep, that's one of those added little benefits of the medicine. Amazing, huh?

PATIENT: Sí, a pensar que viví tantos años con las uñas tan feas.

DOCTOR: Yes. Maybe this is a silver lining. A small one anyway. So are you sexually active these days?

PATIENT: Pues, sí. He estado saliendo con un hombre. Es buena persona. Creo que lo acaba de conocer antes de la última vez que estuve aquí.

DOCTOR: Well, that's great. You deserve a nice man. And he's lucky! It's going well?

PATIENT: Sí, doctora. Estoy contenta.

DOCTOR: And has he been tested?

PATIENT: Sí. Dice que se hizo la prueba hace dos años. Dice que no está preocupado.

DOCTOR: OK, but what about the past two years? I know you are probably very happy, and it's exciting, but Olga, are you using condoms?

PATIENT: Usamos condones, pero...Usted sabe. Se rompió un condón. Es que...A veces la pasión, se rompe el condón y creo que en el momento uno no se da cuenta.

DOCTOR: That's what this epidemic is all about, isn't it? The moment. Passion makes people irrational and blind. Olga, let's talk about this a little bit. OK?

PATIENT: *(lowers her gaze)* Sí, doctora.

PART 2

DOCTOR: Olga, I'm not gonna scold you, I just think it would be good to do a little condom review, so we can keep you alive and healthy for many years. So you know the condom has to be latex, not lambskin, right?

PATIENT: Sí. Siempre uso látex.

DOCTOR: Right, even if he says he has an allergy. It's your life. Now it's important to remember that condoms can break if they get too dry. So if you're having sex and you take a break and go back at it again, it might get dry. Make sure you have lubricant on hand. Keep it near the bed.

PATIENT: Sí, sí.

DOCTOR: Putting the condom on the right way is key—people don't know how to do that. You have to pinch the end of it so there's room in there for the semen. A lot of people think you want to roll it on and have an air bubble, but that can burst too. So pinch the end, or have him pinch the end when he's putting it on, so there's room in there. Got that? Practice, practice, practice!

PATIENT: Sí.

DOCTOR: Make sure they aren't expired. Check the date. If he doesn't, then you do it. And for God's sake, don't use one that's been carried around in someone's back pocket. The heat will also cause them to break.

PATIENT: Bien, doctora. Tiene razón.

DOCTOR: Olga, you know, you're in great health right now, but I'm worried about you being exposed to things that can give you infections. Even drug-resistant HIV strains that you don't have. You understand that, right?

PATIENT: Sí, doctora. Gracias.

DOCTOR: That's OK. I'm not trying to rain on your parade, but like I've said before, it's really up to you to be your best friend and take care of yourself. OK—end of sermon. So what else?

PATIENT: ¡Oh Doctora! ¡Casi se me olvida lo más importante!

DOCTOR: What's that, Olga?

PATIENT: ¡El paciente ese, doctora! Siempre se me olvida preguntarle. Usted sabe, él que estaba en las noticias. Dicen que quizás han encontrado un tratamiento para curar el SIDA y que lo recibió un hombre en Europa o algo. ¡Yo quiero lo mismo doctora, quiero el mismo tratamiento para curarme de una vez! Quiero que usted me dé este tratamiento.

DOCTOR: Hold your horses, Olga. It is very exciting, very promising, but the jury's still out on this one. There's a long way to go before this is something that might actually be available to everyone.

PATIENT: ¿Y por qué, doctora?

DOCTOR: Well, you know his situation was very unique, apart from the headline. I'm not saying it's impossible, but it's still being studied. He underwent really serious treatment with possibly life-threatening side effects. If you're HIV-positive and not healthy, the treatment can kill you.

PATIENT: Pero es posible. ¿No?

DOCTOR: Yes, but it's not really practical right now on a large scale.

PATIENT: Pero es posible.

DOCTOR: That's true, but there's just a lot to it. Are you ready?

PATIENT: Sí.

DOCTOR: Well, first you have to understand how the HIV virus gets into cells to attack them. Most HIV strains use something called a receptor, the CCR5 receptor on the surface of a cell to enter. Are you following me?

> **PATIENT:** Sí, doctora.

DOCTOR: The treatment focuses on this pathway, but it's not for everyone. It's not really practical on a massive scale. Right now there are medicines that people can take to keep things pretty well controlled, but they aren't for everyone either. There are adherence questions.

> **PATIENT:** ¿Como qué, doctora?

DOCTOR: Well, Olga, let's look at your case. You've been doing a good job, you are much better than the first time you walked in here. But in a way, you've had some really good luck. You haven't gotten to that place where we need you to start a whole new regimen. If you did, we might be in trouble.

> **PATIENT:** Pero ¿por qué, doctora? Ahora hay acceso a estas medicinas y tengo mi seguro médico.

DOCTOR: Some of those meds require that you follow a really strict schedule. You're already doing that, but it can be even stricter and less forgiving. You can't miss a dose. If you do, they stop working for you—then you're really screwed.

> **PATIENT:** Si, yo entiendo.

DOCTOR: My patients who are taking those meds wear watches that are set to go off every day at specific times, so they never, never miss a dose. They have to know where they are sleeping every night and where they will wake up. They have to know their medicines will be there too. It takes a lot of responsibility. That's a challenge for a lot of people. It won't work for everybody.

> **PATIENT:** Ah.

DOCTOR: All these factors have to be taken into consideration when we decide which meds will work for which patients—it's not just a decision about the right drug for the right virus. There are lots of social factors. And you can't be putting yourself at risk in other ways. You follow me?

> **PATIENT:** Sí.

DOCTOR: Yes. If you want to start meds like that, you need to be ready to be adherent. If you're not, they'll stop working, you'll have drug resistance. If that happens, you'll have fewer choices and have to deal with possible worse side effects.

> **PATIENT:** Ah, ya entiendo. *(Patient sighs.)* Es lo mismo entonces...El corazón salta cada vez que aparece algo así en las noticias y después uno se queda desilusionado.

PART 3

DOCTOR: Yes, but things are getting better. It's more and more possible to get down to where your viral load is undetectable, and things are really getting better as far as reducing transmission.

PATIENT: Comprendo.

DOCTOR: Well, there's hope, and every time they have success with someone, they learn something that they may be able to apply on a larger scale or something that will help find a cure. You can see, there's still a long way to go, but it's changing all the time. In six months, who knows how things will be?

PATIENT: Sí, doctora.

DOCTOR: The important thing for you, Miss Olga, is that you take care of yourself in the meantime. Just to give you a heads-up, especially with new treatments, a patient has to go through a whole assessment to see if she's a good candidate. If she gets lots of STDs, certain treatments might be too risky. So take care of yourself. "Be here for the cure," as they say. Right?

PATIENT: Sí. Tiene razón.

DOCTOR: See what you think about coming to the next appointment with your partner, and we can talk about how to reduce the risk of transmission.

PATIENT: OK.

DOCTOR: And how's your friend, the one you were worried about?

PATIENT: ¿Cuál de ellos?

DOCTOR: The one who was going to disclose her status to her boyfriend. I remember the last time you did that yourself, you were beaten to a pulp and ended up in the emergency room. And I know you were worried about her. Is she OK?

PATIENT: Sí, su novio tiene su cuchillo, y ella temía que la iba a vestir de corduroy, pero ella está bien. No se puso violento, se puso triste. Luego se separaron. Quién sabe si realmente es que él no supo lidiar con la situación. Pero no le hizo nada a ella.

DOCTOR: Well, I'm glad she's OK. It can be dangerous disclosing, as you well know. I'm glad she's OK.

PATIENT: Yo también.

DOCTOR: So, anything else you want to talk about, Olga?

PATIENT: No, eso es todo.

DOCTOR: All right, then. It was great to see you, Olga. You keep taking good care of yourself. You're doing great. Now, will you make an appointment to come back and see me in three months and get your labs before you do, just like you did this time?

PATIENT: Sí. Muchas gracias, doctora.

DOCTOR: And bring that new man, OK?

PATIENT: Sí. doctora, gracias.

DOCTOR: You're welcome. I'll see you in three months. Take care.

General medicine role play—HIV-positive and AIDS care (English only)

PART 1

DOCTOR: Hi, Olga. How are you? It's nice to see you. It seems like such a long time since you were here, but it was only three months ago. How are you?

PATIENT: Good afternoon, doctor! I'm fine, just fine. Thank you.

DOCTOR: Here Olga, have a seat over here. This is our interpreter today.

PATIENT: Hello.

INTERPRETER: Good afternoon. My name is ___________. I'm your interpreter. I'd like to let you know that everything you say will be interpreted, and everything will be kept confidential. Please speak directly to each other, not to me, and pause when I make this signal *(raises hand)* so I can interpret.

DOCTOR: So, Olga. How are you? Tell me how you've been.

PATIENT: I've been fine, doctor. Everything is fine.

DOCTOR: Well, that's good to hear. I'll just pull up your labs here *(checks computer)*. In the meantime, tell me, how are things at home?

PATIENT: Everything's good.

DOCTOR: Good. I'm glad. How's your son doing?

PATIENT: Really well, much better. The counselor and the support group have really helped him a lot.

DOCTOR: Well, that's great. I'm so glad to hear that. He seems like a wonderful boy.

PATIENT: Yes, thank God things are better. He really IS the light of my life.

DOCTOR: OK. Here are your labs. Thank you for remembering to do the labs last week. That was very helpful.

PATIENT: Oh, doctor. Before I forget, they said my order was expired and I have to get another one from you.

DOCTOR: No problem. Let me do that right now. Here we go. It's all electronic now.

PATIENT: Thanks.

DOCTOR: This looks great, Olga. You know your T-cells look really good right now. Your viral load is really low.

PATIENT: Oh, that's great. It's a miracle.

DOCTOR: Well, don't chalk it all up to miracles. You've been working really hard. How is that fungus?

PATIENT: Oh, look, doctor. My nails look normal again.

DOCTOR: Yep, that's one of those added little benefits of the medicine. Amazing, huh?

PATIENT: Yes, and to think I lived all those years with my nails looking so ugly.

DOCTOR: Yes. Maybe this is a silver lining. A small one anyway. So are you sexually active these days?

PATIENT: Well, yes. I've been seeing a man. He's a good person. I think I'd just met him the last time I was here.

DOCTOR: Well, that's great. You deserve a nice man. And he's lucky! It's going well?

PATIENT: Yes, doctor. I'm happy.

DOCTOR: And has he been tested?

PATIENT: Yes. He says he got tested two years ago. He says he's not worried.

DOCTOR: OK, but what about the past two years? I know you are probably very happy, and it's exciting, but Olga, are you using condoms?

PATIENT: We use condoms, but...You know. A condom broke. It's just that...Sometimes passion gets to you, the condom breaks, and in the moment you don't realize what happened.

DOCTOR: That's what this epidemic is all about, isn't it? The moment. Passion makes people irrational and blind. Olga, let's talk about this a little bit. OK?

PATIENT: *(lowers her gaze)* Yes, doctor.

PART 2

DOCTOR: Olga, I'm not gonna scold you, I just think it would be good to do a little condom review, so we can keep you alive and healthy for many years. So you know the condom has to be latex, not lambskin, right?

PATIENT: Yes, I always use latex.

DOCTOR: Right, even if he says he has an allergy. It's your life. Now it's important to remember that condoms can break if they get too dry. So if you're having sex and you take a break and go back at it again, it might get dry. Make sure you have lubricant on hand. Keep it near the bed.

PATIENT: Yes, yes.

DOCTOR: Putting the condom on the right way is key—people don't know how to do that. You have to pinch the end of it so there's room in there for the semen. A lot of people think you want to roll it on and have an air bubble, but that can burst too. So pinch the end, or have him pinch the end when he's putting it on, so there's room in there. Got that? Practice, practice, practice!

PATIENT: Yes.

DOCTOR: Make sure they aren't expired. Check the date. If he doesn't, then you do it. And for God's sake, don't use one that's been carried around in someone's back pocket. The heat will cause them to break as well.

PATIENT: OK, doctor, you're right.

DOCTOR: Olga, you know, you're in great health right now, but I'm worried about you being exposed to things that can give you infections. Even drug-resistant HIV strains that you don't have. You understand that, right?

PATIENT: Yes, doctor. Thank you.

DOCTOR: That's OK. I'm not trying to rain on your parade, but like I've said before, it's really up to you to be your best friend and take care of yourself. OK—end of sermon. So what else?

PATIENT: Oh, doctor! I almost forgot the most important thing!

DOCTOR: What's that, Olga?

PATIENT: That patient, doctor! I keep forgetting to ask you. You know, the one who was in the news a while back. They say that maybe they found a treatment to cure AIDS, and a man got it in Europe or something. I want the same thing, doctor, I want the same treatment, so I can be cured once and for all! I want you to give me that treatment.

DOCTOR: Hold your horses, Olga. It is very exciting, very promising, but the jury's still out on this one. There's a long way to go before this is something that might actually be available to everyone.

PATIENT: But why, doctor?

DOCTOR: Well, you know his situation was very unique, apart from the headline. I'm not saying it's impossible, but it's still being studied. He underwent really serious treatment with possibly life-threatening side effects. If you're HIV-positive and not healthy, the treatment can kill you.

PATIENT: But it's possible, right?

DOCTOR: Yes, but it's not really practical right now on a large scale.

PATIENT: But it's possible.

DOCTOR: That's true, but there's just a lot to it. Are you ready?

PATIENT: Yes.

DOCTOR: Well, first you have to understand how the HIV virus gets into cells to attack them. Most HIV strains use something called a receptor, the CCR5 receptor on the surface of a cell to enter. Are you following me?

PATIENT: Yes, doctor.

DOCTOR: The treatment focuses on this pathway, but it's not for everyone. It's not really practical on a massive scale. Right now there are medicines that people can take to keep things pretty well controlled, but they aren't for everyone either. There are adherence questions.

PATIENT: Like what, doctor?

DOCTOR: Well, Olga, let's look at your case. You've been doing a good job, you are much better than the first time you walked in here. But in a way, you've had some really good luck. You haven't gotten to that place where we need you to start a whole new regimen. If you did, we might be in trouble.

PATIENT: But why, doctor? Now there's access to those medicines, and I have my health insurance.

DOCTOR: Some of those meds require that you follow a really strict schedule. You're already doing that, but it can be even stricter, and less forgiving. You can't miss a dose. If you do, they stop working for you—then you're really screwed.

PATIENT: Yes, I get it.

DOCTOR: My patients who are taking those meds wear watches that are set to go off every day at specific times, so they never, never miss a dose. They have to know where they are sleeping every night, and where they will wake up. They have to know their medicines will be there too. It takes a lot of responsibility. That's a challenge for a lot of people. It won't work for everybody.

PATIENT: Ah.

DOCTOR: All these factors have to be taken into consideration when we decide which meds will work for which patients—it's not just a decision about the right drug for the right virus. There are lots of social factors. And you can't be putting yourself at risk in other ways. You follow me?

PATIENT: Yes.

DOCTOR: Yes. If you want to start meds like that, you need to be ready to be adherent. If you're not, they'll stop working, you'll have drug resistance. If that happens, you'll have fewer choices and have to deal with possible worse side effects.

PATIENT: Ah, now I understand. *(Patient sighs.)* It's the same thing then...My heart jumps every time I hear something on the news, and then I'm so disappointed.

PART 3

DOCTOR: Yes, but things are getting better. It's more and more possible to get down to where your viral load is undetectable, and things are really getting better as far as reducing transmission.

PATIENT: I get it.

DOCTOR: Well, there's hope, and every time they have success with someone, they learn something that they may be able to apply on a larger scale or something that will help find a cure. You can see, there's still a long way to go, but it's changing all the time. In six months, who knows how things will be?

PATIENT: Yes, doctor.

DOCTOR: The important thing for you, Miss Olga, is that you take care of yourself in the meantime. Just to give you a heads-up, especially with new treatments, a patient has to go through a whole assessment to see if she's a good candidate. If she gets lots of STDs, certain treatments might be too risky. So take care of yourself. "Be here for the cure," as they say. Right?

PATIENT: Yes, you're right.

DOCTOR: See what you think about coming to the next appointment with your partner, and we can talk about how to reduce the risk of transmission.

PATIENT: OK.

DOCTOR: And how's your friend, the one you were worried about?

PATIENT: Which one?

DOCTOR: The one who was going to disclose her status to her boyfriend. I remember the last time you did that yourself, you were beaten to a pulp and ended up in the emergency room. And I know you were worried about her. Is she OK?

PATIENT: Yes. Her boyfriend had a knife and she thought he was gonna dress her in stripes, but she's fine. He didn't get violent; he got sad. Then they broke up. Who knows if it's just that he couldn't deal with the situation. But he didn't do anything to her.

DOCTOR: Well, I'm glad she's OK. It can be dangerous disclosing, as you well know. I'm glad she's OK.

PATIENT: Me too.

DOCTOR: So, anything else you want to talk about, Olga?

PATIENT: No, that's all.

DOCTOR: All right, then. It was great to see you, Olga. You keep taking good care of yourself. You're doing great. Now, will you make an appointment to come back and see me in three months, and get your labs before you do, just like you did this time?

PATIENT: Yes, thank you, doctor.

DOCTOR: And bring that new man, OK?

PATIENT: Yes, thanks, doctor.

DOCTOR: You're welcome. I'll see you in three months. Take care.

What's important to know about this chapter?

"AIDS is a family affair—for ill and for good."

—Michel Sidibé (2010)

Overview

Being infected with HIV is clearly different than it was two decades ago. Depending on your citizenship, your gender, poverty or wealth, where you live in the world and your access to care, you may or may not survive. You may or may not be able to have a family and lead a life where you are not consumed every minute by survival.

Being close to people infected with HIV can also turn the world on its head. Some may seem to deal well with the symptoms and then succumb to the disease; they may find services and care for the first time in their lives; they may remain asymptomatic. They may be men, women and children within groups considered safe, who never imagined they could get HIV. There is a lot to learn. Despite all we know about how to reduce infection, some populations are experiencing a *rise* in the rate of infection.

For purposes of this book we need to ask, "What does the medical interpreter need to know about HIV?" We also need to ask the inextricably linked question, "What does any human need to know about HIV?"

Terminology

See the illustration at the end of this chapter and the terminology that accompanies this dialogue. Here are some basic terms and concepts that may be useful:

Acquired immune deficiency syndrome (AIDS): This syndrome (not a single disease but a collection of symptoms and diseases) is acquired, meaning it is not inherited but contracted after conception. It results in a deficient immune system (the immune system includes all the cells and organs that help fight disease). AIDS is an end stage of HIV infection.

Human immunodeficiency virus (HIV): HIV is a potentially life-threatening virus that today can be treated with effective drugs to reduce the risks. However, failure to treat HIV adequately increases the risk of other opportunistic infections and, if untreated, HIV can lead to AIDS. In countries without general access to treatment, HIV can still be a death sentence. In the United States, the drugs used to treat HIV are expensive, but most are widely available. Many health insurance plans and prescription drug plans cover them. Patients with HIV who receive beneficial treatment can live fairly normal lives.

HIV transmission: [17] Transmission happens when specific fluids from one infected body enter another body: blood, semen, preseminal fluid, vaginal fluid and breast milk.[18]

17 For more detailed information about HIV transmission and body fluids, go to www.cdc.gov/hiv

18 It's interesting to note that in several informational communications about Ebola virus transmission, for example, at major teaching institutions in the United States, when referring to bodily fluids, there is an omission of vaginal secretions. The decision to specifically name, in writing or verbal communiqués, all other bodily fluids but omit mention of vaginal secretions seems to be a decision based not on medical soundness but some kind of social consideration. As with HIV, the fact that such fluids do include vaginal secretions is essential information.

Pre-exposure prophylaxis (PrEP): Medicines to help prevent contracting HIV. Keep in mind that recent research suggests that people with an undetectable viral load are highly unlikely to transmit the virus. This means that opinions about the riskiness of sex without condoms are changing rapidly.

Post-exposure prophylaxis (PEP): Medicines to help prevent the spread after a possible exposure to HIV.

AIDS Drug Assistance Program (ADAP): This government program provides FDA-approved medications to low-income people with HIV.

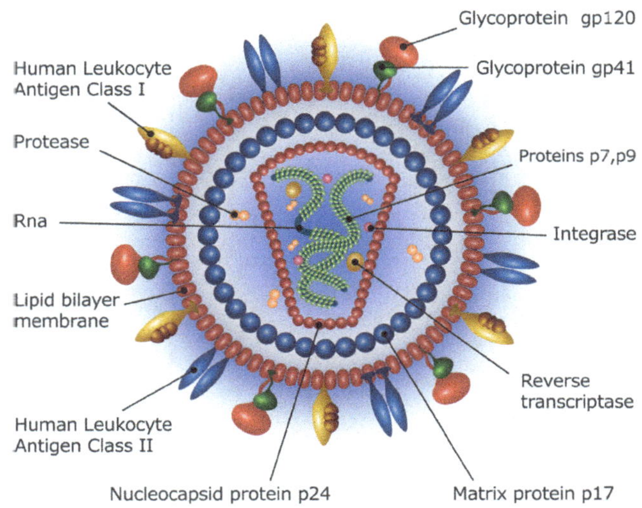

HIV/AIDS is preventable

HIV/AIDS prevention requires avoiding the sharing of any of the above-named bodily fluids. Strategies[19] include the following suggestions:

- Abstinence from sexual relations (between any two humans, in any way where bodily fluids are shared).
- *Proper use* of condoms and barriers.
- Not sharing hypodermic needles.
- Infected mothers avoiding breastfeeding.
- Antiretroviral drugs before, during and after birth for babies with infected mothers.
- PrEP and PEP treatments, reducing an HIV-infected individual's likelihood of transmitting the virus by reducing his or her viral load through use of antiretroviral drugs and treatments.

HIV is treatable

Medicines are available to keep HIV in check and to keep from developing AIDS. Such medications include antiretroviral therapy (ART) and highly active antiretroviral therapy (HAART).

19 Retrieved from www.cdc.gov/hiv or www.aids.gov

Life span variations

People infected with HIV have varied average life spans, depending on their access to treatment, quality of healthcare and socioeconomic conditions (food, water, shelter, support, etc.).

Trauma: Increasingly, research suggests a causal relationship between trauma and sexual diseases and infections.[20]

Staying healthy

It is believed that when the immune system launches an attack against an illness in your body, certain immune cells are more "open" to HIV invasion. Taking good care of your health is an additional strategy for fighting HIV.

Resources: Information on HIV/AIDS is now widely available.[21]

20 Retrieved from www.cdc.gov/hiv/risk/gender/women/facts/bibliography.html

21 For example, see www.cdc.gov

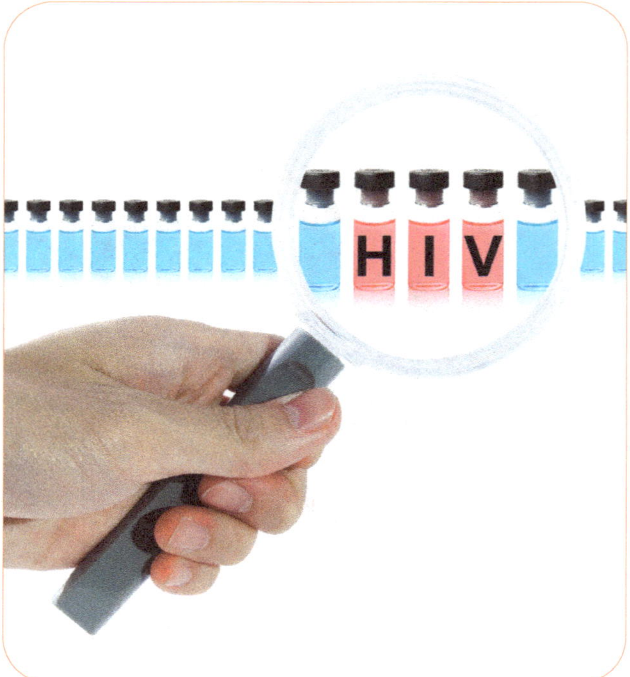

What should an interpreter know about HIV/AIDS?

First: We are *all* at risk. Interpreting for an HIV or STI clinic might feel uncomfortable, if it involves discussion of unsafe behaviors that many people whom we know, often including ourselves, have ever engaged in. Is anyone's behavior always safe? For example, any woman who has ever been pregnant has engaged in unprotected sex (meaning unsafe to a greater or lesser degree), and no one but the father can know the father's sex and drug history for certain. Marriage and monogamy are not alone protection from HIV. Protection requires having a partner who is infection free and has no other partners.

Denial: In addition to knowing how to translate the word "denial," it's helpful to have an understanding of the word as it relates to the psychological and behavioral mindset of someone who is unwilling to recognize a problem or situation. This type of denial could manifest itself in many ways, for example, acquiring a sexually transmitted infection (STI) because of being too timid to do anything to prevent it, being forced to have unprotected sex, willingly having unprotected sex and infecting others, being in an abusive relationship that involves sex, not seeking healthcare, not taking prescribed medications, not adhering to treatment or not believing that HIV causes AIDS, to offer just a few examples.

Women and HIV/AIDS: One in four people living with HIV infection in the United States is female, and most new HIV infections in women are from heterosexual contact (87 percent). Women made up 19 percent (8,328) of the estimated 44,073 new HIV infections in the United States in 2014.[22] "Some women infected with HIV report more than 1 risk factor, highlighting the overlap in risk factors such as inequality in relationships, socioeconomic stresses, substance abuse, and psychological issues."[23] See also Forna et al. (2006) for HIV infection factors among Black women. A woman is significantly more likely than a man to contract HIV infection during vaginal intercourse (European Study Group on Heterosexual Transmission of HIV, 1992).

Behavior and labels: In interpreting the word "behavior," it's important to understand the intent of and meaning of questions about behavior, particularly sexual behavior. If a clinician asks a patient how he or she identifies regarding sexual orientation, for example, "Are you gay? Straight? Lesbian? Bi?" an interpreter should communicate just that. But these are labels. Depending on the context, what might be more relevant and what the clinician really might be asking is, "Do you have sex with men? With women? With both?" Transgender is a label that could also be included here. What does the clinician really want to know?

The answer to that question could be extremely important, since in some cultures, for example, men may be married to women but have sex with men outside their marriage and consider themselves "straight." Men may have sex with men, but depending on the position could identify as "straight" by regarding those on the "receiving end" as "gay." Immigration fears can add an extra layer of social complexity. An immigrant, migrant or refugee with family members in both the home and host countries

22 Retrieved from www.cdc.gov/hiv/group/gender/women/

23 Retreived from www.dabtheaidsbearproject.com/woandhivrifa.html

could have a deep fear of putting a family member's immigration status or ability to enter the United States at risk.

While speaking about Africa and the Middle East, Executive Director of UNAIDS[24] Michel Sidibé (2010) made comments highly applicable to the United States and any nation that depends on an immigrant labor force:

> "Migrant workers and their families, who do so much for the regional economy, are often shut out of basic health services, including those for HIV, upon sero-conversion. Why not take action to help support migrants in avoiding HIV, rather than restricting those who have it. Ensuring migrant families' access to prevention, treatment, care and support is a step in the right direction and one that other countries in the region could be encouraged to take" (Sidibé, 2010).

Labels can drive people away, a risk that no nation can afford in the face of the HIV epidemic.

> "Instead, for the good of the public health, there is a need for understanding—an imperative to draw those most at risk out of the shadows and enable them to protect themselves and by extension, the entire community, from spreading HIV. There is a need to make sure those affected receive care and treatment by offering a hand up rather than a slap down" (Sidibé, 2010).

If the clinician isn't experienced in knowing how to ask a question that will help him obtain the information he is looking for, it is not the interpreter's responsibility to figure it out. On the other hand, if the interpreter knows that people may be hurt by a lack of communication and says nothing, is she "doing no harm"? If you sense there is not full understanding of the intended meaning of or the answer to a question, it might be a professional responsibility to suggest that the clinician or patient clarify what was said or intended.

24 UNAIDS is the Joint United Nations Programme on HIV/AIDS. Its goal is to help countries strengthen their long-term capacity to cope with the epidemic.

Sexual orientation pre- and post-diagnosis

If a clinician asks about sexual orientation for the purpose of assessing risk factors before the diagnosis of an STI, such as HIV, getting past the labels (and possibly tapping into the interpreter's cultural knowledge) may be relevant. If, on the other hand, a clinician asks a patient already diagnosed with HIV about sexual orientation, is it relevant? Does it make any difference in managing care? Is it necessary to ask or an infringement on privacy?

What would you do if, at a dermatology appointment, you were asked if you are sexually active and with whom? How should you proceed? If you believe this type of question to be inappropriate, offensive or objectionable and you sense that some LEP or Deaf/Hard of Hearing patients might not be speaking up about their discomfort, how could you finish the following sentence? "As the interpreter, I want to mention that questions like these might..." Would doing so be professionally appropriate?

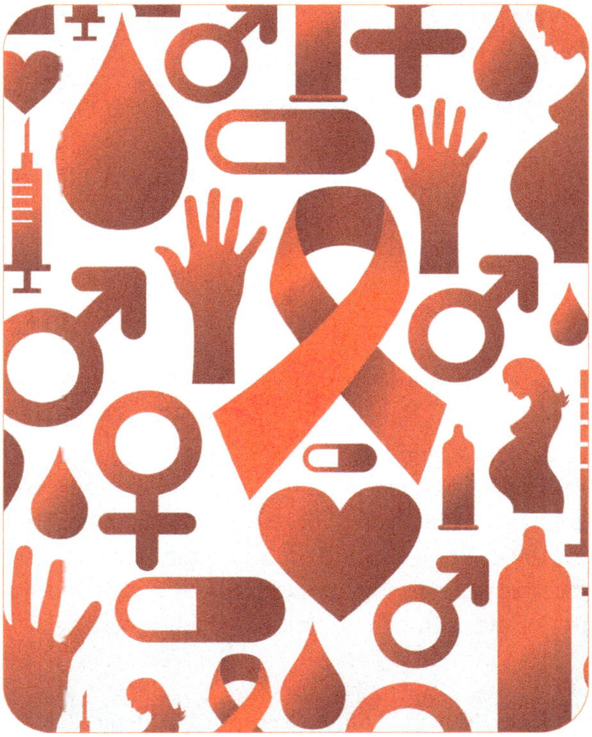

Stigma

Stigma is common regarding sexually transmitted diseases (STDs) and infections (STIs),[25] especially HIV, and questions about sexual identity or orientation. Such stigma might keep clients from communicating honestly with their providers, which can interfere with patient safety and quality care.

Disclosure

Disclosure of HIV status can be life-threatening. In some countries, people are afraid to disclose their HIV status to health practitioners due to the fear of deportation, incarceration, domestic violence, being ostracized or death (at the hands of the government or others). Unfortunately, there are also places where *not* reporting that a person is gay is a crime. In the dialogue above, the patient describes two incidents where people were beat up by intimate partners after disclosing their HIV status. The role play dialogue was inspired in part by an article by Rae Lewis-Thornton (2012), which is dedicated to a young woman who was murdered by her intimate partner after disclosing her HIV status.

Domestic and sexual violence

People, mostly women but also men, are subjected to intimate partner violence the world over. More still are exposed to sexual violence (for example, trafficking and sexual slavery, sexual assault by an intimate partner, child marriage or rape as a weapon of war). A past history of such violence can come up in the course of "normal" and "routine" health appointments: in gynecology or urology and also in arthritis, general medicine, and adolescent and pediatric checkups, among others. If a person is being held against her will, a "relative" will often be present for the entire appointment and often insist on doing the interpreting. Sometimes, the presence of a medical interpreter can help to uncover such problems.

25 While the term STI is often preferred, the term STD is still in common usage in healthcare settings.

Mandatory reporting

In many states and institutions in the United States, interpreters, like teachers, are required to report any suspicion of child abuse or vulnerable adult abuse (but rarely domestic violence). Interpreters are not required to be sure about the abuse but simply to report the suspicion. In many others states, interpreters are required to leave the investigation, judgment and reporting to healthcare professionals. To know the requirements in your state, see Youdelman (2009).

Why interpreters should be informed about HIV/AIDS

The rationale for knowledge

Should a healthcare interpreter know more than relevant terminology, more about HIV/AIDS in general, than he or she knows about other infections and diseases?

Yes. HIV/AIDS is a highly sensitive topic. Preparation in advance, for nearly any session that involves this topic, is always preferable. There are many socially and emotionally charged areas to navigate. Learning about them will help prepare for smoother, higher quality interpreting. That knowledge can also give interpreters a more informed picture of the world and ourselves.

General background

At some point early on in the AIDS epidemic, when it was still being called by some a "gay disease," it was, to a large extent, ignored by the health systems of wealthy nations. Even when heterosexual transmission became widespread in Haiti and Africa, the perception for many years was that the disease was largely restricted to gays. Then it was discovered that those at highest risk and rate of infection in Chile were married women. Why? Because they had unprotected sex with their husbands. Husbands had unprotected sex with men, yet didn't identify as "gay" or as anything other than heterosexual. Gay stigma endangered both these men and their wives.

In addition, at the time, those in Chile most responsible for public education and curbing the rate of infection by teaching about condoms were sex workers. This turned some public perception on its head, but it made practical sense, at least to the sex workers. What is significant about this point for interpreters is that it shows how many people had—and still have—unconscious assumptions about HIV/AIDS that need to be examined.

For years, women were being infected and dying of AIDS, but they went uncounted. Many of the symptoms and conditions resulting in a diagnosis of AIDS were more relevant to men (Kaposi's sarcoma, a cancer of blood vessel walls causing the appearance of skin and mouth lesions). AIDS-related symptoms or diagnoses in women were not yet being looked for (for example, chronic pelvic inflammatory disease or chronic yeast infection). As a result of these blind spots in healthcare, many women who should have received timely diagnoses of HIV or AIDS did not.

As an interpreter, the more aware you become about a disease and its presenting symptoms and risk factors, the more tempting you might find it to offer suggestions or comments. If you feel that ethically it is called for, you need to know how to do so in a professional manner.

Consider being an informed interpreter facilitating a discussion in the following circumstances. Maybe you interpret for a woman at a health clinic who has many signs of compromised immunity or HIV infection and a practitioner dismisses the usefulness of an HIV test because he isn't aware of symptoms that are more common among women (and after all, the patient is married, having sex only with her spouse). As the interpreter, say that you interpreted for the patient's husband at an HIV clinic. Is there anything you could do that might change this woman's life or possibly save it while still maintaining interpreting standards of ethics and professionalism? What action *could* you take? How would you go about it? What about the legal requirements of confidentiality?

This scenario might be hard to imagine today in the United States now that provider awareness has increased and HIV is a more normalized part of healthcare. Many people can now obtain medicines that allow them to live fairly normal lives with this infection. Yet there are important points to consider. Interpreting often requires weighing the situation and making personal decisions. How do you balance impartiality, confidentiality and advocacy? How do you fulfill your role and do no harm? It's important to seriously consider, discuss and try to answer the following questions *before* you find yourself facing similar situations in real life.

How'd you get it?

This question, "How did you get HIV?" is one that a lot of people want to ask those who have been diagnosed with HIV or AIDS, including providers. This question is often offensive. Indeed, the question and the answer are still all too often used to judge, categorize and stigmatize people and to determine who is "innocent" (children) and what degree of "guilt" an infected person carries. There may be valid reasons for asking for this information. If so, what are these reasons, and are they being asked in the appropriate context?

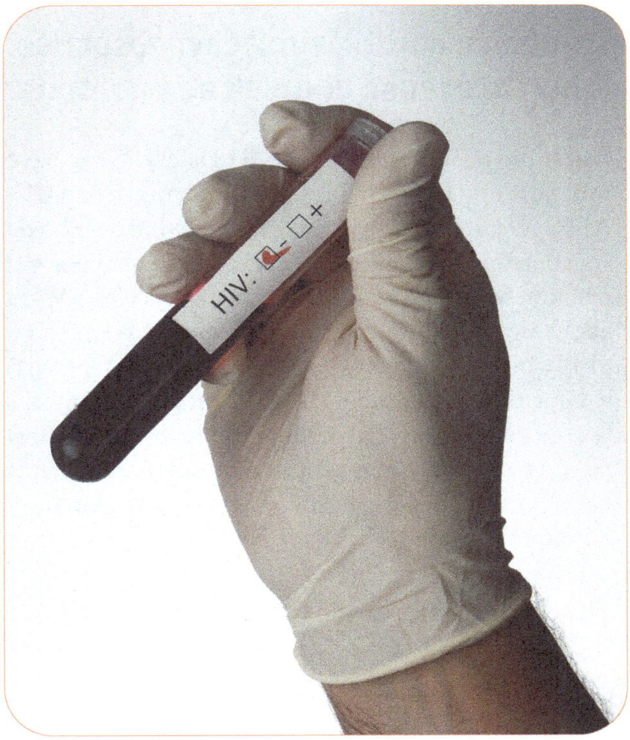

Who has it?

At the 2012 International AIDS Conference, Gail Wyatt, associate director of the UCLA AIDS Institute, offered sobering statistics, for example:

> "3 percent of all residents in Washington D.C. are infected with the HIV virus...7 percent of all black males are HIV-positive; the city has a higher infection rate than African countries like Ethiopia, Nigeria and Rwanda" (Wyatt, 2012).

According to UNAIDS, in 2015 worldwide between 34 and nearly 40 million people were living with HIV, 2.1 million people were newly infected and 1.1 million people died of AIDS.[26] According to the Centers for Disease Control and Prevention (CDC), in 2012 nearly 1.2 million Americans were living with HIV/AIDS, an all-time high, with nearly 50,000 new infections every year; almost 13 percent of those infected did not know they had HIV.[27]

Denial, behavior, stigma and disclosure about HIV/AIDS are still huge challenges that lead to many human tragedies.

Emotional impact, subjective response: When to excuse yourself as interpreter

For some of us, especially if STDs and STIs have touched our lives, it's hard to interpret for HIV/AIDS appointments and not be affected. How do you feel personally about HIV/AIDS? What is your gut reaction when you hear that someone has HIV? What about a woman infected by her husband? What about girls who are raped by men who believe that sex with a virgin can cure their HIV? What about mothers with access to antiviral medicine, which would allow them to bear HIV-free babies, but over 1,700 infants become infected with HIV daily, 90 percent from mother-to-child transmission?[28]

26 Retrieved from www.unaids.org/en/resources/fact-sheet

27 Retrieved from www.cdc.gov/hiv/statistics/overview/index.html

28 Retrieved from www.who.int/reproductivehealth/topics/linkages/pmtct/en/

How do you feel about same-gender sexual orientation (homosexuality)? What about transgender people and transgender sex? Are you sure that your feelings do not show up in your body language, including facial expressions, when you interpret?

An interpreter's emotional state affects her performance. It's important to think about what might impact your interpreting before you confront common situations for the first time. Consider a professional interpreter's responsibility and ask yourself if you are up to the task of interpreting for highly sensitive encounters, including appointments that you know in advance are HIV/AIDS related. Remember, however, that these topics can emerge in nearly any routine encounter. While a great deal of attention is being given to self awareness about attitudes regarding HIV/AIDS, one lesson for interpreters needs to be widely accepted: be aware of *any* subject that might compromise your interpreting so that you can deal with it appropriately. For most interpreters, there are some subjects that are more challenging to interpret. We need to know what they are.

Interpreters need to know when to excuse themselves. It is difficult to be an impartial and focused interpreter if a situation disturbs you deeply. If your emotional state affects your performance and accuracy, you might have to excuse yourself or, with advance notice, arrange for another interpreter to take your place. After all, you don't really want to be in the middle of the session and then ask to speak in private with the provider to excuse yourself. How might the patient feel?

On the other hand, if you are able to provide interpreting that is accurate, respectful, nonjudgmental and professional, you have the opportunity to contribute to an environment that supports quality care to vulnerable patients. Feeling accepted, not judged, helps patients to make informed decisions about treatments, disclosure and risk behaviors in *any* area of health. Patients who feel supported can engage more easily and actively in improving not only their own health outcomes but the well-being of those they love.

Ethics and standards: Reflect and practice

Goal 3: Impartiality

Translation and paraphrasing

1. Look at NCIHC standards of practice related to impartiality (Standards 9 and 10, NCIHC, 2005, p. 6). Working individually, *paraphrase* the objective, its related ethical principle and the two standards.
2. Working individually, *translate* the original text of these standards into your other working language(s) or interpret it into sign language.
3. Find a partner or partners. Compare, discuss and modify your translations and paraphrasing until you are satisfied with your final products as a group.
4. If you can, pick a group representative and discuss your final versions with any other groups that share your working languages. Compare and discuss your differences.

Suggested reading

Downing, B., and Roat, C.E. (2002). *Models for the provision of language access in health care settings.* Washington, DC: National Council on Interpreting in Health Care.[29]

Read the section on using family and friends as interpreters in terms of impartiality. Reflect also on the other standards you are familiar with.

Consider and discuss

1. **Standard 9** An interpreter has lost a sister to AIDS and finds herself interpreting in an HIV clinic. During the encounter, the provider speaks with a patient who is describing how "hard" it is to have safer sex and how annoying it feels to use a condom. The interpreter finds herself upset and angry with the patient. What should she do?
2. **Standard 9** At a reproductive genetics appointment, a pregnant woman learns of severe birth defects, including heart defects and multiple organ damage of her fetus. Clinicians explain the conditions, the likely course of pregnancy and the probability of stillbirth (when a fetus dies in the womb after 20 weeks of pregnancy). Because the appointment takes place in California and is in the second trimester of pregnancy, termination (abortion) is offered as an alternative. When the provider leaves the room, the patient turns to the interpreter and asks, "What should I do? What would *you* do?" How could the interpreter respond in a professional, impartial and yet compassionate way?

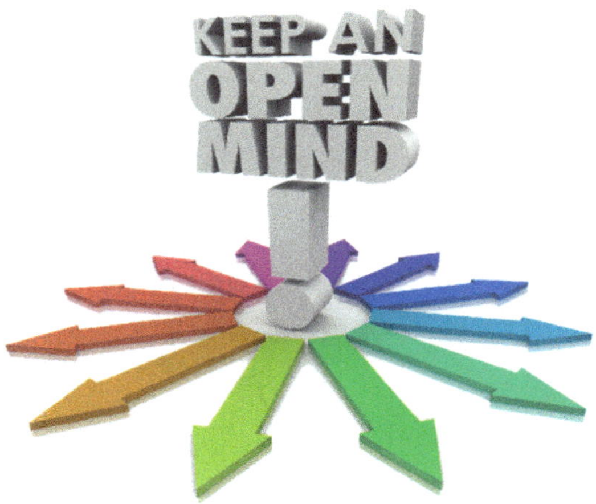

29 Retrieved from www.hablamosjuntos.org/pdf_files/Models_for_the_Provision_of_Language_Access_final_.pdf

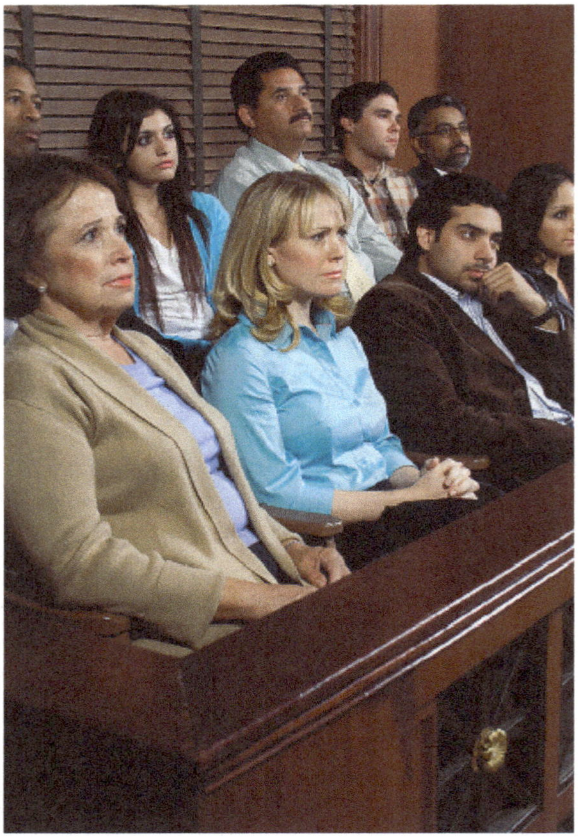

3. **Standard 9** Clearly, this conversation above happened because the interpreter and patient are alone. What if the interpreter has a compelling moral need to tell the patient that abortion is against her (or their) religion and morally unacceptable? What could be done to avoid such a conversation in the first place?
4. **Impartiality and the law:** Depending on federal, state or local laws, can an interpreter legally refuse to interpret at an abortion clinic? Can an employer legally accommodate an interpreter's request not to serve at an abortion clinic? Can an employer legally deny interpreting services to a clinic that provides or assists in arranging abortions? How should such requests be handled by the language service? By the interpreter who feels he or she cannot be impartial enough to interpret there? In what other kinds of clinics, specialties or appointments might the subject of abortion arise?
5. **Consider this scenario:** One interpreter has lost a father to cancer and finds himself interpreting in an oncology ward soon after. A second interpreter has tried for years to have a child, lost many pregnancies and is interpreting for a woman who uses no contraceptives and is discussing her sixth elective abortion. How might the personal experience of each of these interpreters impact their interpreting?
6. **Point for reflection:** How are an interpreter and a member of a jury alike and different in their responsibilities and power?

Occupational therapy for interpreters

EXERCISES FOR THE TONGUE, HEART AND MIND

"HIV/AIDS is one scary-ass illness."

—Rae Lewis-Thornton (2012)

Suggested reading

Lewis-Thornton, R. (2012). The horror of HIV/AIDS: The murder of Cicely.[30]

Note: This article contains strong language, images that some readers might find disturbing or offensive, and a controversial message about sexual assault. Consider carefully if you wish to read this article. Nonetheless, it offers valuable information and frank perspectives about HIV/AIDS from someone who is living with the disease.

Consider and discuss

1. Have you had experience interpreting for patient with HIV or AIDS? Talk about it with colleagues, without violating confidentiality or discussing any private, identifying information. Also discuss the Lewis-Thornton article, if you choose. The following terms and phrases are from that article. Discuss and translate or interpret the phrases.

    a. "HIV/AIDS is one scary-ass illness."
    b. "With those early images of ghostly looking white men who lined the walls of hospitals around the country."
    c. "AIDS hospices."
    d. "People were in panic mode for sure."
    e. "In that [*sic*] five years I had held my infection close to my heart."
    f. "While Magic [Johnson] was being ostracized by his fellow NBA teammates, my upwardly mobile friends were cracking jokes about HIV and I sat in silence and suffered."
    g. "Treatment was mediocre at best and AIDS was a death sentence for sure."
    h. "I was in absolute turmoil."
    i. "If a person knows that they have been exposed to HIV and seeks a prophylaxis treatment with [*sic*] 72 hours it will reverse the HIV. They can take an HIV medication cocktail for 30 days and it will destroy the HIV in their body."

2. Create a glossary of words relevant to HIV/AIDS/STDs/STIs. See how many terms you can list. Check them in the glossaries in Appendix 3. Translate them. Share your terms and translations with colleagues to enhance your personal glossary. If you notice that you feel uncomfortable reading or interpreting certain terms or phrases, examine your feelings. Why do those terms or phrases make you ill at ease? Would those feelings affect your ability to interpret them in real life accurately and impartially? Why or why not? How could you desensitize yourself to them? (Be specific, e.g., practice repeating and/or interpreting them in front of a mirror or to a colleague or friend.) This exercise is a rich learning opportunity, not only to enhance your interpreting but to learn more about yourself.
3. Set aside any questions about interpreting and translation. Based on what affected you most in this chapter, write down two questions or topics that strike you as important regarding any health and social issues related to HIV/AIDS.

30 The easiest way to find and read this article is to do a search for it on the Internet. Just copy the author's name and title into your browser

Medical terminology: The lymphatic system

Below you will find anatomical drawings relevant to the content of this chapter. Follow the instructions found at the end of Chapter 1 to study the terminology in this section.

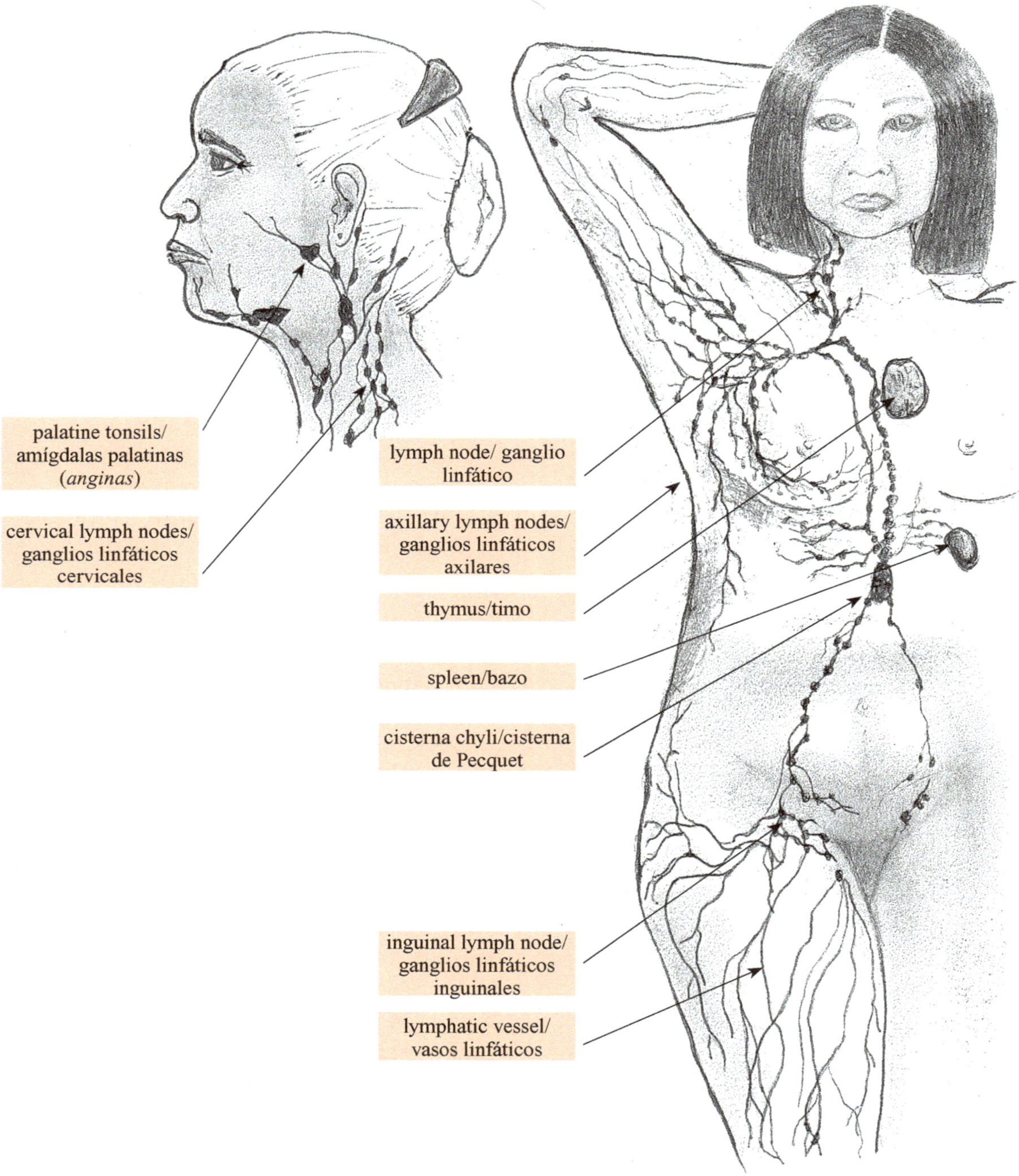

Figure 3-A: The lymphatic system (English and Spanish)

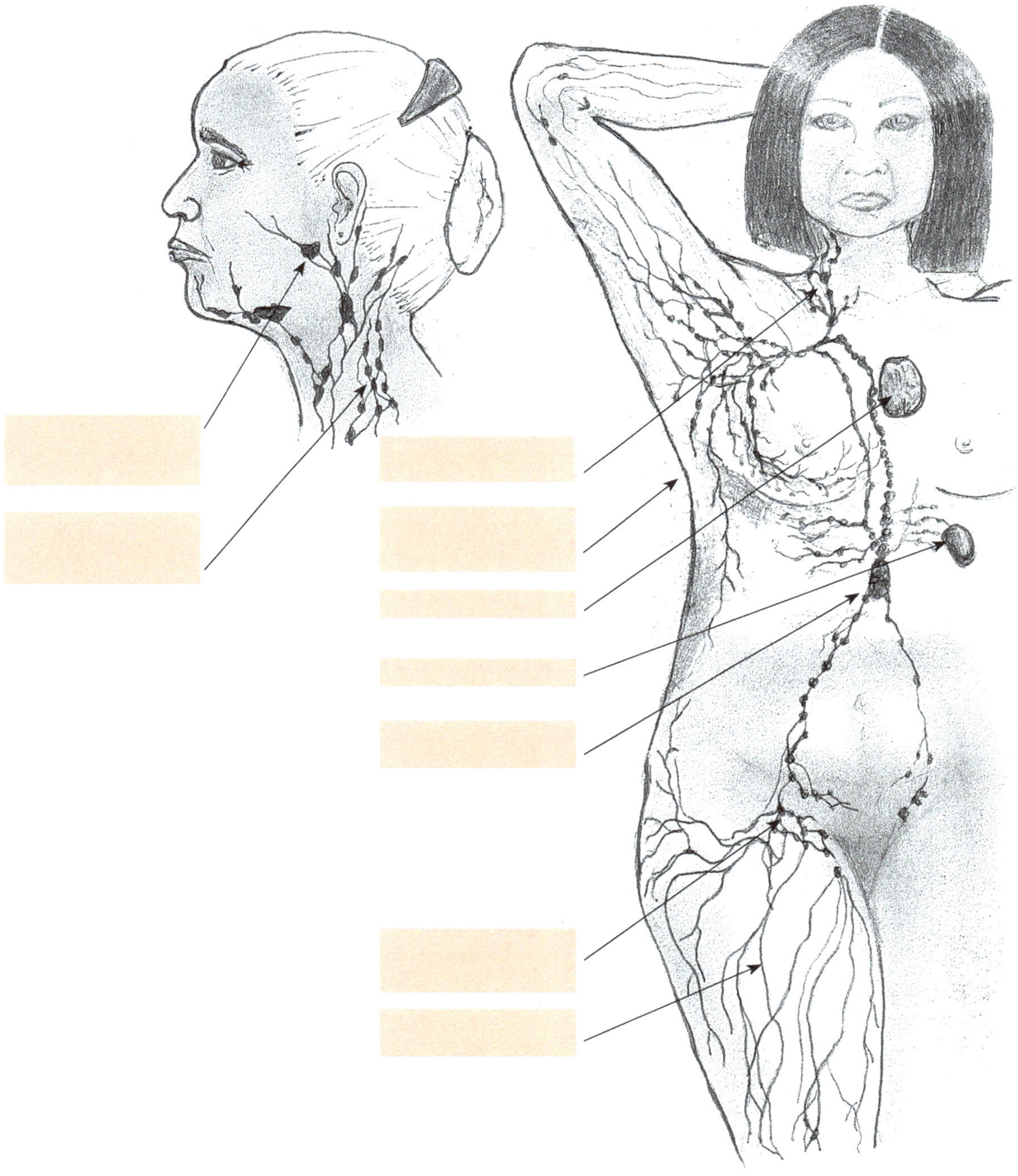

Figure 3-B: The lymphatic system (blank labels)

Medical terminology list

The lymphatic system

VOCABULARY FOR GRAPHIC–IN ENGLISH	VOCABULARY FOR GRAPHIC–IN SPANISH	ANY OTHER LANGUAGE
thymus	timo	
spleen	bazo	
palatine tonsils	amígdalas palatinas (anginas)	
lymph node	ganglio linfático	
axillary lymph nodes	ganglios linfáticos axilares	
cervical lymph nodes	ganglios linfáticos cervicales	
lymphatic vessel	vasos linfáticos	
lymphatic duct	conducto linfático	
cisterna chyli	cisterna de Pecquet	
bone marrow	médula ósea	
inguinal lymph node	ganglios linfáticos inguinales	
lymph	linfa	
lump	protuberancia, bola, bulto, masa	
tonsils	amígdalas (anginas)	
adenoids	adenoides	
OTHER HIV AND IMMUNE VOCABULARY		
CD4 cells (T-cells)	células CD4 (células-T)	
T-cells (CD4 cells)	células-T (células CD4)	
AIDS (Acquired Immune Deficiency Syndrome)	SIDA (Síndrome de inmunodeficiencia adquirida)	
HIV (Human Immunodeficiency Virus)	VIH (Virus de inmunodeficiencia humana)	
PReP (Pre-Exposure Prophylaxis)	Profilaxis preexposición	
undetectable viral load	carga viral indetectable	
non-transmissible		
PEP (Post-Exposure Prophylaxis	PEP (profilaxis posexposición)	
ADAP (AIDS Drug Assistance Programs)	Asistencia De Medicamentos para el SIDA (ADAP)	
Antiretroviral drugs	medicamentos antirretrovirales	
Viral load		
ART (Anti-Retroviral Therapy)	TAR (Tratamiento antiretroviral)	
HAART (Highly Active Anti-Retroviral Therapy)	Tratamiento antirretroviral de gran actividad	
stigma	estigma	
disclosure	divulgación, divulger, notificar	
denial	negación, negarse, no aceptar	

Obstetrics 4

Advisory

This chapter involves material related to gynecology, childbirth, ectopic pregnancy and religious beliefs regarding specific medical practices and blood transfusions.

This patient is a 21-year-old mother with a two-year-old daughter. She has been hospitalized due to an ectopic pregnancy. Her husband is at the hospital with her. They are both Jehovah's Witnesses (a religion with distinctive beliefs). Her sister-in-law is also present and was helping to interpret before the interpreter arrived.

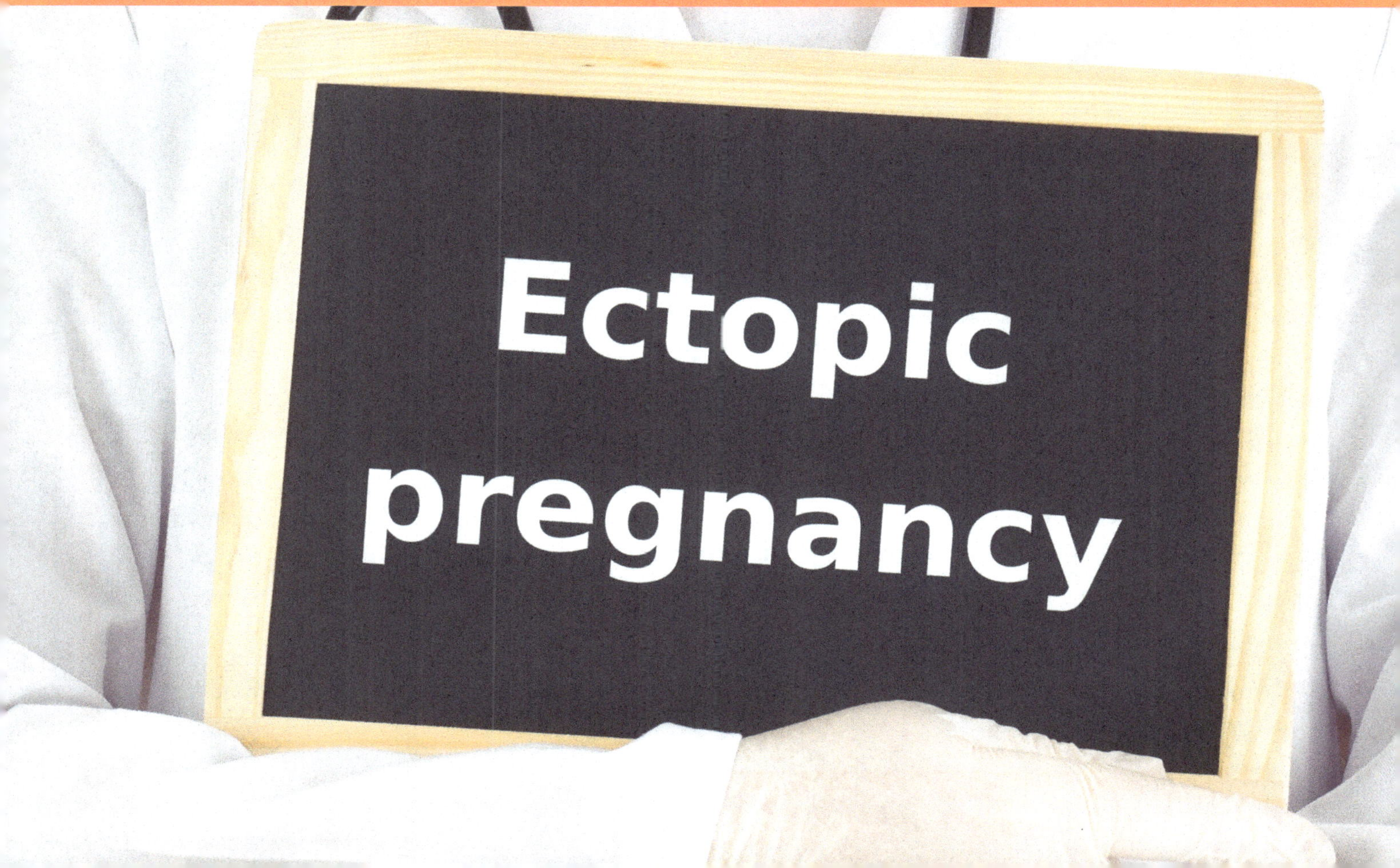

Obstetrics – Ectopic pregnancy role play (English-Spanish)

PART 1

INTERPRETER: Hello. My name is _______________. I'm your interpreter. I'd like to let you know that everything you say will be interpreted, and everything will be kept confidential. Please speak directly to each other, not to me, and pause when I make this signal *(raises hand)* so I can interpret. *(Interpreter repeats this introduction in patient's language.)*

DOCTOR: Good morning, Karla.

PATIENT: Buenos días, doctora.

DOCTOR: I know we talked a little bit about this yesterday, but I wanted to go over it again today with an official translator just to make sure this is all clear. I know your sister-in-law and your husband speak English, and your sister-in-law's been doing a great job translating, but we need to use a hospital translator to get these consents signed, for legal purposes.

PATIENT: Muy bien.

DOCTOR: Yo sabe que entendiste todo ayer, pero voy a repetir. Tu tienes un embarazo *eutópico*, en la, ¿cómo se dice? en la matriz. No, no en la matriz no pero en la salida de la matriz, el *cervix*, *(English pronunciation)*.

INTERPRETER: Cervix o cuello de la matríz.

DOCTOR: OK. So, este *emabarzo* es en el neck, cómo es? I'll just speak in English and let the translator say it. So this pregnancy is in the neck of the uterus. It is a very dangerous situation. We need to take care of this now in order to keep you out of danger. So we are going to go ahead with the ultrasound and make sure that we agree with the doctors you see in Wallace before we do anything. Then, what we'd like to do, if we find that we agree with those doctors, that the pregnancy is still in the neck of the uterus, then we'd like to inject it with some medicine and take care of it that way.

PATIENT: Pero yo no quiero eso. Yo no puedo hacer eso, yo no puedo abortar un bebé.

DOCTOR: I know that because of your religion you are against this procedure. But I need to make sure that you have all the information before you make that decision. I promise we will not do anything without your consent. There are some things I need to tell you about.

PATIENT: Bueno.

DOCTOR: The first thing you need to know is that this is a very unusual situation. This pregnancy is outside the uterus. It is not in a place where it should be. It cannot grow into a baby where it is. It is not a viable pregnancy.

PATIENT: Yo entiendo eso, pero ¿no es posible esperar hasta que salga solito? Eso es lo que yo quiero. Yo entiendo que está fuera de la matriz, pero yo no lo quiero matar.

DOCTOR: Karla, usually un embarazo eutopico está en las tubas de Fallopian.

PATIENT: Si, yo entendí eso.

DOCTOR: When a pregnancy is in the Fallopian tubes, I mean trompas, it also will not survive. This pregnancy cannot survive either. You really need to understand that there is no way that this pregnancy can develop into a baby. But the big difference between you and other women with ectopic pregnancies is the place it's in. Either way it's very dangerous, but in this case, with the embryo in the neck, the cervix, it's worse.

PATIENT: Pero yo no puedo hacer eso, es cruel.

Sister-in-law: Karla, deja que termine. Deja que te explique todo. Tú sabes que yo no estoy aquí para decirte qué debes hacer. Pero quiero que escuches todo antes de que tomes una decisión.

PATIENT: Va, pues.

DOCTOR: All right. Now when a pregnancy is outside the uterus like this, in the Fallopian tubes, if it isn't terminated, it eventually ruptures and there can be a lot of bleeding. If the pregnancy occurs like this and there is a miscarriage in the tubes or in the uterus, there are several things we can do to stop it. We can give medicines to make the muscles contract, or we can put a balloon-type device inside the uterus that will put pressure on it and help stop the bleeding, or in the worst case we can take out the tubes and the uterus.

PART 2

PATIENT: No me importa. Me pueden quitar la matriz.

DOCTOR: Karla, you're a young woman, I imagine you still want to have more children. Is that right?

PATIENT: Bueno pues, sí, yo quería tener éste. Pero si así lo quiere Dios, pues así es, no me importa si me quitan la matriz, pero yo no quiero matar este bebé.

DOCTOR: OK, I understand your point of view, Karla. I'm also not here to tell you what to do. My job is to take care of you and make sure you are safe. I need to finish explaining a few other things about this.

PATIENT: Bien.

DOCTOR: So what makes this unusual, as I was saying before, is that your pregnancy is in the cervix. The cervix is different because there are a lot more blood vessels there, and it isn't composed of muscle. It's mostly fibrous tissue. What that means is that those other remedies I talked about won't work here. If this pregnancy gets to the point where it ruptures, you will have very heavy bleeding and you can die. Your life is in danger.

PATIENT: Pero yo—

Sister-in-law: Karla, deja que termine.

DOCTOR: So do you understand what I mean when I say "rupture"? I'm saying that if you wait for a miscarriage or spontaneous abortion, you could have heavy bleeding and die. ¿Comprendes?

PATIENT: Yo quiero esperar a ver qué sucede.

DOCTOR: Now, Karla, you've waited four weeks since this was diagnosed, so the situation is much more serious. Every day you've waited, those blood vessels have gotten bigger and carry more blood. This could miscarry at any time, and you could bleed to death. If we could have taken care of this four weeks ago, we could've given you an injection in your butt, and it probably would have taken care of the danger, but you waited a long time and now that won't work anymore.

PATIENT: Entonces, ¿está diciendo que tengo que inyectar al bebé con una aguja?

DOCTOR: What we would like to do is go in using ultrasound and if we see the embryo is in the same place, we would inject the water around the embryo with a medicine called methyltrexate. It would cause the tissue to dissolve and be reabsorbed into your body.

HUSBAND: But that's like an abortion. Bueno, mejor voy a hablar en español. No podríamos mirar esto desde otro punto de vista? ¿No podíamos trabajar con esto de otra forma? ¿Qué pasaría si simplemente sacan el bebé de su lugar y lo tratan de mover, de subirlo a la matriz y ponerlo allí más arriba?

DOCTOR: You can't just do that. It would be like tearing a plant out by its roots, it wouldn't work.

HUSBAND: Pero quizás lo podríamos aceptar así, si algo sucediera en el proceso de tratar de moverlo, pues sería diferente.

DOCTOR: I don't think you understand. This pregnancy, this embryo, isn't going to make it. It isn't in a place where it can survive.

PATIENT: ¿Y porqué no podemos esperar a que salga solito, en vez de destruirlo?

DOCTOR: That's the whole point. We don't want you to have a spontaneous abortion. We want it to disintegrate and be reabsorbed so you don't bleed.

HUSBAND: What do you mean by reabsorbed?

DOCTOR: Well, it's like, you know when you have a bruise; maybe sometime you've gotten a big bruise on your arm or leg? First it's very dark, blue and purple. Then after a few days it turns kind of yellowish or green, and then little by little it disappears. That's blood underneath your skin that is being slowly reabsorbed by your body.

PATIENT: De todas maneras, yo prefiero esperar a que se venga solito.

DOCTOR: Karla, the other thing you have to take into account is that this can happen at any time. I'm going to be perfectly frank with you. I'm hoping for the best, but honestly, I don't know if we will be able to save your life. I don't know if the medicine will work anymore because we've waited so long, but it is your only chance. If this pregnancy starts to bleed, I don't know what we'll do. It will cause very heavy bleeding, and you are a Jehovah's Witness and won't accept blood transfusions. Is that correct?

PATIENT: Sí, es correcto, pero me pueden quitar la matriz, eso no me importa. Me pueden quitar la matriz y los ovarios.

DOCTOR: You know, Karla, if you don't accept this treatment and you go home and this happens anywhere else but this facility, *now*, your life will be in serious danger. There may not be time for any of that.

PART 3

PATIENT: Pero no me pueden regresar mi sangre, usar una de esas máquinas que usan donde limpian la sangre o algo así?

DOCTOR: Karla, you are going to bleed very heavily. Where are we going to get that blood? Scrape it off the floor or wring the bed sheets out? In those situations with machines for dialysis, things happen under sterile conditions. We can't do that.

PATIENT: Pues, yo no puedo matar a este bebé. Es cruel.

DOCTOR: Don't you have other children, Karla?

PATIENT: Sí, tengo una niña.

DOCTOR: Have you thought about what will happen to her?

PATIENT: Pues sí, pero si así lo quiere Dios, así tiene que ser. Yo tengo mucha fe en Dios. Yo quiero esperar a ver si viene solito, así no me sentiré tan mal.

DOCTOR: You know, we are here now, we're ready for whatever happens and the appropriate people are here, with the exception of a special doctor I have to call in from another hospital. If this happens close to home or in the night, I'm not going to be here, and neither are the other doctors. It could take hours. Your life is in danger.

PATIENT: Yo no le quiero hacer eso a mi bebé. Si Dios quiere, a lo mejor será diferente y no va a haber tanta sangre.

DOCTOR: You know, we had another woman in here with a similar situation. Not exactly the same, but a similar situation. She bled, had a spontaneous abortion and we had to transfuse her with ten units of blood; it happened very fast. Ten units of blood, and that was in one hour. We saved her life, but just barely, and you refuse to accept blood.

PATIENT: Yo todavía no quiero hacerlo. Yo entiendo lo que me está diciendo.

DOCTOR: All right, but it's against my advice. I have to tell you I think it's very unsafe.

PATIENT: ¿Yo puedo hacer una pregunta?

DOCTOR: Of course.

PATIENT: Yo entiendo lo que usted dijo, que no va a nacer, que el bebé no está en su lugar y todo, ¿verdad? Pero...Si es que nace, ¿qué problemas, o sea, qué trastornos puede tener cuando nazca, qué daño le puede causar la medicina que me dieron ya?

DOCTOR: Karla, you don't understand. There is no way this baby will be born. It cannot grow into a baby in the place it is now. It is not possible. In a little while you will rupture. It's not going to survive.

PATIENT: Yo sé, yo sé lo que me ha dicho. Pero en caso de que sí, ¿cómo puede haberlo afectado la medicina?

DOCTOR: Well, there are two ways. It could have leukemia, or it could die.

PATIENT: Oh.

HUSBAND: *(to patient)* ¿Tienes otra pregunta?

PATIENT: Sí. Usted dijo que voy a tener un aborto espontáneo. Entonces quiero saber si usted va a mandar informes acerca de mi caso a los hospitales cerca de donde vivo explicándoles que me pueden quitar la matriz, para que no pierdan tiempo viendo si pueden parar el sangrado para salvar mi matriz.

DOCTOR: First, I need to clarify something. I didn't say you would have a miscarriage. I said it could happen. You may simply start to bleed and die from the bleeding without miscarrying. Or you may have a miscarriage.

SISTER-IN-LAW: Karla, ¿entiendes todo lo que te está diciendo?

PATIENT: Sí, yo entiendo.

DOCTOR: And no, I won't be sending out any reports. I will, however, document your situation in a letter and make clear what your wishes are, but I will give the letter to you. You will have to take the letter with you to wherever you go, if you go to a hospital.

PATIENT: Está bien.

DOCTOR: All right. Well, you know this pregnancy is not viable, and this is against my advice, but I will respect your wishes. I'll be back in a few minutes with some forms I'll need you to sign. You know we care about what happens to you, so if you change your mind and want to come back for treatment, or if you have questions, you can get a hold of your regular OB and she can get hold of us.

PATIENT, HUSBAND, SISTER-IN-LAW: Gracias.

Ectopic pregnancy role play (English only)

PART 1

DOCTOR: Good morning, Karla.

PATIENT: Good morning, doctor.

DOCTOR: I know we talked a little bit about this yesterday, but I wanted to go over it again today with an official translator just to make sure this is all clear. I know your sister-in-law and your husband speak English, and your sister-in-law's been doing a great job translating, but we need to use a hospital translator to get these consents signed, for legal purposes.

PATIENT: All right.

DOCTOR: *(Tries to speak in patient's language but makes many mistakes. The person playing the doctor should try to sight translate the following text in brackets into the patient's language, if possible, including all the mistakes.)* [I knows that you understand yesterday, but I to repeat. You have a pregnant ectopic, in the how do you say it, in the uter, I mean the uterus. No, no, not the uter, in the opening of the uterus, the cervix.]

INTERPRETER: *(says the words in the patient's language)* Cervix or uterine opening.

DOCTOR: [OK. So this pregnant is in the neck of the uterus, how do you say it?] I'll just speak in English and let the translator say it. So this pregnancy is in the neck of the uterus. It is a very dangerous situation. We need to take care of this now in order to keep you out of danger. So we are going to go ahead with the ultrasound and make sure that we agree with the doctors you see in Wallace before we do anything. Then, what we'd like to do, if we find that we agree with those doctors, that the pregnancy is still in the neck of the uterus, then we'd like to inject it with some medicine, and take care of it that way.

PATIENT: But I don't want to do that. I can't do that, I can't abort my baby.

DOCTOR: I know that because of your religion you are against this procedure. But I need to make sure that you have all the information before you make that decision. I promise we will not do anything without your consent. There are some things I need to tell you about.

PATIENT: All right.

DOCTOR: The first thing you need to know is that this is a very unusual situation. This pregnancy is outside the uterus. It is not in a place where it should be. It cannot grow into a baby where it is. It is not a viable pregnancy.

PATIENT: I understand that, but can't we wait until it comes out by itself? That's what I want to do. I understand it's outside the uterus, but I don't want to kill it.

DOCTOR: *(in patient's language—but filled with mistakes)*[31] Karla, usually an ectopic pregnancy is in the Fallopian tubes. [Karla, usually and eutropica prgancy is in the Fallopian tubas.]

PATIENT: Yes, I understood that.

DOCTOR: When a pregnancy is in the Fallopian tubes it also will not survive. This pregnancy cannot survive either. You really need to understand that there is no way that this pregnancy can develop into a baby. But the big difference between you and other women with ectopic pregnancies is the place it's in. Either way it's very dangerous, but in this case, with the embryo in the [neck], the cervix, it's worse.

PATIENT: But I can't do that, it's cruel.

SISTER-IN-LAW: Karla, let the doctor finish. Let her explain everything. You know that I'm not here to tell you what you should do. But I want you to listen to everything before you make a decision.

PATIENT: OK.

DOCTOR: All right. Now, when a pregnancy is outside the uterus like this, in the Fallopian tubes, if it isn't terminated, it eventually ruptures, and there can be a lot of bleeding. If the pregnancy occurs like this and there is a miscarriage in the tubes or in the uterus, there are several things we can do to stop it. We can give medicines to make the muscles contract, or we can put a balloon-type device inside the uterus that will put pressure on it and help stop the bleeding, or in the worst case we can take out the tubes and the uterus.

PART 2

PATIENT: I don't care, you can even take out my uterus.

DOCTOR: Karla, you're a young woman, I imagine you still want to have more children. Is that right?

PATIENT: Well, yes, I wanted to have this baby. But if God wants it this way, well, then this is the way it is. I don't care if you take out my uterus, but I don't want to kill this baby.

DOCTOR: OK, I understand your point of view, Karla. I'm also not here to tell you what to do. My job is to take care of you and make sure you are safe. I need to finish explaining a few other things about this.

PATIENT: OK.

DOCTOR: So what makes this unusual, as I was saying before, is that your pregnancy is in the cervix. The cervix is different because there are a lot more blood vessels there, and it isn't composed of muscle. It's mostly fibrous tissue. What that means is that those other remedies I talked about won't work here. If this pregnancy gets to the point where it ruptures, you will have very heavy bleeding and you can die. Your life is in danger.

31 Obviously, this is a life-and-death situation with a serious decision to be made based on informed consent. This is not a Spanish class. If the doctor is hindering the process or simply making it impossible for you to interpret effectively, what can you do?

PATIENT: But I—

Sister-in-law: Karla, let her finish.

DOCTOR: So do you understand what I mean when I say "rupture"? I'm saying that if you wait for a miscarriage or spontaneous abortion, you could have heavy bleeding and die. Do you understand?

PATIENT: I want to wait and see what happens.

DOCTOR: Now, Karla, you've waited four weeks since this was diagnosed, so the situation is much more serious. Every day you've waited, those blood vessels have gotten bigger and carry more blood. This could miscarry at any time, and you could bleed to death. If we could have taken care of this four weeks ago, we could've given you an injection in your butt, and it probably would have taken care of the danger, but you waited a long time and now that won't work anymore.

PATIENT: So you're saying I have to inject the baby with a needle?

DOCTOR: What we would like to do is go in using ultrasound, and if we see the embryo is in the same place, we would inject the water around the embryo with a medicine called methyltrexate. It would cause the tissue to dissolve and be reabsorbed into your body.

HUSBAND: *(in English)* But that's like an abortion. Well, I better speak in ______. *(Switches to patient's language.)* Can't we look at this from another point of view? Can't we work with this another way? What would happen if we simply take the baby out from where it is, and try to move it, to put it back in the uterus, to put it up inside?

DOCTOR: You can't just do that. It would be like tearing a plant out by its roots, it wouldn't work.

HUSBAND: But maybe we'd be able to accept it like that, if something happened in the process of trying to move it, well, it would be different.

DOCTOR: I don't think you understand. This pregnancy, this embryo, isn't going to make it. It isn't in a place where it can survive.

PATIENT: And why can't we wait for it to come out by itself instead of destroying it?

DOCTOR: That's the whole point. We don't want you to have a spontaneous abortion. We want it to disintegrate and be reabsorbed so you don't bleed.

HUSBAND: *(in English)* What do you mean by reabsorbed?

DOCTOR: Well, it's like, you know when you have a bruise; maybe sometime you've gotten a big bruise on your arm or leg? First it's very dark, blue and purple. Then after a few days it turns kind of yellowish or green, and then little by little it disappears. That's blood underneath your skin that is being slowly reabsorbed by your body.

PATIENT: Either way, I prefer to wait and let it come out by itself.

DOCTOR: Karla, the other thing you have to take into account is that this can happen at any time. I'm going to be perfectly frank with you. I'm hoping for the best, but honestly, I don't know if we will be able to save your life. I don't know if the medicine will work anymore because we've waited so long, but it is your only chance. If this pregnancy starts to bleed I don't know what we'll do. It will cause very heavy bleeding, and you are a Jehovah's Witness and won't accept blood transfusions. Is that correct?

PATIENT: Yes, that's right, but you can take out my uterus, I don't care. You can take out my uterus and my ovaries.

DOCTOR: You know, Karla, if you don't accept this treatment and you go home, and this happens anywhere else but this facility, *now*, your life will be in serious danger. There may not be time for any of that.

PART 3

PATIENT: But can't you just give me back my blood, use one of those machines where they clean the blood or something like that?

DOCTOR: Karla, you are going to bleed very heavily. Where are we going to get that blood? Scrape it off the floor or wring the bed sheets out? In those situations, with machines for dialysis, things happen under sterile conditions. We can't do that.

PATIENT: Well, I can't kill this baby. It's cruel.

DOCTOR: Don't you have other children, Karla?

PATIENT: Yes, I have a little girl.

DOCTOR: Have you thought about what will happen to her?

PATIENT: Well, yes, but if God wants it like this, then this is the way it has to be. I have a lot of faith in God. I want to wait and see if it comes by itself, I won't feel so bad like that.

DOCTOR: You know, we are here now, we're ready for whatever happens and the appropriate people are here, with the exception of a special doctor I have to call in from another hospital. If this happens close to home or in the night, I'm not going to be here, and neither are the other doctors. It could take hours. Your life is in danger.

PATIENT: I don't want to do that to my baby. If God wills, maybe it will turn out differently, and there won't be so much blood.

DOCTOR: You know, we had another woman in here with a similar situation. Not exactly the same, but a similar situation. She bled, had a spontaneous abortion and we had to transfuse her with ten units of blood; it happened very fast. Ten units of blood, and that was in one hour. We saved her life, but just barely, and you refuse to accept blood.

PATIENT: I still don't want to do that. I understand what you are telling me.

DOCTOR: All right, but it's against my advice. I have to tell you I think it's very unsafe.

PATIENT: Can I ask a question?

DOCTOR: Of course.

PATIENT: I understand what you said, that it's not going to be born, that the baby isn't in the right place and everything, right? But...if it is born, what problems, I mean, what disorders might it have when it's born? What damage can that medicine do that they already gave me?

DOCTOR: Karla, you don't understand. There is no way this baby will be born. It cannot grow into a baby in the place it is now. It is not possible. In a little while you will rupture. It's not going to survive.

PATIENT: I know, I know what you've told me. But in case it is born, how might the medicine have affected it?

DOCTOR: Well, there are two ways. It could have leukemia, or it could die.

PATIENT: Oh.

HUSBAND: *(to patient)* Do you have another question?

PATIENT: Yes. You said that I will have a miscarriage. So then I want to know if you are going to send reports about my case to the other hospitals close to where I live, explaining to them that they can take out my uterus, so that they don't waste time trying to stop the bleeding to save my uterus.

DOCTOR: First, I need to clarify something. I didn't say you would have a miscarriage. I said it could happen. You may simply start to bleed and die from the bleeding without miscarrying. Or you may have a miscarriage.

SISTER-IN-LAW: Karla, do you understand what she is saying?

PATIENT: Yes, I do.

DOCTOR: And no, I won't be sending out any reports. I will, however, document your situation in a letter and make clear what your wishes are, but I will give the letter to you. You will have to take the letter with you to wherever you go, if you go to a hospital.

PATIENT: All right.

DOCTOR: All right. Well, you know this pregnancy is not viable, and this is against my advice, but I will respect your wishes. I'll be back in a few minutes with some forms I'll need you to sign. You know we care about what happens to you, so if you change your mind and want to come back for treatment, or if you have questions, you can get a hold of your regular OB and she can get hold of us.

PATIENT, HUSBAND, SISTER-IN-LAW: Thank you.

What's important to know about this chapter?

Overview

Patients' religious beliefs and their more general beliefs (about healthcare, healing, what is causing a certain issue and broader issues) often conflict with Western biomedical views. The patients' perspectives can also contradict the beliefs of their healthcare providers. As the interpreter, you might find some of these situations difficult or distressing to interpret. You may feel "caught in the middle."

Terminology

The terminology in this chapter is important for any medical interpreter to know. Below you will find definitions (taken from Oxford Dictionaries[32]). The definition of *hysteria* offers you a glimpse into cultural perspectives on women and how it is reflected historically in language:

> ***Obstetrics:*** *The branch of medicine and surgery concerned with childbirth and midwifery.*
>
> ***Gynecology:*** *The branch of physiology and medicine which deals with the functions and diseases specific to women and girls, especially those affecting the reproductive system.*
>
> ***Hysteria:*** *Exaggerated or uncontrollable emotion or excitement.*
>
> > ***Origin of the word:*** *In ancient times, doctors (who were male) regarded hysteria as a disease of women caused by a disturbance of the womb. In the early 19th-century, English pathologists (also male) formed the English name from Greek hustera 'uterus, womb'.*

32 Retrieved from www.oxforddictionaries.com/definition/english/obstetrics

Hysterectomy: Based on the origin of the word "hysteria," try to write your own definition of this word.

Hysterectomy: How would you define this word based on modern medical usage?

Religion

The family in this dialogue is Jehovah's Witnesses. Interpreters will come across a rich variety of religious beliefs among patients. For example, most practicing Jehovah's Witnesses believe, based on their interpretation of the biblical prohibition against eating or drinking blood, that it is forbidden to accept blood transfusions or any of the major parts of blood (red or white cells, platelets or plasma), nor should they donate or store blood for later use. This belief can become problematic in certain cases, for example, for procedures or conditions that lead to excessive bleeding or a need for blood. Interpreting for Jehovah's Witnesses might even involve court orders that allow hospitals to go against the patient's beliefs to save a life, especially if children are involved.

Many religious beliefs become relevant in healthcare settings. Are there certain foods that a Muslim, Jewish, Buddhist, Baha'i, Zoroaster, or Hindu patient must eat or must not eat—or must not eat on certain days or at certain times? Do you know of religious beliefs involving the origins of foods or their preparation? What are some of the religious or cultural practices regarding hot and cold foods or hot and cold drinks? What about other cultural or religious beliefs that affect clothing? Male-female relationships? Prayer? Hygiene? Hands? Discuss some of the religious or cultural misunderstandings that you have observed in healthcare settings.

Translator or interpreter

Are you a translator or an interpreter? In general, interpreters render oral or signed messages from one language into another, while translators render a text into another language in writing. However, many people (perhaps most) see no real difference between the two activities, and they often call interpreters "translators."

The doctor in the dialogue above in fact refers to the interpreter as a *translator*. If you are the interpreter, is it important to point out that you are not a translator (or not acting as one)? If you decide not to explain the difference, should you interpret the doctor's word, *translator* as **translator**, or should you interpret *translator* as **interpreter**?

Formality

In your working languages, are there different pronouns, verb forms or other grammatical differences when speaking to one type of person versus another? (For example, older vs. younger, more educated vs. less educated, male vs. female, etc.) In some languages, the way the doctor is speaking to the patient in this dialogue role play, in the informal mode of address, might impact the patient-provider relationship in a negative way, but perhaps not. How might that situation be perceived in your working languages?[33]

Your sister-in-law is doing a great job interpreting

What qualifications, skills or knowledge would a doctor or anyone else need in order to listen to an interpretation and make the evaluation that a nonprofessional interpreter is doing a "great job"?

Vocabulary

Is "neck of the uterus" an acceptable way to say "cervix" in English? Interpret *ectopic pregnancy* and *Fallopian tubes* into your other working language.

If a doctor states an important medical term in the patient's language incorrectly, should you correct the doctor? Why or why not?

Euphemism

Practitioners sometimes talk about life, death or bodily functions in euphemisms (that is to say, fancy or vague language that isn't clear, instead of using plain words that are easier for the patient to understand). Often, healthcare providers do so in difficult situations to avoid being too blunt or sounding insensitive. However, these providers are often unaware that euphemisms don't "translate" well. Plain language is much easier to interpret.

Paraphrase "a viable pregnancy" in English. Then interpret both "a viable pregnancy" and your paraphrase into your other working language(s). Think: What does "a viable pregnancy" really mean to a parent?

33 This topic is addressed in more detail in the next chapter.

Providers who use "Tarzan Language"

In one part of this chapter's dialogue, the doctor said she needed to use an official interpreter for legal purposes. Before that, the doctor was getting by on speaking the patient's language in a broken way and having the sister-in-law interpret. What reasons might the doctor have had for trying to speak the patient's language when the doctor is not adequately proficient in that language? Name a few possibilities. Depending on your working languages, the problem of the provider who tries to speak the patient's language (but does so badly) even when you are present might be a common or a rare problem. Interpreters in California or Florida, for example, quite often encounter providers who know some Spanish and want to use it. How will you handle this situation? Be prepared!

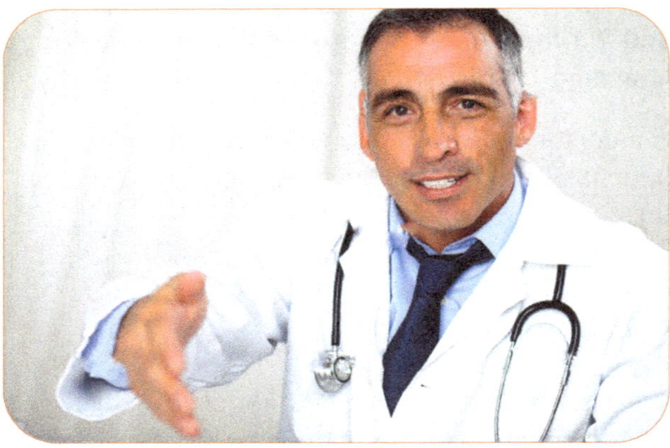

Examples

1. Is the doctor speaking the other language only for greetings and to establish warmth and rapport? Then perhaps you can let it pass without comment.
2. Is the doctor speaking the other language poorly and making mistakes that could lead to medical misunderstandings? You will need to decide if the mistakes are having a negative impact. If not, and the doctor only rarely breaks into the patient's language, will you just let it go?
3. If the doctor is speaking the other language often and these communications represent a risk for the patient's correct understanding of healthcare information, or if the patient has to struggle to understand, you might need to intervene. (Struggling to understand the doctor puts an undue burden on the Deaf, Hard of Hearing or LEP patient in what is often or usually a somewhat stressful encounter for the patient.) If you do intervene, what will you say? How will you address both parties? E.g., you might say, *Excuse me, the interpreter is concerned that the (language, e.g., Spanish) being spoken by the doctor might not be comprehensible. If the doctor wishes to speak English, the interpreter will be happy to interpret.* (Remember that for transparency, whatever you say to one party you must report to the other.)
4. If you cannot fix the problem, you might need to offer to withdraw. For example, you could say, *Excuse me, as the interpreter I'm happy to either interpret for you or withdraw. Please let me know if you'd like me to stay and interpret or leave.* In an extreme case, you might need to be clear that patient safety is at risk—perhaps after the session. You might even need to consider reporting the doctor. (See the introductory section of this book titled "Guide to Advocacy.")

Now consider the specific dialogue in this chapter. Is it appropriate for the practitioner in this dialogue to use the patient's language? This encounter is about a life-and-death situation. There are serious decisions to make based on informed consent. Such decisions are highly emotional. They are stressful. Clarity is essential because the outcomes, based on conversations and communication, might lead to a court order (forcing the patient to get blood against her consent) or death (if the patient refuses blood under circumstances in which only blood may save her life). Either way, the situation could lead to a lawsuit. In short, this is not a language classroom. If the doctor is making it hard for the patient to understand or impossible for you to interpret, what can you do? Every situation is different. Each solution is unique. Discuss with colleagues how you might phrase an intervention to clarify your role and also make clear why the provider should not communicate in the patient's language except to establish a warm relationship.

Ethics and standards: Reflect and practice

Goal 4: Respect

Translation and paraphrasing

1. Look at the three NCIHC standards of practice related to respect (Standards 11, 12 and 13 in NCIHC, 2005, p. 7). Working individually, *paraphrase* the objective, its related ethical principle and the three standards.
2. Working individually, *translate* the original text of these standards into your other working language(s) or interpret it into sign language.
3. Find a partner or partners. Compare, discuss and modify your translations and paraphrasing until you are satisfied with your final products as a group.
4. If you can, pick a group representative and discuss your final versions with any other groups that share your working languages. Compare and discuss your differences.

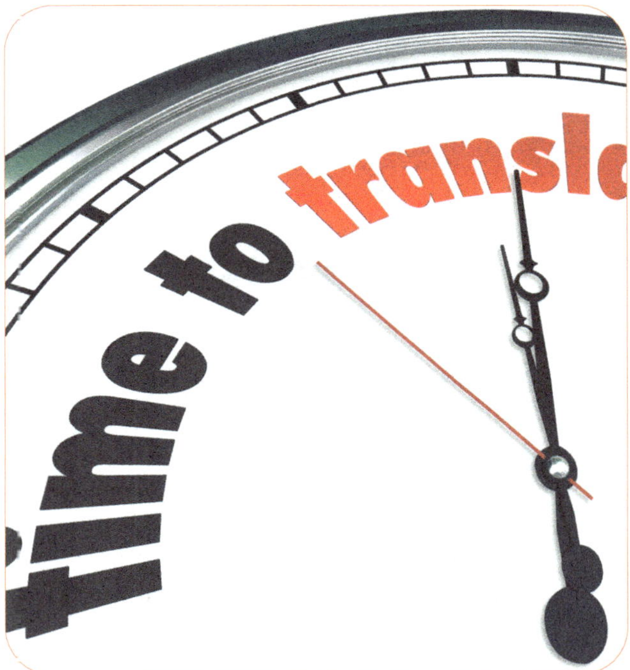

Suggested reading

> Downing, B., and Roat, C.E. (2002). *Models for the provision of language access in health care settings*. Washington, DC: National Council on Interpreting in Health Care.[34]

Read this paper and discuss the section on having family members and friends act as interpreters (pp. 10 and 11). Explore the impact of having family or friends interpret on impartiality.

Consider and discuss

1. **Standard 11** Imagine that a healthcare provider begins by using limited Portuguese (or another language) instead of bringing in an interpreter. The provider addresses the patient using an informal register. When asking an 87-year-old grandfather to sit down, the provider's statement in the other language comes across as, "*You sit down,*" rather than "*Have a seat, sir.*" What is the impact of the doctor's statement on the patient? Imagine that the grandfather did not graduate from elementary school. The provider is a specialist. How might the provider's speech affect the power dynamics? How might those dynamics affect the patient's ability or willingness to communicate symptoms? To ask the doctor questions? To request that the doctor speak in language that is easier to understand?
2. **Standard 11** This standard addresses how the interpreter should use "professional, culturally appropriate ways" of showing respect. List

34 Available at http://www.ncihc.org/publications

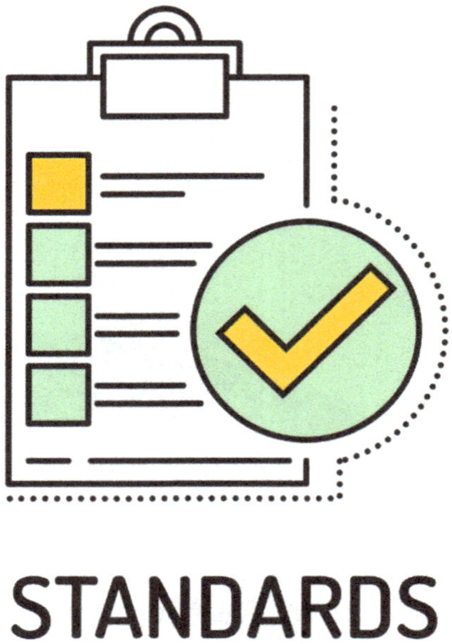

examples of things that interpreters might say to show respect (e.g., addressing a patient as "Mr. So-and-So" or "Mrs. So-and-So" or another formal title in the other language). What if providers speak in culturally disrespectful ways to patients, how might an interpreter open a discussion on this topic with a provider? Offer some strategies for interpreters to gently educate providers on helpful ways to address patients without stereotyping them. (Be aware of cultural differences within groups.)

3. **Standard 11** If a doctor introduces himself as "John" to the patient, rather than "Dr. Smith," and refers to other colleagues with their first names and without titles, will you simply interpret this information? Among patients from other countries, is it common to refer to professionals by their first name? How might this practice affect the patient's perception of the provider and his or her competence? Discuss whether or not to speak to providers about this type of situation. If so, do you think it is better to do so formally or in an informal "water cooler chat" (by speaking colleague-to-colleague in a relaxed way)?
4. **Standard 11** Some guides for practitioners suggest that familiarity is important with "Latino" patients and that they "may want to feel comfortable with physicians as friends" (Smith, Sudore, & Pérez-Stable, 2009). Do you agree? Why might a practitioner who reads cultural information in books or articles need to be careful about acting on that information? What is your experience when doctors try to be "familiar" or personal with patients of your language group?
5. **Standard 12** This standard addresses the interpreter's role in promoting direct communication between parties in the health encounter. How can the interpreter encourage direct provider-patient communication in a *nonverbal* manner? In other words, what can the interpreter do nonverbally to help prevent the provider and/or patient from looking at, and speaking to, the interpreter?
6. **Standard 12** What can an interpreter do when a practitioner continually refers to the patient in third person, for example "Ask *her* if *she* got the flu shot last year." Mention at least three different strategies (not including those in your answer to the previous question).
7. **Standard 13** A patient's mother is a seasonal cannery worker with little formal education who is raising three children. The mother asks how to apply for free state health insurance for her child with disabilities. She is told "just download it from the Internet" by a social worker. How does the social worker's comment relate to this standard (13)? What possible problem might the social worker be missing?
8. **Standard 13** A social worker directs a patient's parents to obtain the fax number for the U.S. Embassy in San Salvador so that a letter can be sent asking for a grandparent's visa to see a dying grandchild. From previous experience, the interpreter knows that for the family this request will involve (a) several long-distance telephone calls, (b) a trip to the embassy by a family member, (c) lost work by that family member in order to wait in line to speak to a front-gate security person at the embassy and (d) possible repeat calls or hardships if the first number provided is wrong. This family is extremely poor. There is a high probability that

the family has no direct access to computers or knowledge about how to use them in a local library. The fax number is easily accessible via the Internet for the social worker but not the family. The social worker wants this family to be "self-sufficient." Is the request appropriate? As the interpreter, how would you handle this situation? How does it relate to the concept of respect?

9. **Standard 13** In the two situations described above, suppose you have carefully considered what to do and you have decided to take action. Write an example for each situation of what an interpreter might do and say during or after the encounter.
10. **Standard 13** Legal requirements aside, how might a lack of visible signs to inform patients of their rights to an interpreter (and how to request one) be related to the concept of respect for patients?
11. **Standard 13** A patient has terminal cancer. After a discussion about possible next steps, the patient and providers decide on some chemotherapy that may give the patient a few more months with his family. The doctors promise to do their best for the patient. He responds. Interpret the text below.

For Spanish speakers, try not to look farther down at the English text. If you are not a Spanish interpreter, interpret the following English adaptation of the text into your other language.

Spanish

Gracias, doctor. Espero que hagan sus mejores esfuerzos. Yo me he esforzado mucho en este país y he trabajado duro para que usted tenga buena comida en su mesa todos los días. Muchos de nosotros trabajamos todos los días para que vivan bien.

English

Thank you, doctor. I hope you'll try your hardest. I've made every effort to do my best in this country, and I've worked hard so that you have good food on your table every day. Many of us work every day so that all of us can live well.

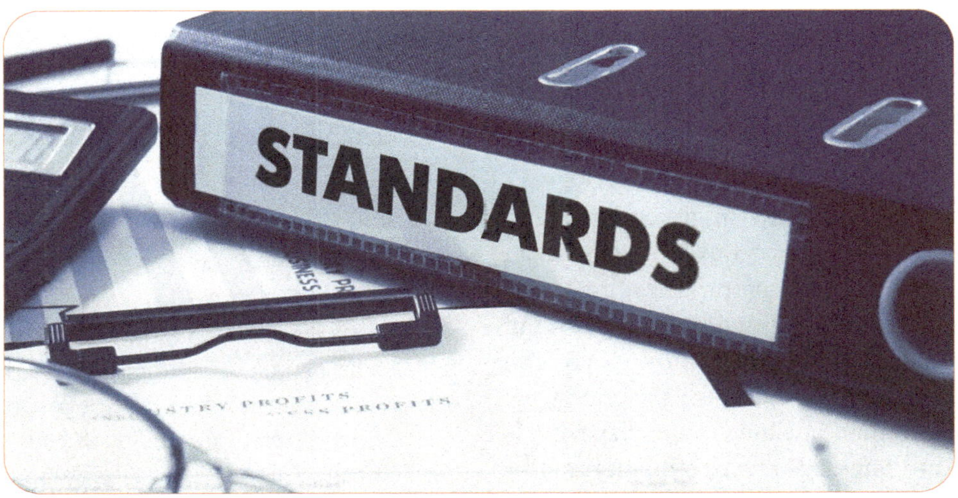

Occupational therapy for interpreters

EXERCISES FOR THE TONGUE, HEART AND MIND

Suggested reading

Diamond, L.C., and Jacobs, E.A. (2010). Let's not contribute to disparities: The best methods for teaching clinicians how to overcome language barriers to healthcare. *Journal of General Internal Medicine* 25(2), 189-193.

Consider and discuss

1. The authors of this article discuss popular public health topics: health equity and health disparities. What do they mean by these two terms?
2. In general, is there a difference between a "disparity" and an "inequity"? Does one of them imply human behavior, nature or responsibility more than the other?
3. Can you think of a health disparity involving diabetes among Latinos/Hispanics and whites? Describe what you think might contribute to the disparity. Is it related to language, race, ethnicity, economics and/or culture?
4. Can you think of a health disparity involving breast cancer survival among African Americans/Blacks and whites? Describe what you think might contribute to the disparity. Is it related to language, race, ethnicity and/or culture?
5. The authors of this article document that, "Having limited English proficiency (LEP) is a risk factor for health disparities" (p. S189). They offer specific examples of the consequences of language barriers, such as:

    a. Decreased access to preventive health services
    b. Decreased satisfaction with care
    c. Poor understanding of instructions or medications
    d. Longer hospital stays
    e. Increased risk of medical errors and misdiagnoses

    Which of these consequences do you believe might pose the most serious risk for health? Which might lead to the patient not following the treatment plan?
6. The authors cite research that demonstrates how providing professional interpreters for health appointments or proficient communication with bilingual providers can lead to:

    a. Fewer errors in communication
    b. Reduced disparities in utilization of services
    c. Improved clinical outcomes

    Which of these improvements might help LEP patients avoid a huge hospital bill or another serious problem that could cost them money? Which of these improvements might make compliance with their treatment plan easier?
7. The article mentions how studies show that doctors still often do not call in professional interpreters, "frequently substituting their own limited non-English language skills during clinical encounters, even when they are aware of their non-English language limitations and their potential impact on quality of care" (p. S189). Why do you think health professionals might not want to call in professional interpreters when they are needed?

8. The authors caution that some educational practices intended to reduce health disparities "may actually increase the likelihood that LEP patients will experience disparities" (p. S189). How could a six-week language course for health providers (e.g., *Medical Spanish* or *French for Doctors*) cause problems in healthcare?
9. How would you explain to an administrator why health professionals who say they speak another language should be tested for their language skills before being allowed to provide care in another language?
10. Will it be easy to convince health professionals who believe they speak another language adequately to take a standardized language test? If not, why not? How could you help convince them?
11. Do "native" language speakers (e.g., doctors who grew up in the United States with Arabic-speaking parents at home or doctors who spent the first 12 years of life in an Arabic-speaking country) also need to take such tests? Why or why not? (Note that language specialists refer to someone who grew up speaking a non-English language in this country as a "heritage speaker" of that language.)
12. How can letting family and friends interpret for patients contribute to health disparities?
13. Imagine an 11-year-old boy whose father has a debilitating neurological condition. The neurologist asks him to help his father fill out a form and interpret the answers (as follows):

    Q: Do you ever have thoughts of harming yourself or ending your life?
    A: Yes.
    Q: Have you ever tried to harm yourself or end your life?
    A: Yes.

    Describe how the child might feel. Point out any potential problems for accuracy when asking family members or friends—especially children—to interpret.
14. Imagine a 13-year-old adolescent girl with a serious heart condition. Describe what challenges she might face in interpreting to her mother that she needs a life-saving surgery that includes a 50 percent risk of stroke or death.
15. The Institute of Medicine says that specific educational measures are essential in order to reduce disparities. Such measures would address the following:

    1. Cultural competence
    2. The legal rights of LEP patients
    3. The need to provide qualified interpreters

    Chose one of these three issues and outline the main points that you would want to include, if you were making a presentation on that topic to a group of health professionals.

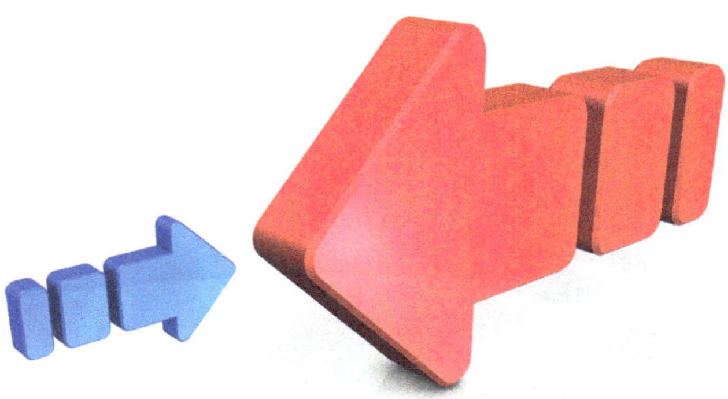

Medical terminology: Ectopic and normal pregnancy

Below you will find anatomical drawings relevant to the content of this chapter. Follow the instructions found at the end of Chapter 1 to study the terminology in this section.

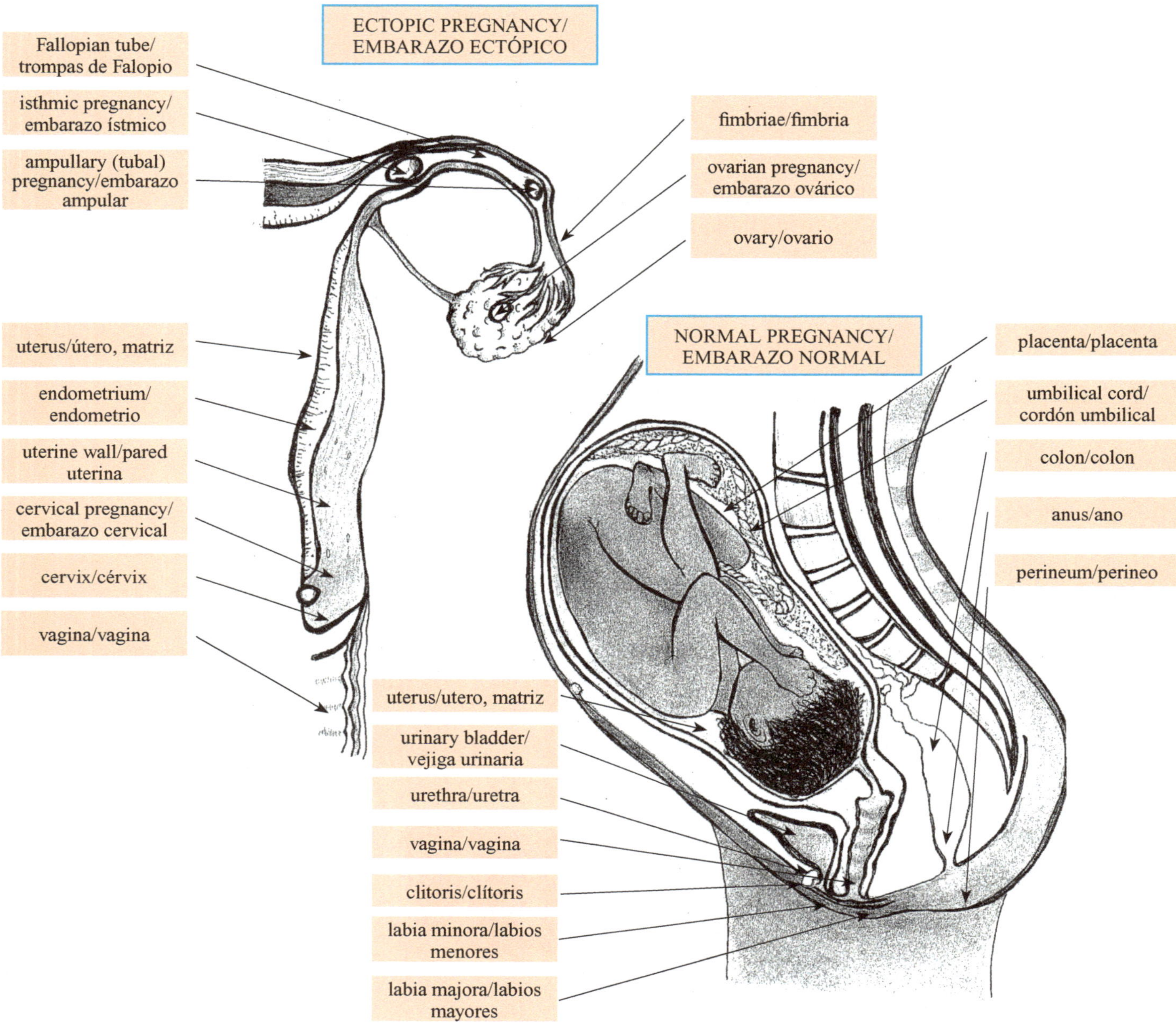

Figure 4-A: Ectopic and normal pregnancy (English and Spanish)

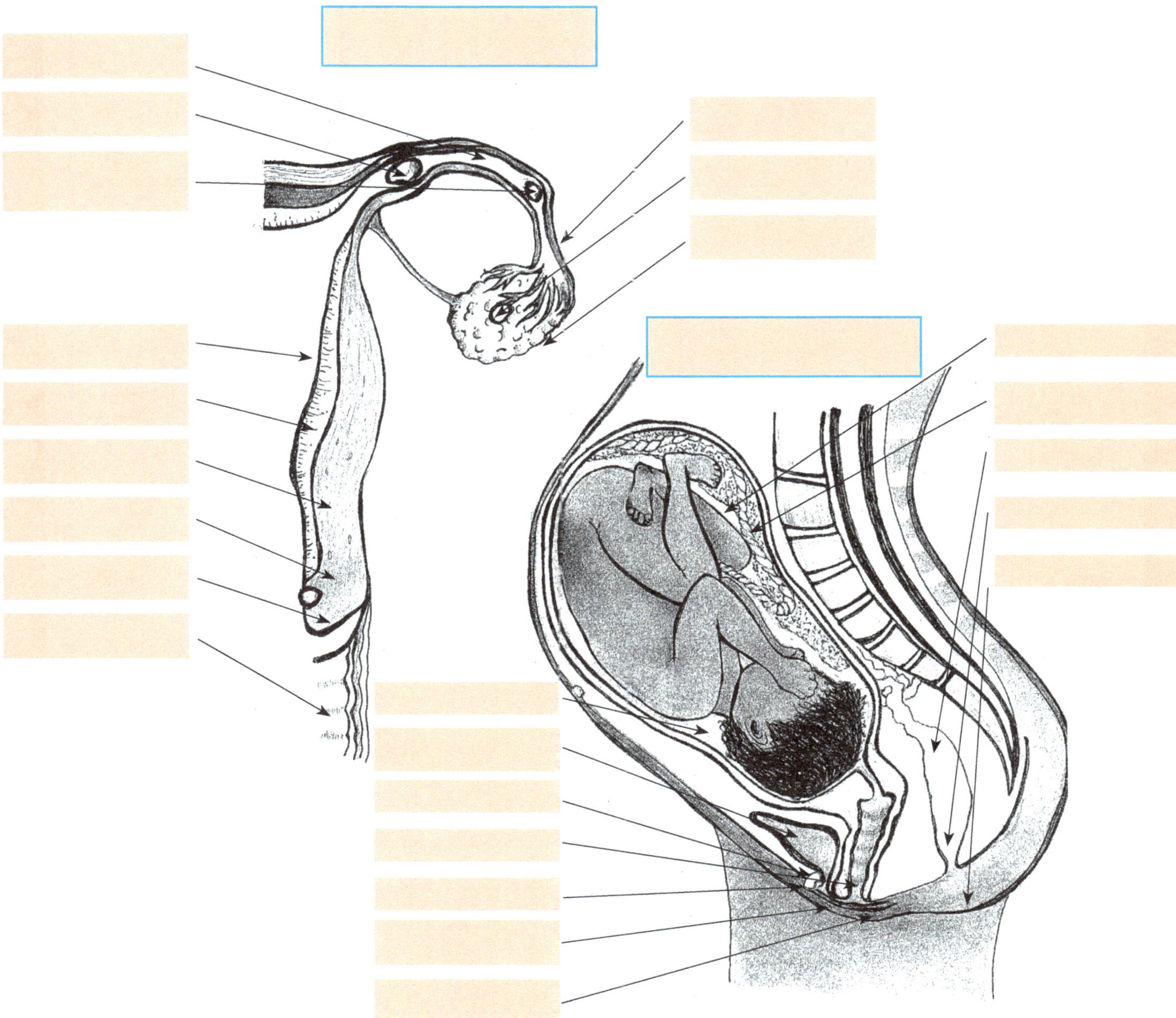

Figure 4-B: Ectopic and normal pregnancy (blank labels)

Medical terminology list

Ectopic and normal pregnancy

VOCABULARY FOR GRAPHIC–IN ENGLISH	VOCABULARY FOR GRAPHIC–IN SPANISH	ANY OTHER LANGUAGE
Amniotic fluid	Líquido amniótico	
ampullary (tubal) pregnancy	embarazo ampular	
anus	ano	
cervical pregnancy	embarazo cervical	
cervix	cervix	
clitoris	clítoris	
colon	colon	
ectopic pregnancy	embarazo ectópico	
endometrium	endometrio	
Fallopian tube	trompas de Falopio	
fimbriae	fimbria	
isthmic pregnancy	embarazo ístmico	
labia majora	labios mayors	
labia minora	labios menores	
normal pregnancy	embarazo normal	
ovarian pregnancy	embarazo ovárico	
ovary	ovario	
perineum	perineo	
placenta	placenta	
umbilical cord	cordón umbilical	
urethra	uretra	
urinary bladder	vejiga urinaria	
uterine wall	pared uterina	
uterus	utero, matriz	
vagina	vagina	

Endocrinology—Adult 5

Advisory

This chapter involves information about endocrine and hormonal conditions and infertility.

The patient is a young married woman who is accompanied by her husband. The doctor knows a little Spanish (or it could be another language spoken by the patient) and wants to practice speaking it. The doctor is also mixing up English and the other language in the same sentences. This can be one of the more frustrating situations for an interpreter, because the doctor interferes with the role of the interpreter. It is also just hard to interpret when the speaker is switching between two languages and committing many mistakes, whether the speaker is the provider or the patient. As discussed in the previous chapter, such practices can undermine clear communication, quality care and patient safety.

Note: This is a shorter role play, so it is not divided into three parts. Shorter role plays in this book will not be divided into smaller sections.

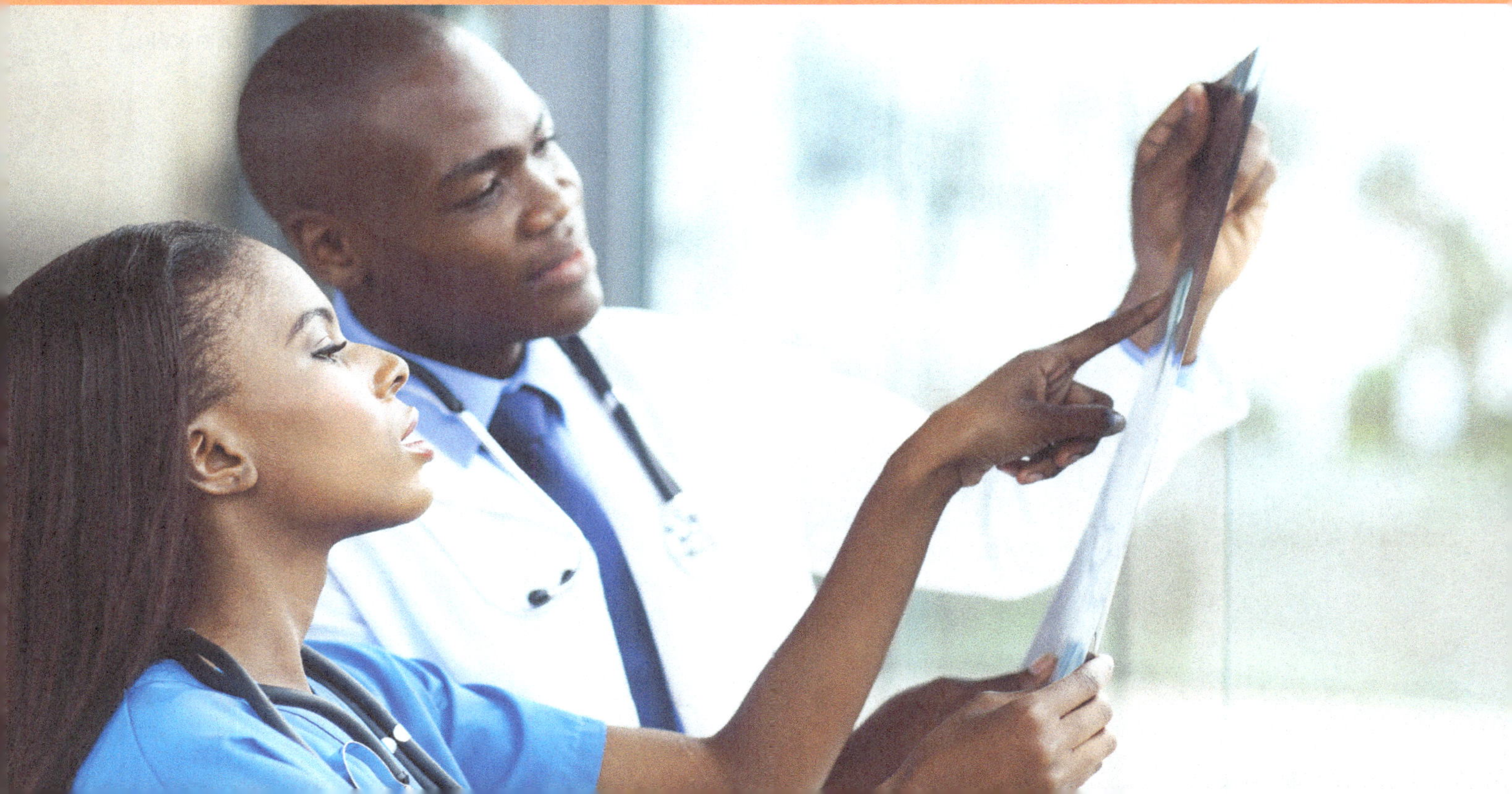

Adult endocrinology role play (English-Spanish)

DOCTOR: Buenas días Paulina. Yo estoy el doctor Johnson. Estoy un doctor de resident.

PATIENT: Hola, doctor.

HUSBAND: Buenas tardes.

DOCTOR: So, how have you been?

PATIENT: Bien, he estado bien.

DOCTOR: ¿Tu tienes alguna problema since pasado vez que we saw you here? ¿Tienes dolor de cabeza still?

PATIENT: Siempre tengo dolores de cabeza, pero no son tan severos como antes.

DOCTOR: How frequent are they, and how long do they last?

PATIENT: Pues, antes duraban más tiempo, como cuatro o cinco días. Ahora solamente duran como uno o dos días y son cada 15 días, no cada 8 días como antes.

DOCTOR: ¿Y tú tomas la misma medicina que tú were taking before?

PATIENT: Si, aquí las traigo. Son éstas dos.

DOCTOR: And are you taking them the same way, uno de éstos en la mañana y uno otro en la noche y dos de un otro of these en la mañana?

PATIENT: Sí.

DOCTOR: So then these are working out?

PATIENT: Pues, siempre me duele la cabeza, pero no como antes. Pero yo me siento mucho mejor que antes de comenzar el tratamiento. Pero no me he podido embarazar.

DOCTOR: *(Doctor responds without waiting for the interpretation.)* Well, that's good. How's your mood been?

HUSBAND: Está muy bien.

PATIENT: Diría que estoy mejor que nunca, feliz, con mucha energía.

DOCTOR: Good. And you're eating?

PATIENT: Ei! ¿Cómo no? Estoy subiendo de peso.

DOCTOR: All right, so there's no problem with your appetite. How has your menstruation been? Are your periods regular?

PATIENT: Pues, acaba de terminar. Los primeros días, como...Cuatro días era apenas una manchita y como color cafecito. Después se me vino normal, cinco días fuertes, o sea normales. Pero no entiendo porqué no me embarazo.

DOCTOR: *(Doctor doesn't allow the interpreter to interpret and puts his hand up to her.)* That's OK, I'm pretty sure I got it. *(turns to the patient and her husband)* Good, good. That's fine. Your period's fine. Now, the last time you were here, you said you were interested in getting pregnant. Are you still thinking about that? Are you still working on trying to get pregnant?

HUSBAND: *(a little irritated)* Sí, como dijo ella, por eso venimos, es que queremos información acerca de eso.

PATIENT: No entendemos porqué me está tomando tanto tiempo embarazarme.

HUSBAND: ¿Y la medicina podría dañar al bebé? ¿La tiene que seguir tomando?

DOCTOR: OK. Hold on. First of all, you're doing very well and the tumor is shrinking.

PATIENT: Entonces se está encogiendo, estoy mejorando?

DOCTOR: Yes. Now, some patients later need to undergo surgery, but sometimes they don't. Also, some people need to take this medicine forever, and others just a few years. It is all right for you to get pregnant. This medicine won't hurt, but we need to know when you are pregnant so we can take care of you properly and make any changes if necessary.

PATIENT: Oh, qué bien. ¿Pero por qué me está tomando tanto tiempo?

DOCTOR: Well, here's the situation. The medicine is working for the tumor, which is what we want, but it affects the pituitary gland in such a way that it causes a decrease in production of the hormone that causes you to ovulate, so this is why you're having so much trouble getting pregnant. But I believe there's something we can do about that. I'm going to talk to my attending. He'll probably want to come back and have a look at you, and then he'll also talk to you about what we can do next.[35]

35 Consulting with another physician often takes a long time. What can an interpreter do when she is under time constraints?

Adult endocrinology clinic role play (English only)

It is afternoon. This doctor is mixing up English and the patient's other language, often in the same sentence. Words in italics in this dialogue are those that the doctor attempts to say in the second language, leaving other (non-italics) in English. Interpret them as they are and be sure to insert many errors into the second language. Sometimes what the doctor says should sound like nonsense to the patient!

DOCTOR: *Good morning*, Paulina. *I am being the* doctor Johnson. *I am in the moment a doctor of* resident.[36]

PATIENT: Hi, doctor.

HUSBAND: Good afternoon.

DOCTOR: So, how have you been?

PATIENT: Good, I've been good.

DOCTOR: *You has some priblem from the time last that* we saw you here? *You has headache* still?

PATIENT: I still have headaches, but they aren't as severe as before.

DOCTOR: How frequent are they, and how long do they last?

PATIENT: Well, before they lasted longer, about four or five days. Now they only last one or two days. And it's every 15 days, not every 8 days like before.

DOCTOR: *And you the same medicine took that you* were taking before?

PATIENT: Yes, here they are. These two.

DOCTOR: And are you taking them the same way, *one of these in morning and one other in night, and two of one other* of these in *one morning*?

PATIENT: Yes.

DOCTOR: So then these are working out?

PATIENT: Well, I always have headaches, but not like before. But I feel a lot better than before starting the treatment. But I haven't been able to get pregnant.

DOCTOR: *(Doctor responds without waiting for the interpretation.)* Well, that's good. How's your mood been?

[36] Should the interpreter correct and/or interpret any of these sentences? How would correcting and/or interpreting them affect the rest of this session?

HUSBAND: It's fine.

PATIENT: I'd say I'm happier than ever, happy, with a lot of energy.

DOCTOR: Good. And you're eating?

PATIENT: Yes, and how! I'm gaining weight.

DOCTOR: All right, so there's no problem with your appetite. How has your menstruation been? Are your periods regular?

PATIENT: Well, I just finished. The first days, like, four days were just barely a spot, and coffee-colored. After that it came normally, five days of heavy bleeding, in other words, normal. But I don't understand why I haven't been able to get pregnant.

DOCTOR: *(Doctor doesn't allow the interpreter to interpret and puts his hand up to her.)* That's OK, I'm pretty sure I got it. *(turns to the patient and her husband)* Good, good. That's fine. Your period's fine. Now, the last time you were here, you said you were interested in getting pregnant. Are you still thinking about that? Are you still working on trying to get pregnant?

HUSBAND: *(a little irritated)* Yes, like she said, that's why we came here, we are here to get information about that.

PATIENT: We don't understand why it's taking so much time to get pregnant.

HUSBAND: And could the medicine hurt the baby? Does she have to keep taking it?

DOCTOR: OK. Hold on. First of all, you're doing very well and the tumor is shrinking.

PATIENT: So then it's shrinking, I'm getting better?

DOCTOR: Yes. Now, some patients later need to undergo surgery, but sometimes they don't. Also, some people need to take this medicine forever, and others just a few years. It is all right for you to get pregnant. This medicine won't hurt, but we need to know when you are pregnant so we can take care of you properly, and make any changes if necessary.

PATIENT: Oh, that's great. But why is it taking so long?

DOCTOR: Well, here's the situation. The medicine is working for the tumor, which is what we want, but it affects the pituitary gland in such a way that it causes a decrease in production of the hormone that causes you to ovulate, so this is why you're having so much trouble getting pregnant. But I believe there's something we can do about that. I'm going to talk to my attending. He'll probably want to come back and have a look at you, and then he'll also talk to you about what we can do next.[37]

---

37 Consulting with another physician often takes a long time. What can an interpreter do when she is under time constraints?

Get the gist?

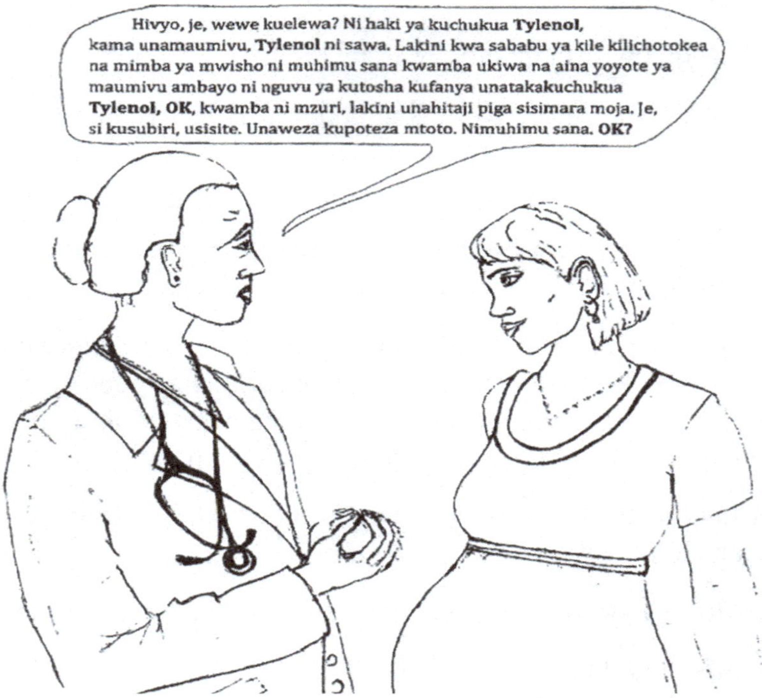
Hivyo, je, wewe kuelewa? Ni haki ya kuchukua **Tylenol**, kama unamaumivu, **Tylenol** ni sawa. Lakini kwa sababu ya kile kilichotokea na mimba ya mwisho ni muhimu sana kwamba ukiwa na aina yoyote ya maumivu ambayo ni nguvu ya kutosha kufanya unatakakuchukua **Tylenol, OK**, kwamba ni mzuri, lakini unahitaji piga sisimara moja. Je, si kusubiri, usisite. Unaweza kupoteza mtoto. Nimuhimu sana. **OK?**

Guess what message is being conveyed here by the doctor. Write it in the space below what you think the doctor is saying. (If you are a Kiswahili speaker, please don't tell anyone in your class or group.)

Turn the page for a translation.

Translation

> "So, do you understand? It is all right to take Tylenol if you have pain. Tylenol is OK. **But because of what happened with your last pregnancy, it is extremely important that if you have any kind of pain that is strong enough to make you want to take Tylenol,** OK, that's fine, but **you need to call us immediately. Don't wait, don't hesitate. You could lose the baby.** It's very important, OK?"

Comprehension is key to patient adherence!
Comprehension is key to health outcomes!
Comprehension is key to patient safety!
Comprehension saves lives!

What's important to know about this chapter?

Overview

Endocrinology is the medical specialty that deals with the endocrine system. This system includes glands in different parts of the body that produce hormones influencing many organs and functions in the body. For example, they influence development, growth, organ and tissue function, sleep, mood, sexual libido, secondary sexual characteristics, movement, reproduction, thirst, sweat, urination and metabolism.

People with diabetes or thyroid conditions often see endocrinologists. In this dialogue, the patient is taking medicine to shrink a benign tumor in the pituitary gland. Her treatment is causing a reduction in levels of hormones that affect fertility and conception. The patient is having difficulty becoming pregnant. Vocabulary regarding menstruation and conception are part of the dialogue.

Calling time

When is a week seven days? When is it eight days? In U.S. English, a week is seven days. A little farther south, a week can refer to eight days. In different languages, we can say "a week" differently. If, for example, it's Thursday, a week away in U.S. English can be "in a week" or "next Thursday" but not "in eight days," as it could be in Spanish and some other languages. "In 15 days" (two weeks away) in one language can mean "in 15 days" in English, but it can also mean "in 14 days," "in two weeks," "in two Thursdays," or "the Thursday after next." In the United States, many native speakers don't even know what a "fortnight" is (two weeks).

In some places, people use calendars different from the U.S. calendar, which is the Gregorian calendar (also called the Western calendar and the Christian calendar). For example, if you ever translate an Ethiopian birth certificate, beware: due to the differences between the Western and Ethiopian calendars, your translation could make that person sound several years older than is really the case. The year in an Islamic calendar might be about 622 years different from the Western calendar!

Are there other differences in the way people around the world refer to periods such as a week, a month or the day of rest? For example, on what day does a week generally start? Does a day begin at sunrise? Or at the disappearance of the last star?

Time constraints

Depending on work conditions and policies, an interpreter might have to leave an appointment before it is over. It can be hard to do so if you've already sensed communication problems. In this dialogue, the provider has already missed important health information by not working effectively with the interpreter. Now the provider is stepping out to consult a senior physician right when the interpreter has to leave.

If you are under time constraints, announce at the beginning of the session what time you have to leave. If that time arrives, is there a coordinator or dispatcher you can ask for an extension or a replacement? Is there telephone or video interpreting available? If you have to leave early and you are uncomfortable doing so, try to provide options. Offering two or three options is ideal.

In dire circumstances, weigh the consequences for everyone involved if you leave (including the consequences for you), and then make your decision to stay or go.

Missed information by provider

Sometimes health providers will ask questions more than once and as the interpreter, trained to pay close attention, you remember the answer. In some cases the repetition is intentional, important and necessary. Depending on circumstances, however, when the same question is asked repeatedly, it can be irritating and feel disrespectful and offensive to patients. It can negatively impact trust and confidence in the care, and it can also feel dismissive of the interpreter's careful, professional efforts to be as accurate with the interpreting as possible. It can be tempting (sometimes extremely tempting!) to answer the question without reinterpreting it, especially the third time around, but, of course, doing so is unacceptable.

If you are interpreting for a series of providers (doctor, nurse, coordinator, social worker, financial counselor on the same day for the same patient), depending on the degree of duplication and information sharing, you can find yourself interpreting the same question and the same answer many times.

In this dialogue, the doctor has twice missed the patient's concern about not being able to get pregnant. He believes that he understands the patient's language when he does not. He even stops the interpreter from doing her job. That behavior has an impact. It leads to tension and frustration for the patient, her spouse and the interpreter. It seems to undermine the trust of the patient and her spouse in the doctor. What are some other possible consequences? What should the interpreter do?

Patients speaking up

In the dialogue, the spouse is becoming annoyed. Will he say anything? There are many reasons why, in general, patients hesitate to speak up when something is awry. Perhaps they can't understand the provider's broken language or become irritated about not being listened to. Perhaps they are being asked a question for the third or fourth time. Maybe they would feel more comfortable with an interpreter but are hesitant to ask. Some of the reasons may be social hierarchies in country of origin, lack of education, poverty and entitlement, immigration status and/or inability to speak or read the language of service. It may feel intimidating to challenge or complain about a person when you depend on that person for care.

In this dialogue, we see a formally educated, professional patient and spouse, yet still, they might not speak up. If a patient does speak up, it is sometimes in the form of a private comment to the interpreter because the patient does not want to complain to the provider. Transparency is important, however: it is important to interpret these comments to the provider.

Providers who practice medicine in a second language

From the beginning of the role play, the interpreter is faced with a challenging situation; in reality, the provider who wants to speak the patient's language when the provider is not qualified to do so is creating a potentially dangerous situation with many possible avenues for things to go wrong and be misunderstood. When a physician wants to practice his second language skills in the patient appointment, he is practicing medicine in a second language. Think about it.

Why do they do it?

Many providers use a language they don't speak proficiently to treat patients because they have a sincere desire to foster a warm patient-provider rapport. Often, such providers want to show a patient their sincere interest and appreciation of culture or the provider values the patient as a person. It may be that some providers want to learn about another culture or language (though sacrificing the patient's quality of care is a poor trade-off!) or they identify with the patient's national heritage. Some may take offense at being told they should be tested for language proficiency before providing care in another language because they assume their language skills are much better than they are. "Convenience" might be a factor in some situations. Being uncomfortable with having an interpreter present could be another.

Despite the proven benefits of having trained medical interpreters, many providers prefer to do without them. The reasons for this preference are complex (Reiss-Končar, 2010). For further reading about possible motivations (since understanding them is important for getting to solutions), see Appendix 2.5, "Why Do They Wing It?"

Outcomes

The implications for medical errors are serious. As discussed in previous chapters, when it comes to health outcomes, patient participation, patient satisfaction and reducing health inequities based on language, one thing is clear: interpreters are often necessary.

Handling mixed-up language

What are some ways that an interpreter can manage a situation where a doctor is speaking more than one language, and speaking the one he knows less well with many mistakes? There are various options.

One solution is for the interpreter to listen to the English portion of the message and the incorrect other language, then render a comprehensible Spanish interpretation of the whole segment.

This would certainly be better than having the interpreter interpret from source to target language, e.g., "Do you have a problem *geroztik* last time that *ikusi dugu hemen*? Do you *oraindik* have a headache?" That would clearly be hard for the patient to understand.

What else might an interpreter do to handle the situation? Would you ask the provider to speak only in English? If so, what would you say? How might you, as an interpreter, find some other way to address the situation with the provider—and what arguments would you use?

Professional considerations

When a provider insists on using a nonproficient language and makes mistakes, will an interpreter say anything? Perhaps not. It can be difficult to tell a doctor that he is mistaken. Challenging a physician's language skills can feel as if the interpreter is challenging his medical expertise. These attitudes might explain why, in one study, 42 percent of the errors committed by clinicians in the presence of interpreters went uncorrected (Flores et al., 2003).

A medical interpreter would need to speak up if patient safety is at risk. But the ethical requirement to do so (discussed later in this book) doesn't make it easy to challenge authority. The fact that the interpreter and patient usually have a lower socioeconomic status or less education than the provider shouldn't matter. But it does.

Practicing what to say and how to say can help. So you might want to practice suggesting that a provider speak only English to help you feel more comfortable. Try practicing in front of a mirror.

Formal vs. informal register

Many doctors, when using a language other than English, use the informal rather than the formal register (for example, tú vs. usted) with patients of all ages and socioeconomic backgrounds, even if using the familiar form can be rude.

Modern standard English usually only has one form of the second person singular (you), so native English speakers do not always understand the difference between formal and informal pronouns and speech. This can help explain why some native English-speaking health professionals don't use the formal style of address with patients when the providers try to speak the patient's language.

However, the fact is that many doctors address their native English-speaking patients by first name while expecting that their patients will address the providers as Dr. So-and-So. This informality of providers reveals important attitudes that can offend some native speakers of English.

Yet it is also true that a branch of linguistics explores the reasons why English has no formal register for addressing people. In the United States, the lack of a formal mode of address might be related to reaching for "the American dream" and breaking down barriers between social classes. Most other languages are different: they have pronouns and verb forms to address someone who is older, has more authority or is unfamiliar, or to show respect. Some languages, such as Japanese, have other complex ways of addressing a person's social status.

If a provider insists on speaking in the patient's language and uses a mode of address that seems rude (due to ignorance of the language), should the interpreter use the formal style of speech for politeness, or just leave things as they are said? What are the doctor's intentions? Perhaps they can guide your decision.

For example, if a practitioner insists on using the patient's language, you might want to mention, as the interpreter, that it is inappropriate in the patient's language for a provider to use the informal pronoun with the patient (but you would have to report this intervention for the patient).

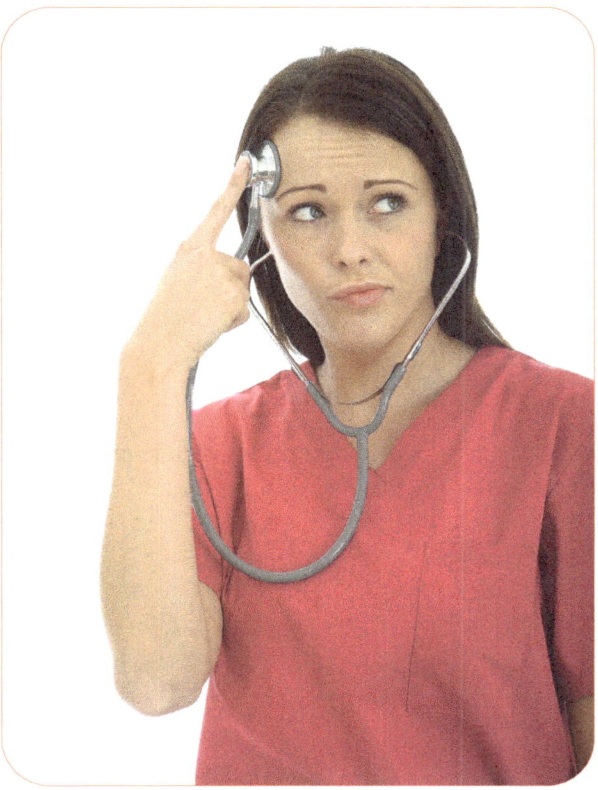

When in doubt, a blogger, Meghan, gives some handy if perhaps controversial advice:

> You can seriously offend people by addressing them informally but you will offend no one if you address them formally. I have not encountered a single language save English that forgoes formal/informal. I know it is the English state-of-mind to be informal with everyone...but not every culture is that low-key. Be respectful of the culture whose language you are learning.[38]

An interpreter sometimes has to use judgment in order to handle these delicate situations. Try to see if a patient is appreciative of the provider's efforts and takes no offense at mistakes—or perhaps feels upset, hurt or offended. Remember too that many patients are already at a social disadvantage. They may be undocumented or illiterate in their own language. They may come from a region where providers (especially doctors) are highly respected and not to be questioned.

Mistakes in the patient's language can increase inequity and unfairness.

Provider proficiency testing

Consider this situation: An interpreter goes to an OB/GYN high-risk clinic for women with histories of difficult pregnancies. The patient is at 30 weeks in this pregnancy and has thyroid problems and diabetes. She lost her previous pregnancy at an early stage and is nervous about this one. The doctor speaks some of the patient's language and wants to use it in the encounter. The doctor has even passed a bilingual provider proficiency test with an 80 percent rating, but her command of certain grammatical tenses isn't complete:

38 Retrieved from https://averagelinguaphile.wordpress.com/2012/06/28/formal-vs-informal-speech/

Here's what the doctor wants to say.

> *If you **were going to lose** this baby, you **would have lost it** by now.*

Here's what the doctor says instead.

> *If you **lose** this baby, you **lose** it now.*

Put yourself in the mother's position. Describe how you might feel on hearing these different sentences.

In this real-life scenario, the provider saw the look of panic on the mother's face and realized she couldn't really express herself. She asked for the interpreter to say what she *really* meant, but the patient was briefly frightened.

Consider this situation

A doctor at a top teaching university passes a bilingual proficiency test with an 80 percent score and is permitted to provide services in that language. The doctor does so with the family of a child undergoing serious, life-threatening treatment for a cancerous brain tumor. However, despite his language proficiency score in the language, he doesn't have complete command of it.

Here's what the doctor *wants* to say:

> **Your child is worse.**

Here's what the doctor *says*:

> **Your child's condition is progressing.**

Here's what the family *hears*:

> **Your child's condition is improving.**

In this context, to "progress" in English means to worsen; in the other language it means to improve. When will this misunderstanding be fixed? By the time the parents learn the truth, how will they feel? What are the human costs of such a misunderstanding?

Provider proficiency testing and plan B

If an interpreter realizes that miscommunication is having a negative impact on the quality of care, she needs to say something. She can ask the provider for a word outside the room and explain what she is seeing. She can politely and firmly address the situation in the room, making sure to introduce herself, "As the interpreter, I would like to let you know that I am concerned about an apparent miscommunication about..." or, "The interpreter is concerned about a possible miscommunication regarding..." If you explain that your concern is for assuring complete and accurate understanding, participants may be receptive.

Sometimes situations like this can get serious, especially when some or all parties assume they understand each other when they do not. If you have intervened but the parties will not address a serious misunderstanding, you might have to excuse yourself or state why you feel you must do so. If the misunderstandings could lead to medical error or health risks, it is important that the interpreter not be blamed for inaccurate interpreting when he or she has done everything possible to support clear communication.

Be transparent

Each and every time you intervene, make sure that whatever you tell one party you communicate to the other. Transparency is not only a standard of practice but an ethical requirement under accuracy.

Transparency applies not only to interpreting what all the other parties say or sign. It also applies to whatever *you* say or sign when you speak up as the interpreter.

Ethics and standards: Reflect and practice

Goal 5: Cultural awareness

Translation and paraphrasing

1. Look at the two NCIHC standards of practice related to cultural awareness (Standards 14-15, NCIHC, 2005, p. 7). Working individually, *paraphrase* the objective, its related ethical principle and the two standards.
2. Working individually, *translate* that same text into your other working language(s) or interpret them into sign language.
3. Find a partner or partners. Compare, discuss and modify your translations and paraphrasing until you are satisfied with your final products as a group.
4. If you can, pick a group representative and share your final versions with other groups that share your working languages. Compare and discuss your differences.

Suggested reading

Bancroft, M.A. (2015). Strategic mediation. In M. A. Bancroft (Ed.), *The Community Interpreter®: An International Textbook* (pp. 191-270). Columbia, Maryland: Culture & Language Press.

Consider and discuss

"Another Western aid group, trying to improve the hygiene and health of Afghan women, issued them bars of soap—nearly causing a riot. In Afghanistan, washing with soap is often associated with post coital activity, so the group was thought to be implying that the women were promiscuous."

—Kristof and WuDunn (2009, p. 162)

"A clinician's knowledge can be made useless in the face of a communication or cultural barrier and all of the scientific acumen in the world won't suffice without cultural competence."

—Ochoa, Evans and Kaiser (2003)

1. **Standard 14** A quiet, reserved Indigenous Mexican (whose primary language is Mixteco, not Spanish) is the parent of a pediatric patient. This parent tends not to make much eye contact during discussions with health providers. A social worker and several nurses repeatedly ask if the parent is "slow" or developmentally challenged, and about the parent's "flat" emotional demeanor. What might be going on from a social or cultural perspective? How might an interpreter educate or talk about this topic with providers?
2. **Standard 14** The parent mentions that the child was given corn silk tea. Is it your job to know that corn silk tea is sometimes given to children to prevent bedwetting? Or the cultural history of its use? If you do know, should you mention this fact to the provider? Or have the provider ask the reason for using corn silk tea (if the nurses, in this case, do not ask)? Where do the cultural knowledge responsibilities of a medical interpreter begin and end, and what should the interpreter do with that knowledge?
3. **Standard 15** During that session, the interpreter interrupts to tell the social worker and the nurses, "No, she's not developmentally challenged. In her culture, you just don't make eye contact with professionals. It's seen as disrespectful. She's doing what is considered respectful in her culture." Then she turns to the parent and says, "I just clarified something with the social worker and nurses." What do you think of this interpreter's behavior? Was it transparent? Could

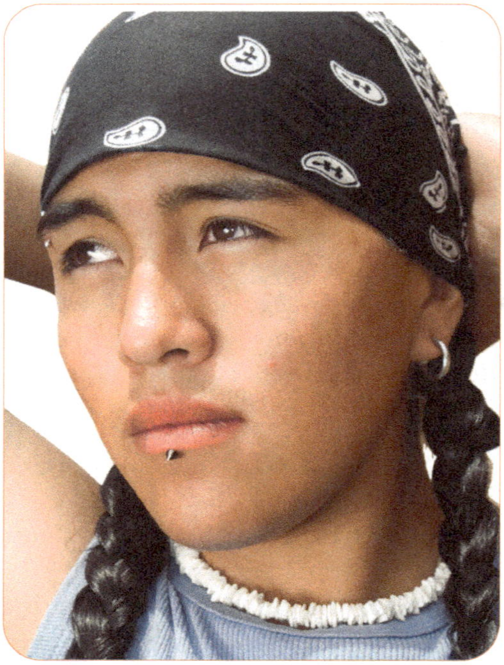

you handle this situation differently? What are the dangers of sharing information that suggests everyone in a certain culture is the same? How might the social worker and nurses view Indigenous patients after this interpreter's speech? (Remember that many Indigenous patients *are* professionals!)

4. **Standard 15** While speaking with this parent, the social worker contorts her body and neck in an effort to force eye contact. On what assumptions about the significance of eye contact is the social worker acting? What is the social worker's goal for behavior modification and for whom? Is this appropriate? How might the social worker modify her own behavior or expectations?

Interpreters, like anyone, can learn how to say a word in another language. But what does that word *mean*, or rather, what meaning does it have? Sometimes, there is tremendous cultural complexity in a single word. No provider and no interpreter can ever be proficient in all cultures, but sharpening one's sensibilities may allow for a way to sense what one doesn't know. As an interpreter, you can then help guide the provider or patient (or parent), if that is helpful, *to ask helpful questions.*

Consider the following scenarios.

Scenario 1: An interpreter conveys to a patient that the doctor will be ordering morphine to help control pain. The patient becomes extremely upset and anxious and bursts into tears. While the interpreter may convey the words, what message might be conveyed that health providers may not be aware of? Under what circumstances is morphine administered in other parts of the Americas or of the world? If the patient fears she or he is dying, and the interpreter is aware that the patient might have this fear, what should the interpreter do?

a. Nothing. Simply continue to interpret.
b. Tell the provider the patient might be afraid of dying.
c. Suggest that the provider ask what morphine is used for in the patient's country.
d. Explain the underlying cultural issues.
e. Something else (specify an appropriate action).

Scenario 2: A mother whose baby has severe birth defects comments that while she was pregnant, she went out at night during a lunar eclipse. The doctor responds with a snort and continues the conversation with questions about something else. What cultural concept might the mother be trying to convey that is not apparent without cultural familiarity? And if so, what should the interpreter do about it?

a. Explain what fears a pregnant woman might have about a lunar eclipse in the patient's country.
b. Tell the provider the patient is afraid her baby's birth defects are the mother's fault.
c. Suggest that the provider ask why she is concerned about the lunar eclipse she saw.
d. Simply continue to interpret.
e. Something else (specify an appropriate action).

Scenario 3: A child with a debilitating neurological condition is repeatedly hospitalized with respiratory distress, which develops into pneumonia and requires intubation. Usually the child recovers from the acute illness but not the underlying, incurable condition. Each episode is worse, longer and more damaging to the child's health and well-being. Eventually painful procedures will be required to sustain life after the child stops breathing (chest compressions that can break ribs). Practitioners repeatedly approach the parents about the subject of a do-not-resuscitate (DNR) order. The child's parents understand but will not sign it, and ask the "doctors who know best" to decide. Doctors will not make this decision for the parents, and this cycle repeats itself each time the child gets ill and someone calls 911. What cultural factors might have led to this situation? If the interpreter has an idea what they might be, what should the interpreter do?

a. Tell the parents about patient autonomy, DNRs and how end-of-life care takes place in U.S. hospitals.
b. Report the doctors for lack of cultural sensitivity.
c. Suggest that the provider make the decision for the parents.
d. Request that a social or hospice worker explain to parents the importance of DNRs and end-of-life care and how they can help support their child.
e. Simply continue to interpret.
f. Something else (specify an appropriate action).

Across many disciplines, efforts to rethink cultural awareness are taking place. Timely efforts to rethink cultural competency and its integration into training are encouraging.

1. Write down a definition for and differences between each of the following terms: **cultural competence, cultural appropriateness, cultural responsiveness, cultural humility**. A quick search on the Internet can be helpful.

2. Which of these terms are you most comfortable with and why? Is there another term you would prefer? Explain.

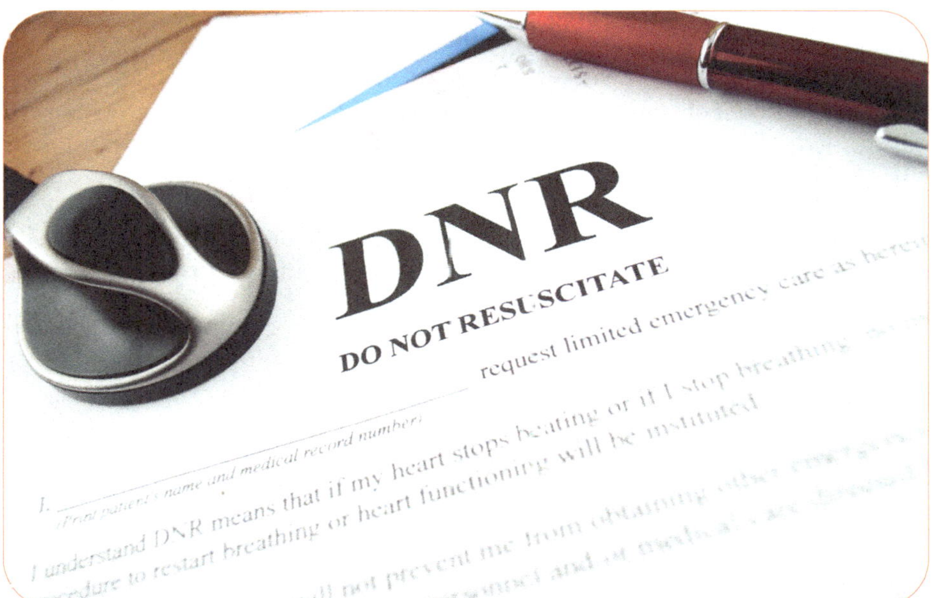

Occupational therapy for interpreters

EXERCISES FOR THE TONGUE, HEART AND MIND

Intention, nuance, variety, culture

Most healthcare providers try hard to communicate with their patients. Often, their efforts fall short. This can sometimes be true for patients who share the same language as the provider. However, clear communication is almost always a problem if a qualified interpreter is needed but not present.

Think about the richness of language. In the first moments of a conversation, you can often guess with fair accuracy the other person's age, gender, social class, educational level and where that person comes from. What else can you guess about that person? The next time you stand in line for a movie or at an automated teller machine (ATM), listen to the conversations and make a mental list of what you think you know about the speaker.

Of course, you could be wrong. Languages express cultural, psychological, emotional, social, spiritual and economic complexity. In each message, there are many layers to "interpret."

A professionally trained interpreter can help the health practitioner understand certain information in the "linguistic envelope" and in the social cues and context that are obvious to the interpreter—but not to the provider. A competent interpreter can help reduce misunderstandings and communication errors that could have an impact on health outcomes.

The professionally trained interpreter will often understand what a practitioner wants to say and how to say it. When she can't do so without changing the provider's message, at least she usually knows there is a problem. That awareness is *critical*. For at that point the interpreter can intervene to request a clarification of what was meant instead of speaking for the provider or patient or taking over anyone's role.

Often, without an interpreter, both providers and patients can get confused. Small mistakes can lead to bigger ones and serious consequences. Such mistakes and miscommunications can affect the patient's understanding, diagnosis, treatment plan and adherence to the plan.

Anything less than clear and complete communication can also alter the patient-provider relationship that is so critical to effective healthcare and beneficial outcomes.

In the table on the next page are 17 examples of potential areas of misunderstanding among patients from around the globe. Mark each example with an indicator of the factor(s) at play that can influence communication and understanding.

(L) Language
(C) Culture
(S) Social class
(E) Educational attainment

Try to add items to the list based on your knowledge and life experience.

1		A patient doesn't understand an explanation of a genetic disorder; he's been a farm worker since the age of eight, had no schooling after second grade and never learned about chromosomes, genes, cells or DNA.
2		A recently emigrated, well-educated dentist from an industrializing nation understands the risks of surgery presented by the provider in the language used in medical research.
3		A nonliterate transplant patient with a complicated drug regimen needs a color-coded system for managing his medications.
4		A former nursing student from an agricultural nation does not have the habit of taking a single penicillin tablet for a sore throat, although most people from her small, rural hometown do.
5		A Native American/Indian/Indigenous/First Nation patient from a neighboring country, who has no proficiency in the provider's language and limited proficiency in the interpreter's language, is unfamiliar with the concept of a vascular system. He does not know what a "lung" is in his native language.
6		A patient is taking the antidepressants prescribed for her but is taking them only on her "bad days." She did not understand the explanation about a waiting period of about three weeks on a full dosage before her medication is likely to take effect.
7		A neurologist comments to a Peruvian patient that he loves Peruvian food, especially *tortillas.* (Tortillas, unleavened corn cakes, are not commonly eaten in Perú.)
8		A dietician works with parents of a child who isn't gaining weight. He eats small corn *tortillas*, typical to his country. The dietician assumes a tortilla is a large wheat (white) *tortilla* with a specific number of calories, fiber and specific nutrients.
9		A doctor assumes that his patient is tired because she complains about *fatiga* and her interpreter reports she has "fatigue." However, the patient means that she has asthma and she is quite well-informed about her condition.
10		A patient sometimes exhibits seemingly schizophrenic behavior, including depositing copper pennies and alcoholic beverages in corners of the room and singing or praying to spirits.
11		Giving a mother sedatives when she screams after her brain-dead child stops breathing would violate her culturally appropriate grieving process.
12		A mother doesn't "discipline" her child in the hospital. The child runs, laughs and plays "inappropriately" there. Hospital staff members become irritated with the mother, who strongly believes, as she was taught and according to her minority culture in her country of origin, that children under two should never be spoken to harshly or allowed to cry.
13		The term "Latino" is an accepted but erroneous description applied to more than 100,000 *non-Spanish-speaking* Mexican nationals presently living in California and Oregon.
14		A physician with a little bit of Spanish tries to explain to a mother that her newborn will have a gastric feeding tube surgically placed into his abdomen, secured by a balloon. Should the doctor say *popa, vejiga* or *globo* (regional alternatives for balloon)? He can't decide so he points to a party balloon. The mother stares at him in shock.
15		*Bomba*: bomb or pump in Spanish. A Spanish-speaking immigrant keeps asking for a "*pompa,*" a term that the interpreter cannot find in a dictionary.
16		A female doctor offers her left hand to shake when she meets a patient, who retracts his hand in alarm.
17		A patient lives in crowded substandard housing and is refusing to eat. He is unable to prepare food washed in the same sink where roommates bathe, brush teeth, etc.

Create your own list of examples like the ones above and share it with interpreters, especially those who speak or sign your working languages.

Medical terminology: The endocrine system

Below you will find anatomical drawings relevant to the content of this chapter. Follow the instructions found at the end of Chapter 1 to study the terminology in this section.

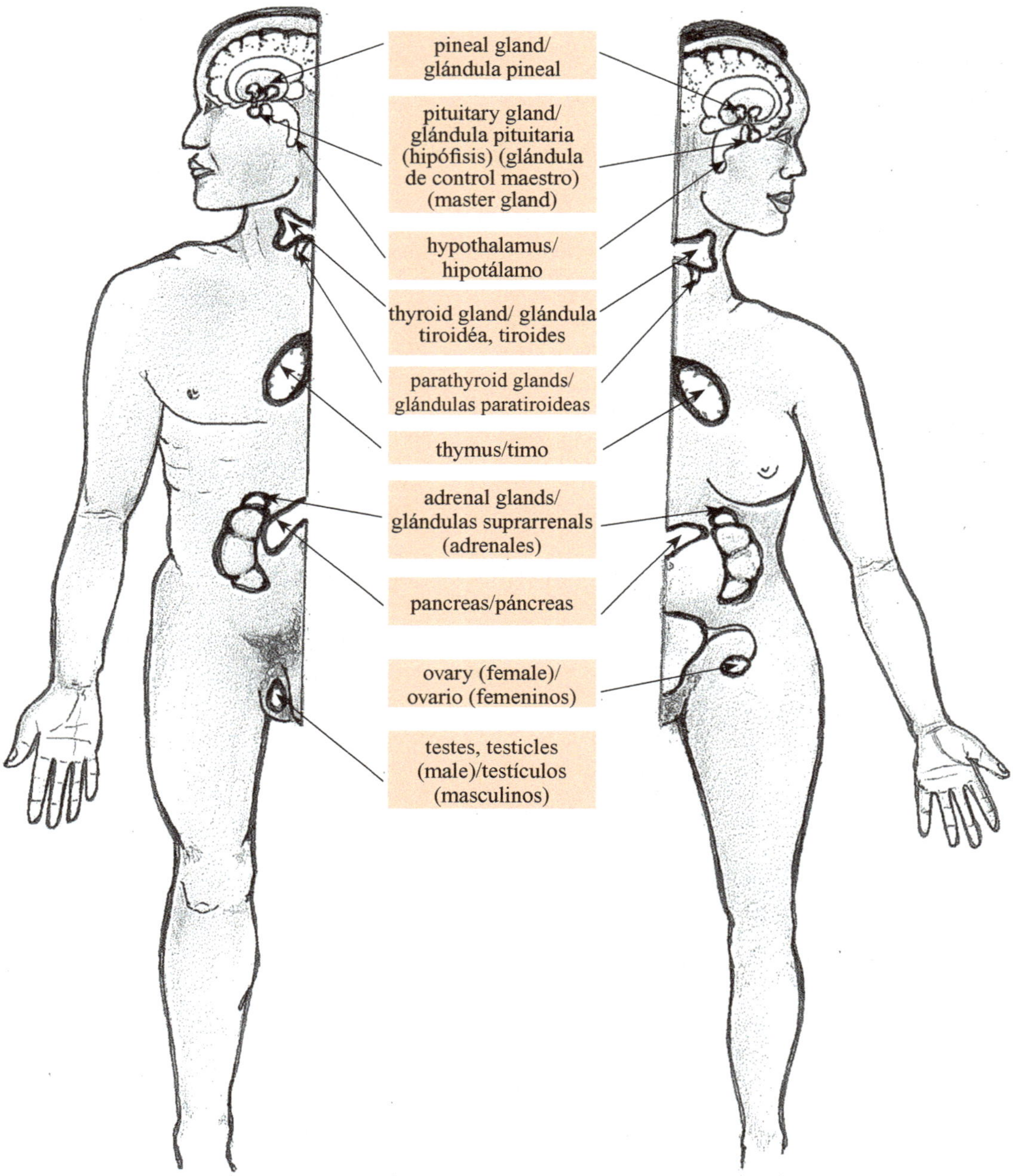

Figure 5-A: The endocrine system (English and Spanish)

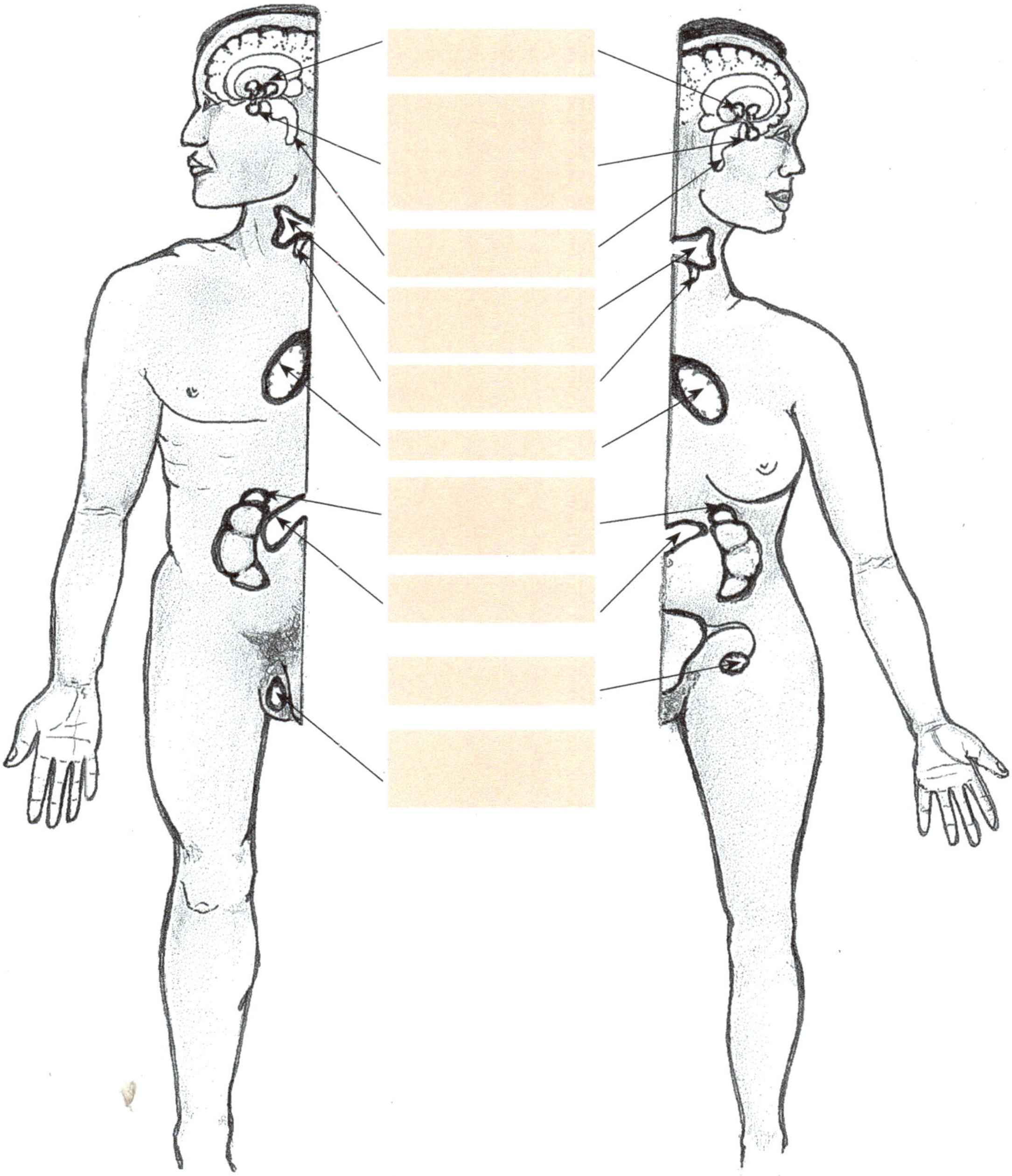

Figure 5-B: The endocrine system (blank labels)

Medical terminology list

The endocrine system

VOCABULARY FOR GRAPHIC—IN ENGLISH	VOCABULARY FOR GRAPHIC—IN SPANISH	ANY OTHER LANGUAGE
Adrenal glands	Glándulas suprarrenals (adrenales)	
Hypothalamus	Hipotálamo	
Kidneys	Riñones	
Ovary (female)	Ovarios (femeninos)	
Pancreas	Páncreas	
Parathyroid glands	Glándulas paratiroideas	
Pineal gland	Glándula pineal	
Pituitary gland (master gland)	Glándula pitutitaria (hipófisis) (glándula de control maestro)	
Testes, testicles (male)	Testículos (masculinos)	
Thymus	Timo	
Thyroid gland	Glándula tiroidéa, tiroides	

Neurology 6

Advisory

This chapter involves some material about endocrine and hormonal conditions, libido, brain tumors, cancer and treatment options.

The patient is a 20-year-old man who appears much younger. He is at an appointment in an endocrinology clinic. He has been coming to this clinic for treatment of a tumor in his pituitary gland for several months. It is early December and he seems to be in low spirits.

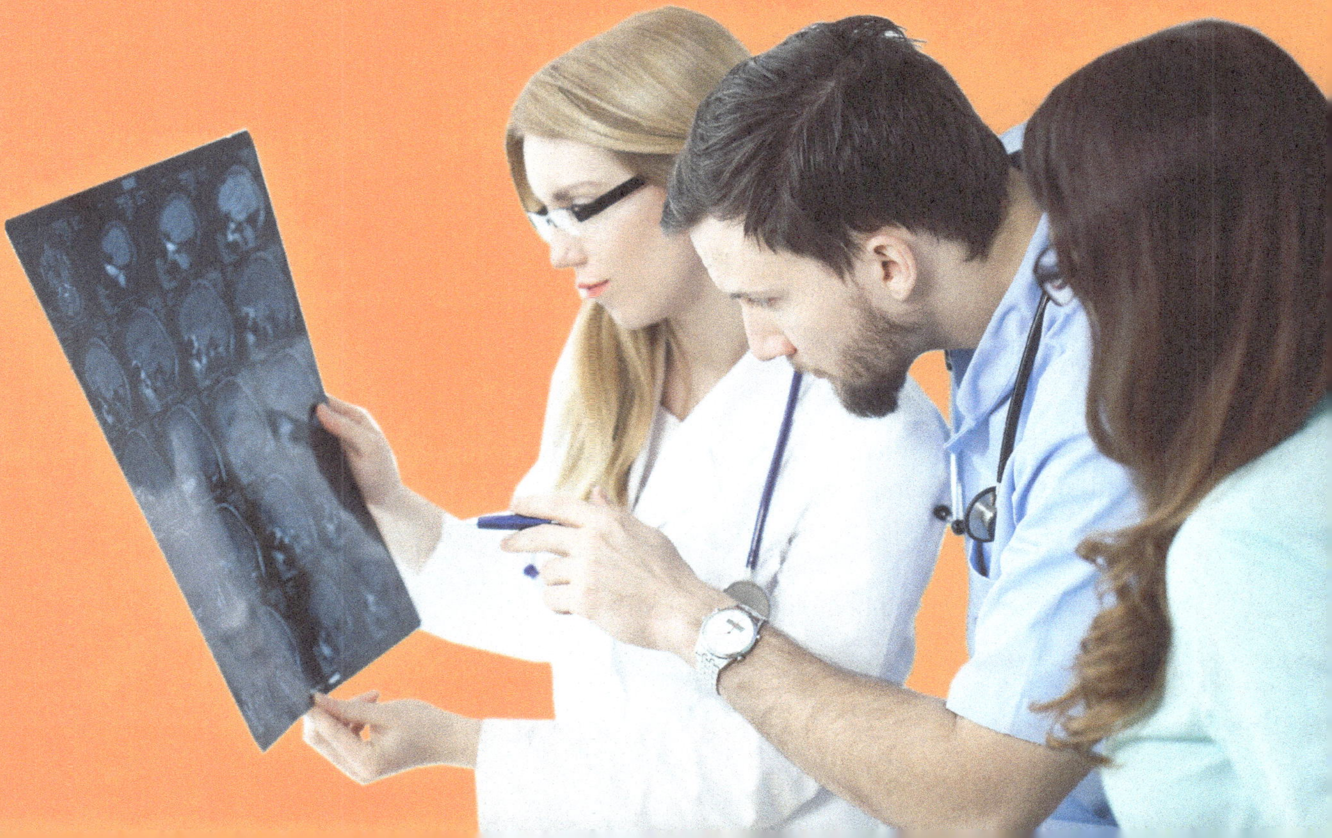

Brain tumor role play (English-Spanish)

Note: *Some of the patient's grammar and syntax reflect a regional variety of Spanish spoken by people in southeastern México.*

PART 1

DOCTOR: Hello, Doroteo, I'm so sorry I'm late. I got really backed up. I know you've been waiting. *(to the interpreter)* Thank you for waiting.

PATIENT: No hay problema.

DOCTOR: So, Doroteo, how have you been feeling?

PATIENT: *(replies despondently)* Pues, algo bien.

DOCTOR: Have you noticed any changes?

PATIENT: Nada.

DOCTOR: No changes at all?

PATIENT: No.

DOCTOR: Have you noticed any weight loss or weight gain?

PATIENT: No mucho.

DOCTOR: Has there been any change in your energy level?

PATIENT: No, me siento igual.

DOCTOR: Has there been any change in your face; are you seeing more facial hair or hair on your body?

PATIENT: No, no he visto ningún cambio.

DOCTOR: How about with your sexual feelings? You're a young man now, we talked about this a little bit the last time you were here. Are you feeling any interest or having any thoughts about sex, or are you interested in anyone?

PATIENT: Pues, no. No tiene mucho sentido.

DOCTOR: OK. Well, maybe we'll talk about that in a minute. In the meantime, were you able to get ahold of that medicine from the pharmacy?

PATIENT: No. Tengo ido como tres veces y no me la quieren dar.

DOCTOR: And have you been taking it at all?

PATIENT: Sí. Estoy tomando la misma cantidad. No he podido subir.

DOCTOR: Well, I'll call the pharmacy to find out what the problem is. Can you go again this afternoon?

> **PATIENT:** Sí. Doctor, perdí la caja con las cajitas donde guardaba las medicinas. He mirado en todas partes y no la busco.

DOCTOR: I'll see if I can get you another one.

> **PATIENT:** Muchas gracias.

DOCTOR: And have you noticed any change in urination? Are you peeing a normal amount, or less or more than before?

> **PATIENT:** Pues, yo creo que ya estoy orinando una cantidad normal o igual que antes.

DOCTOR: Well, after we straighten out the new dose it may get better. And did you have your MRI?

> **PATIENT:** *(looks at interpreter, confused)* No entendí. ¿Qué es eso de resonancia?

DOCTOR: Your MRI of the head, like you had before.

> **PATIENT:** Oh, sí. Sí, me lo hicieron ya. Tengo ido en San Jacinto el mes pasado.

DOCTOR: Good, now let's see here *(looking for results on the computer)*. Here we go. Yes, it looks good. It says the tumor hasn't grown. It may even be a little smaller than before. That's good. It seems like it's responding to the medicine...So I think things are going well. We may have to change the dose of the medicine a little bit and we may want to start you on some testosterone, but I'm going to consult with the attending and I'll come back in a few minutes.

> **PATIENT:** *(appears anxious)* Doctor, quisiera saber como más o ménos cuántos meses, o sea, cuánto tiempo me queda.

DOCTOR: *(brightly)* Oh, OK then, I'll be right back.

PART 2 (a few minutes later)

DOCTOR: Oh, my God! You poor thing! No, no, no. Did you think this was a malignant tumor? This is a benign tumor. You're not going to die.[39]

> **PATIENT:** ¿No? ¿No tengo cáncer? ¿No me voy a morir?

DOCTOR: Oh, no, Doroteo, I'm so sorry you had that impression. You're not going to die. You have a tumor, but it's not the bad kind. I mean, you don't want it to grow, if it gets huge it can affect you, like it has been, but it's not a bad tumor. It's not malignant. It isn't cancer, and it doesn't spread to the rest of your body. Do you understand?

> **PATIENT:** Sí. *(The patient is, tearful and smiling slightly, clearly affected by the news, but trying not to cry.)*

---

[39] How does a person with a benign tumor get through months of treatment and studies and have this misunderstanding? What factors could be responsible?

DOCTOR: So I'm just going to check with my attending and I'll be right back. *(The doctor leaves to consult with the attending physician, and the interpreter and patient wait in the room. The patient is quiet and clearly overwhelmed. The intern and attending physician return a few minutes later.)*

ATTENDING PHYSICIAN: Hello, Doroteo.

PATIENT: Buenos días.

ATTENDING PHYSICIAN: Dr. Walsh was just catching me up about how you're doing. I understand you were under the impression that this was a malignant cancer.

PATIENT: Sí.

ATTENDING PHYSICIAN: So this is great news for you, Doroteo. I'm so sorry you've been living all this time these past six months with the wrong idea. That must have been very hard.

PATIENT: Sí. Yo ya tengo comprado mi boleto para ver a mi familia y decirles adiós. Me estaba preparando para el otro lado.

ATTENDING PHYSICIAN: Well, let me assure you this is not the case. Your tumor is benign, and you aren't going to die, not that we know of in the near future anyway. I mean, we never know if we'll get hit by a car or something else, but as far as we know, you won't die because of a cancer. This tumor is not the dangerous kind.

PATIENT: Bueno.

ATTENDING PHYSICIAN: Now, I was just talking with Dr. Walsh and I think we do need to get your testosterone level up a bit. I think that will help you feel a lot better and have more normal development and drive for a man your age. Though the tumor isn't the bad kind, it does affect the body, and this is one of the ways it does. It affects the production of testosterone. Do you know what that is?

PATIENT: Sí. Un poco.

ATTENDING PHYSICIAN: Well, that's the male hormone that makes the difference between being an adolescent and growing into a man. How does that sound to you, Doroteo, if we go ahead and prescribe some testosterone?

PATIENT: Bien.

ATTENDING PHYSICIAN: All right, then. Dr. Walsh will come right back with a prescription and a lab slip that he'll explain, and I'd like to see you in about two months, OK? And again, I apologize if we weren't clear before about the tumor.

PATIENT: Está bien.

ATTENDING PHYSICIAN: Well, then, we'll see you in about eight weeks. Happy holidays. This will be a wonderful surprise for your family for Christmas.

PATIENT: Gracias.

Brain tumor role play (English only)

PART 1

DOCTOR: Hello, Doroteo, I'm so sorry I'm late. I got really backed up. I know you've been waiting. *(to the interpreter)* Thank you for waiting.

PATIENT: No problem.

DOCTOR: So, Doroteo, how have you been feeling?

PATIENT: *(replies despondently)* Well, a little bit OK.

DOCTOR: Have you noticed any changes?

PATIENT: Nothing.

DOCTOR: No changes at all?

PATIENT: No.

DOCTOR: Have you noticed any weight loss or weight gain?

PATIENT: Not much.

DOCTOR: Has there been any change in your energy level?

PATIENT: No, I feel the same.

DOCTOR: Has there been any change in your face; are you seeing more facial hair or hair on your body?

PATIENT: No, no change.

DOCTOR: How about with your sexual feelings? You're a young man now, we talked about this a little bit the last time you were here. Are you feeling any interest or having any thoughts about sex, or are you interested in anyone?

PATIENT: Well, no. No, there's really no point.

DOCTOR: OK. Well, maybe we'll talk about that in a minute. In the meantime, were you able to get ahold of that medicine from the pharmacy?

PATIENT: No. I have went there some three times and they do not want to give it to me.

DOCTOR: And have you been taking it at all?

PATIENT: Yes. I am taking the same amount. I haven't been able to go up on dose.

DOCTOR: Well, I'll call the pharmacy to find out what the problem is. Can you go again this afternoon?

PATIENT: Yes, doctor. I lost the box with the little boxes inside where I kept the medicines. I have looked everywhere, I can't find it.

DOCTOR: I'll see if I can get you another one.

PATIENT: Thank you very much.

DOCTOR: And have you noticed any change in urination? Are you peeing a normal amount, or less or more than before?

PATIENT: Well, I think I am urinating about right, or the same as before.

DOCTOR: Well, after we straighten out the new dose it may get better. And did you have your MRI?

PATIENT: *(looks at interpreter, confused)* I didn't understand. What did he say? Emarrái?

DOCTOR: Your MRI of the head, like you had before.

PATIENT: Oh, yes, yes. They did that to me already. I have been gone to San Jacinto last month.

DOCTOR: Good, now let's see here *(looking for results on the computer)*. Here we go. Yes, it looks good. It says the tumor hasn't grown. It may even be a little smaller than before. That's good. It seems like it's responding to the medicine...So I think things are going well. We may have to change the dose of the medicine a little bit and we may want to start you on some testosterone, but I'm going to consult with the attending and I'll come back in a few minutes.

PATIENT: *(appears anxious)* Doctor, I wanted to know about, well, more or less, how many months, or in other words, how much time do I have left?

DOCTOR: *(brightly)* Oh, OK then, I'll be right back.

PART 2 (a few minutes later)

DOCTOR: Oh, my God! You poor thing! No, no, no. Did you think this was a malignant tumor?! This is a benign tumor. You're not going to die.

PATIENT: No? I don't have cancer? I'm not going to die?

DOCTOR: Oh, no, Doroteo, I'm so sorry you had that impression. You're not going to die. You have a tumor, but it's not the bad kind. I mean, you don't want it to grow, if it gets huge it can affect you, like it has been, but it's not a bad tumor. It's not malignant. It isn't cancer; it doesn't spread to the rest of your body. Do you understand?

PATIENT: Yes. *(The patient is, tearful and smiling slightly, clearly affected by the news, but trying not to cry.)*

DOCTOR: So I'm just going to check with my attending and I'll be right back. *(The doctor leaves to consult with the attending physician, and the interpreter and patient wait in the room. The patient is quiet and clearly overwhelmed. The intern and attending physician return a few minutes later.)*

ATTENDING PHYSICIAN: Hello, Doroteo.

PATIENT: Good morning.

ATTENDING PHYSICIAN: Dr. Walsh was just catching me up about how you're doing. I understand you were under the impression that this was a malignant cancer.

PATIENT: Yes.

ATTENDING PHYSICIAN: So this is great news for you, Doroteo. I'm so sorry you've been living all this time these past six months with the wrong idea. That must have been very hard.

PATIENT: Yes, I have bought my ticket to travel and see my family and say goodbye. I was preparing myself for going over to the other side.

ATTENDING PHYSICIAN: Well, let me assure you this is not the case. Your tumor is benign, and you aren't going to die, not that we know of in the near future anyway. I mean, we never know if we'll get hit by a car or something else, but as far as we know, you won't die because of a cancer. This tumor is not the dangerous kind.

PATIENT: That's good.

ATTENDING PHYSICIAN: Now, I was just talking with Dr. Walsh, and I think we do need to get your testosterone level up a bit. I think that will help you feel a lot better and have more normal development and drive for a man your age. Though the tumor isn't the bad kind, it does affect the body, and this is one of the ways it does. It affects the production of testosterone. Do you know what that is?

PATIENT: Yes, a little.

ATTENDING PHYSICIAN: Well, that's the male hormone that makes the difference between being an adolescent and growing into a man. How does that sound to you, Doroteo, if we go ahead and prescribe some testosterone?

PATIENT: Good.

ATTENDING PHYSICIAN: All right, then. Dr. Walsh will come right back with a prescription and a lab slip that he'll explain, and I'd like to see you in about two months, OK? And again, I apologize if we weren't clear before about the tumor.

PATIENT: Good.

ATTENDING PHYSICIAN: Well, then, we'll see you in about eight weeks. Happy holidays. This will be a wonderful surprise for your family for Christmas.

PATIENT: Yes. Thank you.

Boundary Issues

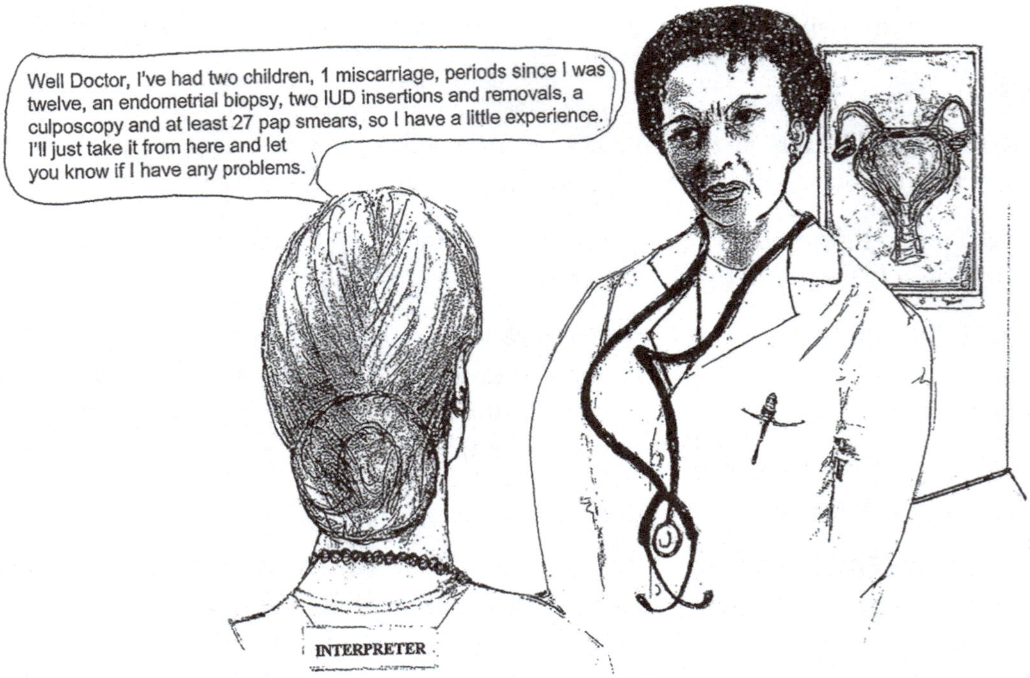

What's important to know about this chapter?

Terminology

It might be helpful to review the endocrinology-related vocabulary presented in Chapters 2 and 5.

What does the medical interpreter need to know?

If an interpreter is competent and knows the appropriate terminology and vocabulary, it might not be necessary to study the specifics about endocrinology or any other specialty. Yet when you first begin interpreting for a particular specialty, it certainly helps to "read up" and be prepared.

Having background information about the medical specialty or a patient's diagnosis can improve accuracy, but be careful. Having knowledge doesn't give you license to disagree with the provider.

If, for example, an interpreter has diabetes and manages it well, she might disagree with how a provider is educating a patient about diabetes. However, the interpreter in this case cannot intervene because the problem here is not accurate communication. The interpreter simply does not agree with the provider.

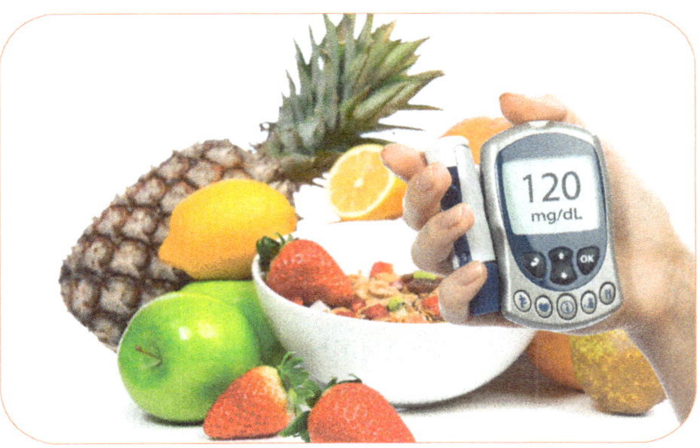

It can be appropriate to inform a provider about any significant misunderstanding or confusion that you notice, but you may not change what the provider is saying or how she or he is saying it. That said, having some information about a specialty could help the interpreter make an important and meaningful difference in another human being's life.

Statements in nonstandard grammar

At some point this patient says, "No. I have went there some three times, and they do not want to give it to me." The patient is not speaking standard grammar. Such statements are difficult to interpret. How do you manage them? How did you interpret this one?

Regional language variety

In the Spanish version of this role play, the patient speaks a regional dialect. His speech is influenced by grammatical and linguistic patterns from another, first language. He uses some words in a less common fashion and it is helpful for the interpreter to notice this because it might make the interpreter aware of the need to pay careful attention to see if the patient is understanding the provider. Take the word "lift" in English. In the United States, it can mean "to pick something up," but does not mean "an elevator," as it does in England. What does it mean to be "pissed" in the United States? And what does it mean in Australia?

In this role play, the speaker substitutes the verbs "to have" or "to possess" ("*tener*" in Spanish) for "have" as an auxiliary verb ("*haber*" in Spanish). This is a common feature of Spanish spoken by Yucatec

Mayans in México, many of whom no longer speak Yucatec but only Spanish. The patient does something similar with other words, for example, "to look for" and "to find," which are often used interchangeably. Which dialects or varieties of your other-than-English working language are you familiar with? Where are they spoken? (E.g., Is Quebec French the same as Dakar French? Is Moroccan Arabic different from Lebanese Arabic? What about Mozambican Portuguese vs. the Portuguese spoken in Bahia, Brazil?)

This patient has transferred features of his first language to the language he is speaking at the health appointment. It is a clue to possible problems: the interpreter should pay particular attention to see if the patient understands the provider.

In the mini-dialogue below, two speakers of the same language variety or dialect understand each other perfectly without the "(translation)." They use ***to look*** to mean ***to look, to look for, to search, to see and to find*** interchangeably, which may be a transference of word usage or structures from their first (other) language.

> **Speaker 1:** I can't look for my keys. (I can't find my keys.)
> **Speaker 2:** Have you looked for them? (Have you looked for them?)
> **Speaker 1:** Yes, I looked for them but I can't look for them. (Yes, I looked for them but I can't find them.)
> **Speaker 2:** Keep looking, you'll look for them. (Keep looking, you'll find them.)
> **Speaker 1:** But I can't look for them. (But I can't find them.)

Assumptions about speech styles

U.S. health professionals working with Indigenous patients from Latin America and other regions often ask the interpreter if the patient has a developmental problem due to a flat style of speech, for example. However, other patients who *do* have developmental delays are sometimes not correctly diagnosed because educators and healthcare providers miss the cues, assuming that the lack of understanding is caused by language or cultural barriers.

Children from families who speak less common languages at home can have special needs that are also often overlooked. Classroom teachers who suspect a cognitive or language delay in a child are sometimes discouraged from pursuing it and instead encouraged to "give the child a chance to learn English first." When children have speech delays, audiologists sometimes suggest that hearing two languages is the cause, or at least one important cause. This is controversial. We are learning more about neurolinguistics and new information about neural pathway development, which may lead to astonishing discoveries about language acquisition.

What if the patient seems unfamiliar with important medical terms?

What is your reaction to this situation where a patient has now had two MRIs, but doesn't seem familiar with the terminology? What could some explanations be? Hearing the patient's history coupled with this unfamiliarity might suggest a serious concern about the level of understanding of the patient's own medical situation and language barriers—but what, if anything, should the interpreter do about such a concern? Also, under what circumstances might a patient with a brain tumor be seen in endocrinology as opposed to neurooncology or neurosurgery specialty clinics?

The patient thinks he is going to die!

At a certain point in the role play above, it should be clear to the interpreter that the patient clearly believes he is going to die—but the doctor has not understood that situation. What should the interpreter do?

In addition, when the anxious-appearing patient says, "Doctor, I wanted to know about, well, more or less, how many months, or in other words, how much time do I have left?" the doctor cheerfully responds, "Oh, OK then, I'll be right back." The doctor plans to leave! Should the interpreter try to stop the doctor from leaving? If so, how?

Ethics and standards: Reflect and practice

Goal 6: Role boundaries

Translation and paraphrasing

1. Look at the three NCIHC standards of practice related to confidentiality (Standards 16, 17 and 18, NCIHC, 2005, p. 8). Working individually, *paraphrase* the objective, its related ethical principle and the three standards.
2. Working individually, *translate* the original text of these standards into your other working language(s) or interpret it into sign language.
3. Find a partner or partners. Compare, discuss and modify your translations and paraphrasing until you are satisfied with your final products as a group.
4. If you can, pick a group representative and discuss your final versions with any other groups that share your working languages. Compare and discuss your differences.

Suggested reading

Roat, C. E. (2010). *Healthcare Interpreting in Small Bites: 50 Nourishing Selections from the "Pacific Interpreters Newsletter," 2002-2010*. Victoria, British Columbia: Trafford, pp. 25-28.

Consider and discuss

Note: You can find suggested answers to each question after question 5.

1. **Standard 16** According to this standard, which of these activities would be acceptable?
   - Go out to coffee with a patient after an appointment.
   - Give a patient in difficult circumstances a ride home.
   - Tell your family what a difficult and distressing day of interpreting you had.
   - Give your personal telephone number to a patient in case they have a question at night or over the weekend.
   - Make arrangements to have carpentry done by the patient's brother.
   - Attend a memorial service for a child patient who died.
2. **Standard 17** A patient and provider review a list of current medications. The patient reports not using insulin for more than a week because she ran out of needles. The doctor provides a refill prescription. The patient then reports her blood sugar levels. The provider commends her on the low, well-controlled numbers. He advises her to continue with her usual regimen. The interpreter worries that if the patient goes back to her usual insulin use with these new low glucose levels, the patient might cause a low drop in blood sugar and go into a diabetic coma. The doctor has left the room temporarily. How can the interpreter maintain professional boundaries and do no harm, yet also help to avoid harm to the patient?
3. **Standard 17** A mother tells the pediatrician about her child's nosebleeds during cold, dry weather when the heat is on. The provider tells the mother it's normal and not to worry and that there is nothing she can do. In many other appointments, the interpreter has heard both pediatricians and otolaryngologists tell parents

they can put a little Vaseline on a cotton swab[40] and put it in the child's nose to moisturize it and help prevent nosebleeds. The interpreter has tried this technique with his nephew and knows it works well. Should he, or may he, tell the mother?

4. **Standard 18** A bilingual social worker organizes and participates in a family meeting. She decides to interpret. How could she explain the difference between her acting as an interpreter and as a social worker? Give an example of what she might say.
5. **Standard 18** A bilingual geneticist conducts her patient's health and family history interview in the patient's other language. A group of healthcare colleagues attend that meeting. How will the monolingual English-speaking providers on the team learn all the information from the patient interview?

Answers

1. **Standard 16** According to this standard, which of these activities would be acceptable?
    - Go out to coffee with a patient after an appointment.
    - Give a patient in difficult circumstances a ride home.
    - **Tell your family what a difficult and distressing day of interpreting you had.**
    - Give your personal telephone number to a patient in case they have a question at night or over the weekend.
    - Make arrangements to have carpentry done by the patient's brother.
    - Attend a memorial service for a child patient who died.
2. **Standard 17** A patient and provider review a list of current medications. The patient reports not using insulin for more than a week because she ran out of needles. The doctor provides a refill prescription. The patient then reports her blood sugar levels. The provider commends the patients on the low, well-controlled numbers. He advises her to continue with her usual regimen. The interpreter worries that if the patient goes back to her usual insulin use with these new low glucose levels, the patient might cause a low drop in blood sugar and go into a diabetic coma. The doctor has left the room temporarily. How can the interpreter maintain professional boundaries and do no harm, or help avoid harm to the patient?

The interpreter in this case might not be able to maintain professional boundaries. Due to the question of patient safety, the interpreter might need to engage in advocacy. How to advocate is discussed in the introductory section of this book, "Guide to Advocacy." Please study that section closely.

Also, be aware that a great deal of the interpreter's decision in a case like this will be affected by his or her employment status. Is the interpreter self-employed, an agency staff interpreter, a staff interpreter working for the hospital or healthcare organization or a bilingual employee pulled in to interpret? The answer can affect what kind of advocacy the interpreter might choose to do—if any.

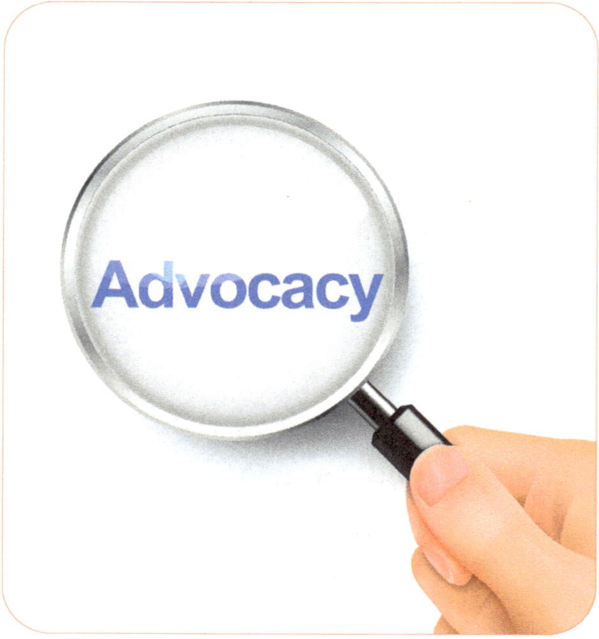

40 The most common brand of cotton swabs sold in the United States is called Q-tips.

3. **Standard 17** A mother tells the pediatrician about her child's nosebleeds during cold, dry weather when the heat is on. The provider tells the mother it's normal and not to worry and that there is nothing she can do. In many other appointments, the interpreter has heard both pediatricians and otolaryngologists tell parents they can put a little Vaseline on a cotton swab and put it in the child's nose to moisturize it and help prevent nosebleeds. The interpreter has tried this technique with his nephew and knows it works well. Should he, or may he, tell the mother?

   No. If the interpreter is a contract interpreter, he or she should say nothing during or after the appointment. If the interpreter is employed by the healthcare organization, he or she could perhaps find the occasion to ask the doctor's opinion about the Vaseline technique. After all, the doctor might have had medical reasons for not recommending it. For example, many people put cotton swabs inside their ears to clean their ears—and that is a common yet dangerous practice! Remember: you are not a doctor. You are an *interpreter.*

4. **Standard 18** A bilingual social worker organizes and participates in a family meeting. She decides to interpret. How could she explain the difference between her acting as an interpreter and as a social worker? Give an example of what she might say.

   The social worker should simply make clear she is switching roles and that while she is acting as an interpreter, she can no longer act as a social worker. In that case, she would need another social worker to conduct her part of the meeting.

   By the way, if you are a bilingual employee in healthcare who interprets, you are often called a "dual role" interpreter. You are also often *expected* to do your job and interpret at the same time. You might have to educate your colleagues, providers, supervisors and administration about why you should not do so. They might not care much about the relevant NCIHC standard, Standard 18 (although, of course, they should). So perhaps you could mention these concepts:

   - **Interpreting is a highly complex skill that requires immense focus and concentration to help assure accuracy.**
   - **One cannot be sure of safely performing another job while interpreting.**
   - **Roles can be blurred when someone tries to interpret and perform another job at the same time. (For example, if the patient asks the social worker a question, suddenly the social worker is expected both to participate in the meeting and interpret it, leading to confusion.)**
   - **The interpreter cannot act impartially while also performing in another role.**

5. **Standard 18** A bilingual geneticist conducts her patient's health and family history interview in the patient's other language. A group of healthcare colleagues attend that meeting. How will the monolingual English-speaking providers on the team learn all the information from the patient interview?

   First, the bilingual geneticist should not interpret the meeting! Instead, an interpreter with a high level of competence in *simultaneous* interpreting skills should attend. Failing that, such an interpreter could be brought in by telephone or video. If there are no provisions for interpreter services, the bilingual geneticist might have to interpret everything that is said: the patient's utterances in the interview, the utterances of colleagues and everything that the geneticist says. However, interpreting accuracy is likely to be at risk, and so is the geneticist's ability to perform his or her own work well, since interpreting will almost certainly interfere with the geneticist's usual cognitive skills during such a session.

Occupational therapy for interpreters

EXERCISES FOR THE TONGUE, HEART AND MIND

Suggested reading

Diamond, L.C., Wilson-Stronks A., and Jacobs, E.A. (2010). Do hospitals measure up to the national culturally and linguistically appropriate services standards? *Medical Care,* 48(12): 1080-1087.

This article contains important information. It is clearly written and is easy to read. Medical interpreters will benefit from understanding how federal standards can directly influence LEP patients and work environments. If you are unable to access the full article, read the abstract, which usually appears online even if the whole article is not available online (or available only at a cost). Even the abstract can be informative.

Consider and discuss

The authors describe the setting or background for their study as follows:

> "Federal regulations require that healthcare organizations provide language services to patients with limited English proficiency. The National Standards for Culturally and Linguistically Appropriate Services in Healthcare (CLAS standards) provide guidance on how to fulfill these regulations. It is not known how U.S. hospitals have incorporated them into practice" (p. 1080).

The authors then discuss their intent in this article to "assess how U.S. hospitals are meeting federal regulations requiring provision of language services using CLAS as a measure of compliance" (p. 1081). In their results and conclusions, the authors of this article state the following:

> "Results: Many hospitals are not meeting federal regulations. The majority reported providing language assistance in a timely manner in their first, but not their third, most commonly requested language. Although hospitals reported that they informed patients of their right to receive language services, many did so only in English. A majority of hospitals reported the use of family members or untrained staff as interpreters. Few reported providing vital documents in non-English languages. Overall, 13% of hospitals met all 4 of the language-related CLAS standards, whereas 19% met none.
>
> Conclusions: Our study documents that many hospitals are not providing language services in a manner consistent with federal law. Enforcement of these regulations is inconsistent and thus does not motivate hospitals to comply. Compliance will likely come with new guidelines, currently being written, by many of the regulatory organizations. Our study reinforces the importance of these efforts and helps target interventions to improve the delivery and safety of care to limited English proficient patients" (p. 1080).

The federal regulations and law referred to by the authors is Title VI of the Civil Rights Act of 1964, 42 U.S.C.§2000d. Section 601 of Title VI states that no person shall "on the ground of race, color, or national origin, be excluded from participation in, be denied the benefits of, or be subjected to discrimination under any program or activity receiving federal financial assistance." ("National origin" has been defined as *language,* and an example of "federal financial assistance" is *Medicaid payments.*)

Now try to answer the following questions.

1. What are culturally and linguistically appropriate services (CLAS) standards? (Try to find this information online.)
2. When were they first published?
3. In which year were the National CLAS Standards revised and republished?
4. How many standards are listed in the most recent version?
5. How do the National CLAS Standards differ from professional standards of practice, such as the NCIHC standards of practice?
6. Are all the National CLAS Standards federal *requirements*? If not, which National CLAS Standards are voluntary, and which are legally required?
7. Which National CLAS Standards address language?
8. In your opinion, which are the three most important National CLAS Standards? Why?

You will now revisit part of the original role play dialogue from this chapter. In this version, the interpreter takes action. Each time the interpreter speaks or acts, decide if you agree with what the interpreter did by answering the questions that follow each excerpt.

Then read the commentary that follows the seven excerpts and see if you want to change any of your answers.

PART 1

DOCTOR: Well, after we straighten out the new dose it may get better. And did you have your MRI?

PATIENT: *(looks at interpreter, confused)* I didn't understand. What did he say? Emarrái?

DOCTOR: Your MRI of the head, like you had before.

INTERPRETER: It's the study where they put you inside a big tube and you have to be still and not move for a while when they take images or photos.

Do you agree that the interpreter here did the right thing to explain an MRI to the patient? Circle your answer.

YES NO MAYBE

Why did you agree or disagree with the interpreter's intervention?

PART 2

PATIENT: *(appears anxious)* Doctor, I wanted to know about, well, more or less, how many months, or in other words, how much time do I have left?

DOCTOR: *(brightly)* Oh, OK then, I'll be right back.

INTERPRETER: *(intervening in the communication)* Dr. Walsh, as the interpreter I'd like to clarify, I'm not sure you understood the question. The patient may have been asking how much time he has left to live, or in other words, he may be under the impression that he is going to die. *(Interpreter interprets this intervention to the patient.)*

DOCTOR: *(stops, looks a bit puzzled, pauses)*

Do you agree that the interpreter's intervention was appropriate? Circle your answer.

YES NO MAYBE

Why did you agree or disagree with the interpreter's intervention?

PART 3

In this case, the interpreter intervened with the doctor.

INTERPRETER: Doctor, the interpreter would like to clarify. Is that a correct impression? Should he be under the impression that he is dying and has a limited time left to live? *(repeats the intervention in the other language for the patient)*

Do you agree that the interpreter's intervention was appropriate? Circle your answer.

YES NO MAYBE

Why did you agree or disagree with the interpreter's intervention?

PART 4

DOCTOR: Oh, my God! You poor thing! No, no, no. Did you think this was a malignant tumor?! This is a benign tumor. You're not going to die.

> **INTERPRETER:** *(After interpreting the doctor's statement, the interpreter reconfirms)* Did you understand what the doctor said? You are not going to die, your tumor is not malignant.

Do you agree that the interpreter's intervention was appropriate? Circle your answer.

YES NO MAYBE

Why did you agree or disagree with the interpreter's intervention?

PART 5

PATIENT: No? I don't have cancer? I'm not going to die?

> **INTERPRETER:** Doctor, can you repeat that again? I'm not sure if he's familiar with "malignant" and "benign." He just knew he has a brain tumor, and without much other knowledge, he just assumed he was dying.

Do you agree that the interpreter's intervention was appropriate? Circle your answer.

YES NO MAYBE

Why did you agree or disagree with the interpreter's intervention?

PART 6

DOCTOR: Oh no, Doroteo, I'm so sorry you had that impression. You're not going to die. You have a tumor, but it's not the bad kind. I mean, you don't want it to grow, if it gets huge it can affect you, like it has been, but it's not a bad tumor. It's not malignant. It isn't cancer; it doesn't spread to the rest of your body. Do you understand?

PATIENT: Yes. *(The patient is, tearful and smiling slightly, clearly affected by the news, but trying not to cry.)*

INTERPRETER: Wow, I guess this is really great news then, no? *(repeats in the patient's language)*

PATIENT: Yes.

Do you agree that the interpreter's intervention was appropriate? Circle your answer.

YES NO MAYBE

Why did you agree or disagree with the interpreter's intervention?

PART 7

DOCTOR: So I'm just going to check with my attending and I'll be right back.

INTERPRETER: So he can call his family and give them the good news for Christmas?

DOCTOR: Oh, yes! *(The doctor leaves to consult with the attending physician, and the interpreter and patient wait alone in the room.)*

Do you agree that it was appropriate for the interpreter to remain alone with the patient? Circle your answer.

YES NO MAYBE

Why did you agree or disagree with the interpreter's intervention?

Commentary

Now read the commentary on each of the seven excerpts above and see if you want to change any of your answers.

PART 1

Beyond comprehension: Here, the physician asks the patient if he's had a follow-up MRI (magnetic resonance imaging). The patient looks at the interpreter, confused, and says, "I didn't understand. What did he say? Emarrái?" The interpreter responds by explaining to the patient what an MRI is.

Interpreters are not permitted to provide medical information. Doing so is the provider's job. The interpreter in this case (a) violated ethical requirements related to role boundaries; (b) gave a medical description that might be inaccurate, confusing and/or inappropriate; (c) was not transparent with the doctor, violating the ethical requirement related to accuracy (and giving the doctor a chance to tell the interpreter not to engage in practicing medicine without a license); (d) risked causing consequences the interpreter could not predict by stepping out of role.

This action by the interpreter could even be considered to be providing medical advice, crossing another boundary. In some states, it might be illegal to provide such explanations without an appropriate license as a healthcare provider.

Still, if the doctor isn't clear, what should the interpreter do instead? If an interpreter fears that a patient does not understand information that is critical to his or her health or well-being, the interpreter can intervene to request a clarification from the *doctor*. Here are a few examples:

Interpreter: *(to the doctor) Excuse me, the interpreter requests you clarify the meaning of MRI.*

or

As the interpreter I'm concerned that the meaning of MRI might not be clear.

or

The interpreter feels there could be a misunderstanding about what an MRI is.

These are just examples. Whatever you say, be sure to repeat or report that message to the other party. Also, you should not state that the "patient doesn't understand MRI." After all, that might not be true, and saying so might offend, or be condescending to, the patient.

Do be alert. This patient has now had two MRIs, yet doesn't seem familiar with the term itself. The misunderstanding might be easy for you to address. But what might the real underlying problem be? For the patient who has had two MRIs, not to know what an MRI is sends up another red flag for the interpreter. Perhaps the patient has a cognitive problem. Maybe the term "MRI" was never used with the patient. Possibly the informed consent process was not done properly. There may be other important parts of the health situation that have not been explained or made clear to the patient. A situation like this should make the interpreter pay close attention to see how well the patient understands the doctor.

PART 2

Look at what happened in this scenario.

> **PATIENT:** *(appears anxious)* Doctor, I wanted to know about, well, more or less, how many months, or in other words, how much time do I have left?

DOCTOR: *(brightly)* Oh, OK then, I'll be right back.

At this point, the interpreter realizes the doctor didn't understand that the patient meant, "So how long until I die?" Clearly concerned for the patient, the interpreter interrupts before the doctor has left the room.

> **INTERPRETER:** *(intervening in the communication)* Dr. Walsh, as the interpreter I'd like to clarify, I'm not sure you understood the question. The patient may have been asking how much time he has left to live, or in other words, he may be under the impression that he is going to die. *(Interpreter interprets this intervention to the patient.)*

DOCTOR: *(stops, looks a bit puzzled, pauses)*

Did the doctor's first response seem like an appropriate response to the patient's question? Clearly not. So this interpreter chose to inform the doctor, "I'm not sure you understood the question" and then explained what the patient meant—or rather, what the *interpreter* thought the patient meant.

Say that the interpreter was, in fact, correct. In general, barring emergencies or special exceptions, what the interpreter did here is still not the best course of action. First, in most cases you might not want to tell a doctor, "I'm not sure you understood"—the doctor might not appreciate the comment, depending how it is delivered (some doctors, if you say it professionally, might be fine with such a comment). Second, instead, you want the *patient* to explain what he meant, if possible—not what you thought he meant. How could you make that happen? One simple way is to intervene with both parties to say something like the following.

> *The interpreter is concerned there is a serious misunderstanding about what the patient just said.*

Then the doctor could ask questions to find out what the *patient* meant—and not what *you* assumed the patient meant. Always remember that you could be wrong. You are not a mind reader.

PART 3

In this part of the dialogue, after the interpreter intervened to suggest the patient thought he was going to die, the doctor didn't answer right away. So the interpreter stepped in again and said:

> **INTERPRETER:** Doctor, the interpreter would like to clarify. Is that a correct impression? Should he be under the impression that he is dying and has a limited time left to live? *(repeats the intervention in the other language for the patient)*

In this case, the interpreter was probably reacting from the heart, not from the head. In other words, the interpreter probably felt compassion and concern for the patient and spoke up to address that feeling.

Yes, the situation was serious. Yes, the doctor needed to do something about it. But the doctor was caught off guard and still thinking about what to do when the interpreter interrupted to speak again.

Your primary job is interpreting. You intervene only if you truly need to do so. When it comes to intervening, a simple rule applies: *When in doubt, stay out.* Simply monitor the situation. You can always step in later—but first, give the parties a chance to speak to each other and fix the misunderstanding themselves.

Now, if the doctor was still trying to exit without addressing what the patient said first, the interpreter might have to speak up. But in this case, the doctor didn't leave. The doctor is simply taking time to absorb and understand the situation.

Intervening always carries a risk. By intervening when you don't need to, you might cause more problems than you fix. Your job is interpreting, not getting involved. Intervene only when doing so is truly necessary.

PART 4

Now the doctor *has* understood the situation and lets the patient know he is not going to die:

DOCTOR: Oh, my God! You poor thing! No, no, no. Did you think this was a malignant tumor?! This is a benign tumor. You're not going to die.

> **INTERPRETER:** *(after interpreting the doctor's statement, the interpreter reconfirms)* Did you understand what the doctor said? You are not going to die, your tumor is not malignant.

Why did the interpreter ask the patient if he or she understood? And then, before even waiting for a reply, why did the interpreter repeat the doctor's information? Again, most likely the reason is that the situation for the patient was so painful and extreme that the interpreter wanted to be sure the patient really understood the good news. However, here are two things to remember.

1. Please, wherever possible, *do not ask the patient, "Did you understand?"* That is the doctor's job. Instead, alert the *doctor* about any need for him or her to check for understanding.
2. You are not normally supposed to repeat statements. Again, there might be emergency or other special circumstances when doing so might make sense, but in essence when you repeat and rephrase statements, you are changing the message.

Is this a case where repeating the message is the right thing to do? If not, what could you do instead? Here is an answer: *Wait to see if the patient understands the doctor*. After all, in this case the doctor was clear. Why jump to conclusions that the patient didn't understand? It's true the patient may be in shock, there have been serious lapses in communication so far and in addition there may be low health literacy. Even so, give the patient a moment to recover. Wait and see.

If, as the exchange continues, you see that in fact the patient *doesn't* seem to understand and *does* still *seem* to be afraid he is going to die, then you could intervene again to suggest you are concerned that what you interpreted about the diagnosis might not be clear.

So wait and see. *When in doubt, stay out.* You can always step in later.

PART 5

Now the patient is responding to the doctor's good news:

> **PATIENT:** No? I don't have cancer? I'm not going to die?

> **INTERPRETER:** Doctor, can you repeat that again? I'm not sure if he's familiar with "malignant" and "benign." He just knew he has a brain tumor, and without much other knowledge, he just assumed he was dying.

Several mistakes were made here—the interpreter:

- Was not transparent with the patient.
- Engaged in "mind reading"—made assumptions (possibly false) about what the patient believed.
- Sounded condescending.
- Showed paternalistic behavior by taking action on the patient's behalf that the patient did not ask for and that might not be necessary.

Instead, the interpreter in this case should *wait* to make sure the doctor and the patient sort this out on their own. If not, the interpreter can intervene, but here there was no need to do so. In addition, the interpreter—even with less-educated patients—should never speak up on the patient's behalf this way without getting the patient's request or permission to do so unless compelling circumstances make it absolutely necessary (for instance, in an emergency department).

After the session the interpreter might have a right to file a critical incident report, but speaking up on the patient's behalf is a serious step, discussed in the "Guide to Advocacy" introductory sections of this book. In cases like this, it certainly could be justified.

Finally, consider the problem that in many places in the world even to hear a diagnosis of cancer can be traumatic to most patients, as it was in the United States 30 years ago (and is still today, for many U.S. patients. Yes, treatments exist now that did not exist years ago. Yet many patients—particularly those coming from outside the United States or not literate in English—are unaware of those treatments. Or perhaps they have heard that such treatments exist but they assume they would have no access to them due to poverty or lack of resources (such as health insurance).

PART 6

Consider what happened here.

DOCTOR: Oh no, Doroteo, I'm so sorry you had that impression. You're not going to die. You have a tumor, but it's not the bad kind. I mean, you don't want it to grow, if it gets huge it can affect you, like it has been, but it's not a bad tumor. It's not malignant. It isn't cancer; it doesn't spread to the rest of your body. Do you understand?

> **PATIENT:** Yes. *(The patient is, tearful and smiling slightly, clearly affected by the news, but trying not to cry.)*

> **INTERPRETER:** Wow, I guess this is really great news then, no? *(repeats in the patient's language)*

> **PATIENT:** Yes.

Perhaps it made the interpreter feel better to share this joyful moment with the patient. But doing so was not necessary or part of the interpreter's job. As you will see below, violating one's impartiality can have subtle but important consequences. The interpreter here should simply have interpreted the exchange, not participated in it.

Yes, we are human. Yes, sometimes it can feel difficult, unnatural, cold or even painful not to share in moments of great tragedy or joy. In some extreme cases, it might be appropriate for the interpreter to make a personal remark, or for an interpreter to cry or pray with a patient.

But in this situation, the circumstances were not exceptional enough to justify interfering with professional boundaries or interpreter impartiality.

In general, as difficult and unnatural as it might feel, you are expected *not* to hug or engage in personal conversation with a patient or family. In reality, as you well know, sometimes that is impossible. But try hard.

PART 7

In this case, the doctor left to find the attending physician, and the interpreter remained alone with the patient—which raises the question: *Should* interpreters be alone with patients?

The usual answer is no. When interpreters are left alone with patients, problems happen. For example, consider the following examples:

- The patient shares important medical information with the interpreter—not the doctor.
- Sometimes the patient says, "Don't tell the doctor I said that."
- The patient might share other personal, embarrassing or distressing information with the interpreter.
- The patient often asks the interpreter personal questions ("Are you married?" "Why don't you have children?" "How much money do you make doing this?" "What church do you go to?"), putting the interpreter in an awkward situation.
- The patient sometimes harasses the interpreter, even sexually, or exposes body parts. ("Look at my scar here!")
- The patient develops a closer relationship with the interpreter than the provider, perhaps undermining trust for the provider.
- If something goes wrong, such as the patient falling or having another type of accident, the interpreter might be liable for what happens.
- Some patients with mental health problems, or histories of violence, have been left alone with interpreters and caused them physical injury.

In short, being alone with the patient can undermine interpreter impartiality, professional boundaries, the patient-provider relationship, interpreter safety and much more.

That said, it is often difficult for interpreters to avoid being alone with a patient. No "blanket rules" of this kind can apply easily to every situation. More and more hospitals now have rules stating that interpreters must not remain alone with patients.

Until such rules are universal, each interpreter will have to make a practical decision about whether or not to be alone with a patient.

Medical terminology: The brain and brain tumors

Below you will find anatomical drawings relevant to the content of this chapter. Follow the instructions found at the end of Chapter 1 to study the terminology in this section.

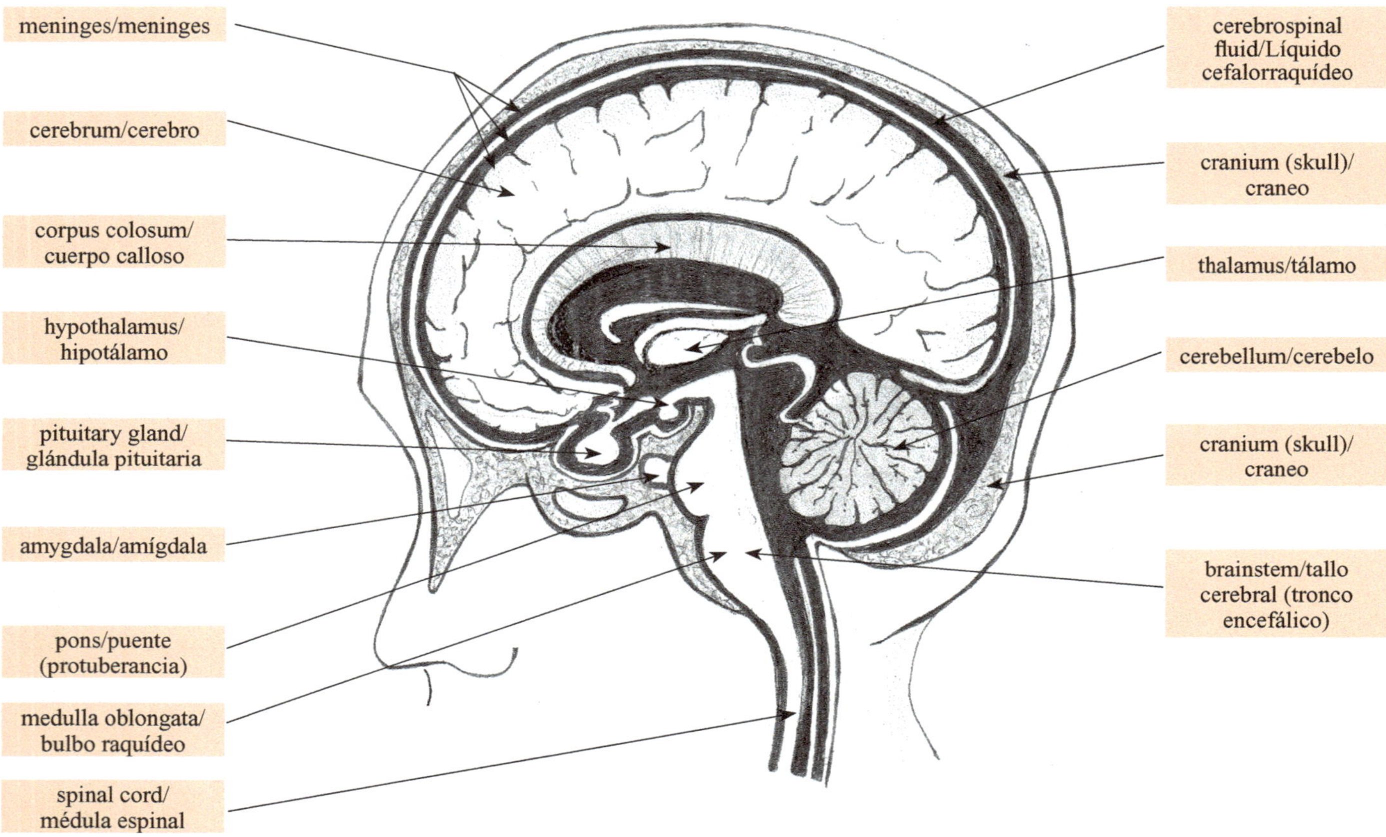

Figure 6-A: The brain (English and Spanish)

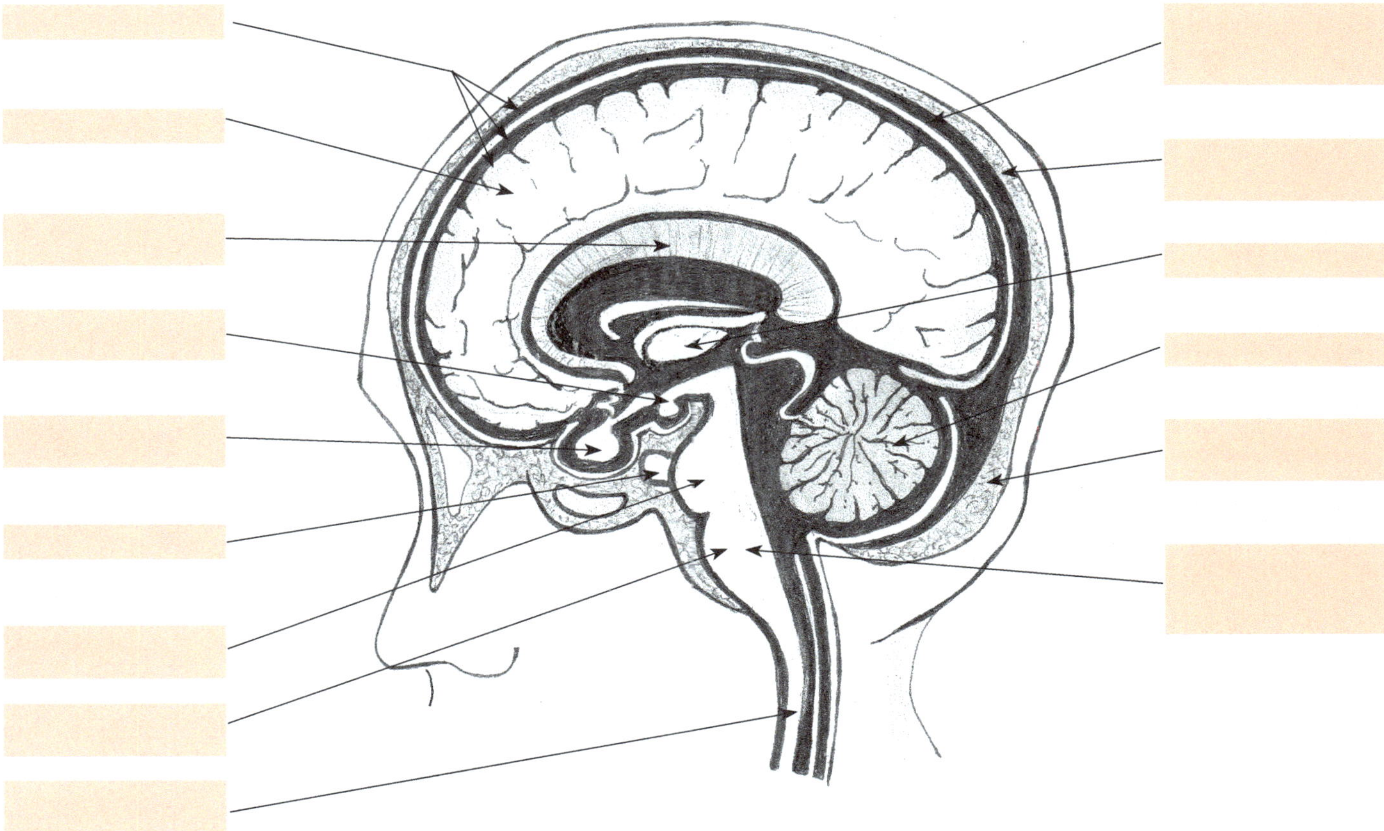

Figure 6-B: The brain (blank labels)

The most common primary brain tumors

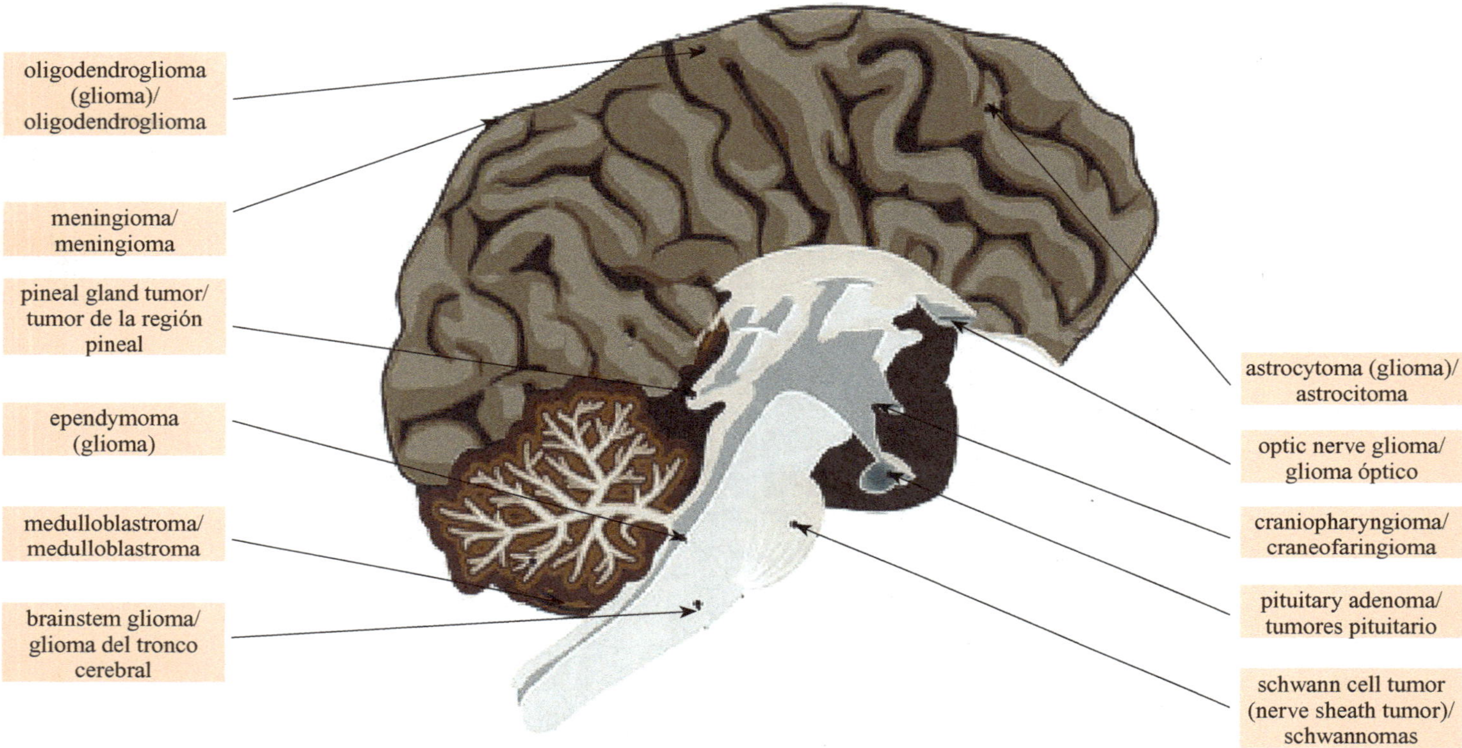

Figure 6-C: Common brain tumors (English and Spanish)

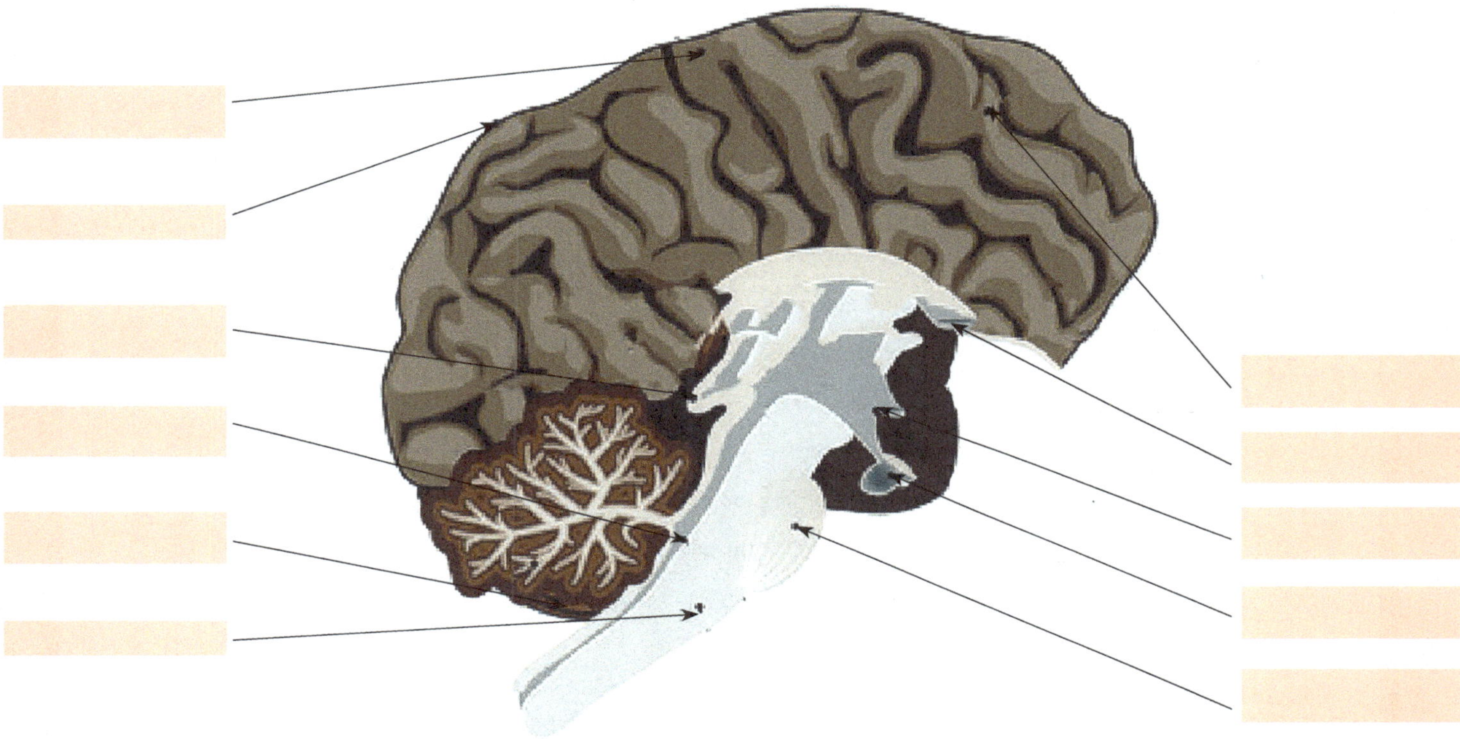

Figure 6-D: Common brain tumors (blank labels)

Medical terminology list

The brain and brain tumors

VOCABULARY FOR GRAPHIC–IN ENGLISH	VOCABULARY FOR GRAPHIC–IN SPANISH	ANY OTHER LANGUAGE
Amygdala	Amígdala	
Brainstem	Tallo cerebral (tronco encefálico)	
Cerebellum	cerebelo	
Cerebrospinal fluid	Líquido cefalorraquídeo	
Cerebrum	cerebro	
Corpus colosum	Cuerpo calloso	
Cranium (skull)	Craneo	
Hypothalamus	hipotálamo	
Medulla oblongata	bulbo raquídeo	
Meninges	meninges	
Midbrain (brain stem)	Cerebro medio (tronco cerebral)	
Pituitary gland	Glandula pitutitaria	
Pons	Puente (protuberancia)	
Spinal cord	Medulla espinal	
Thalamus	Tálamo	

Urology 7

Advisory

This chapter involves some material about genetics, gender, gender identity, gender assignment and human genitalia.

The patient is a seven-year-old child who was born with an undetermined gender. Mom and dad, both emigrants from a country with traditional gender-assigned roles, have come to the appointment with their child. When the baby was born, the parents were overwhelmed with clinical information about their baby. Throughout the years they have become more accustomed to their situation. However, learning about gender identity and gender assignment has opened them up to a whole new world with many new challenges as the child grows older.

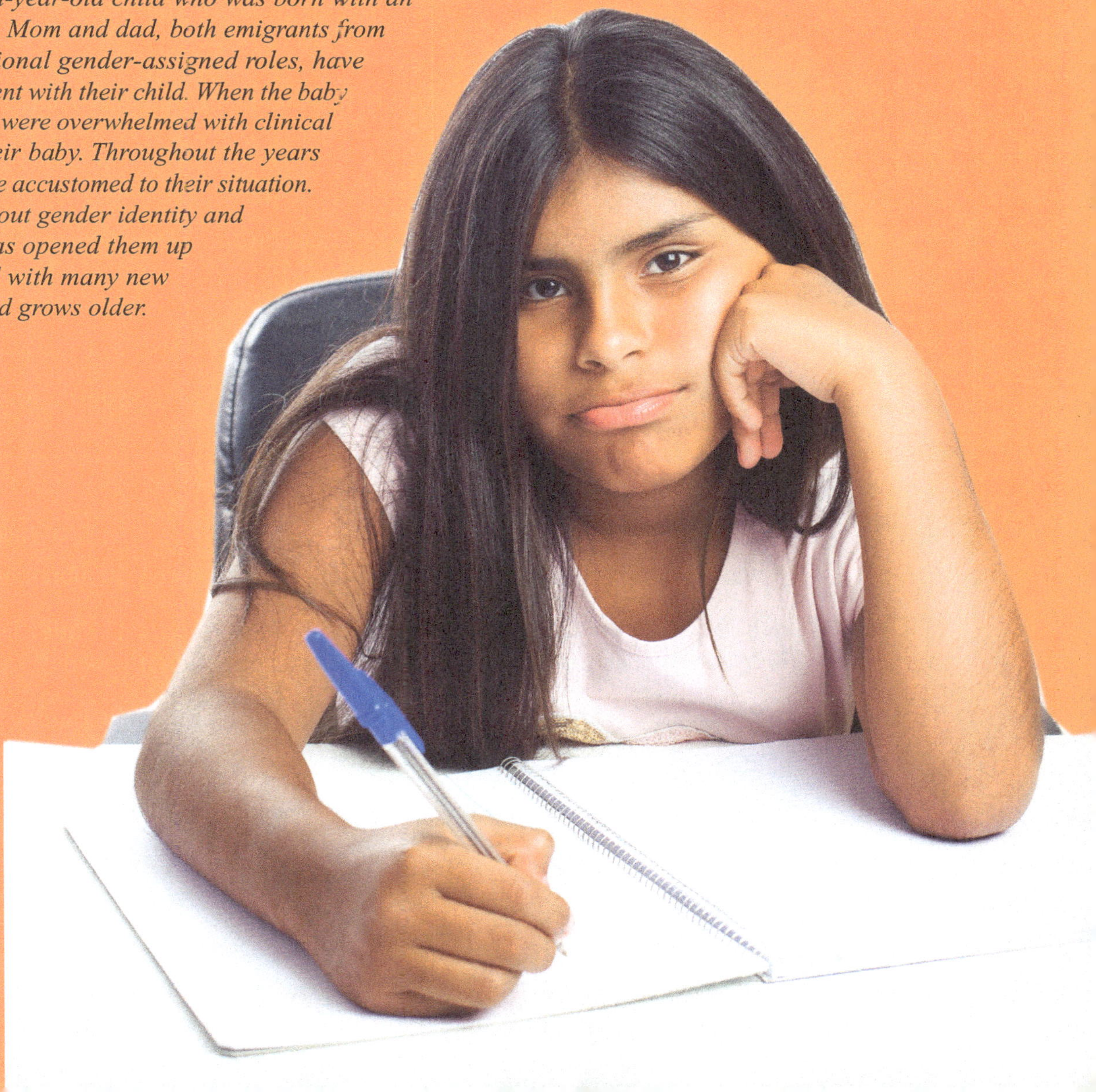

Pediatric urology and genetics—gender identity role play (English-Spanish)

DOCTOR: *(to the interpreter)* Great, you're here. *(to the parents)* I do understand quite a bit of Spanish but I can't speak it. Hi, I'm Dr. Pavignani, how are you?

MOM: Bien, estamos bien.

DOCTOR: And how has Jessica been?

MOM: Bien.

DOCTOR: You're just here for a regular checkup, right?

MOM: Sí.

DOCTOR: So how's she doing? Have there been any problems or changes since the last time we saw you?

MOM: No. Todo está igual.

DOCTOR: Have you noticed any change in the size of her clitoris? Does it seem to be growing?

MOM: Sí, parece que ha crecido un poco.

DOCTOR: Has she noticed it? Does she know she's different? Has anyone at school noticed?

MOM: Pues yo creo. Era muy pequeña antes, pero sí, ya ella nos está preguntando. Hemos empezado a hablar con la psicóloga también.

DOCTOR: Well, that's good. We have a lot to talk about today, then. Do you have any specific questions to start with?

MOM: Pues, no. Las preguntas que tenemos son las de siempre y siempre nos dicen lo mismo.

DOCTOR: Oh, well, what are the questions you have? But before we start, would Jessica like to wait out in the waiting room, or would you rather have her stay here while we talk?

DAD AND MOM: Mejor que se quede en la sala de espera. ¿Yesi, quieres esperar donde la televisión?

DOCTOR: Jessica, how about if I talk to your mom and dad a little while and then one of us will come get you and talk? *(Jessica leaves the room.)*

MOM: Bueno, las preguntas que siempre tenemos... ¿Por qué sucedió esto? ¿Qué es lo que pasa con ella exactamente? Y ¿qué podemos esperar?

DOCTOR: All right. *(silence)*

MOM: Nos preguntamos siempre si hemos hecho todo lo correcto. Los doctores nos dijeron que según toda su experiencia, deberíamos criarla como niña y eso es lo que hemos hecho, pero nos preguntamos si esto es lo que deberíamos hacer. Es que vimos un programa en la televisión y ¿qué tal si más adelante ella quiere ser hombre?

DOCTOR: Well, first of all, if the other doctors you've seen haven't made it clear to both of you yet, this has nothing to do with anything you could or couldn't have done. Your child was born with a condition that was determined before you probably even knew you were pregnant. It's a chromosomal condition, a condition called partial androgen receptor insensitivity. Did the genetics doctors explain all this to you?

DAD: Pues, más que nada nos confundieron.

DOCTOR: Did they explain about the genetic condition?

DAD: Pues, algo.

MOM: Pero como dijo mi esposo, estuvimos tan afligidos y con tantas cosas que más bien nos confundimos.

DOCTOR: Well, I'm not a geneticist, but let me see. In every cell in our bodies we have what we call genetic instructions, like a blueprint for development.

DAD: Sí, sí. Todos consistimos de células, me acuerdo de algo así de una clase de ciencia.

DOCTOR: And each cell has 46 chromosomes. Chromosomes are strings of instructions. If something is different about them, then it causes a change, so for example, if your blueprint called for 6-inch steel bolts and someone were to use 4-inch steel bolts, or mix the cement wrong, the building might not be as strong.

DAD: *(Both parents turn to the interpreter, looking more puzzled and anxious.)* Ya me perdió con eso de planos y cemento y pernos.

DOCTOR: I'm sorry. Let's start with the pregnancy. I imagine you know that it starts with conception when the sperm and egg get together.

MOM AND DAD: Sí, sí.

DOCTOR: Let's say we start out with this fertilized egg, which is like a library. There are millions and millions of cells in the body and they are all copies of that first one. So, let's say that each cell has a library, and in the library there are two copies of each of 23 volumes. So that's 46 books, or 23 pairs of books. Do you understand? Every cell has the library.

MOM AND DAD: Sí.

DOCTOR: Well, the sex cells, the ovum and sperm are different. They have only half the set of instructions each, or one of the two volumes in each pair. They each have half the necessary information for development. Does that sound familiar?

MOM: Sí, sí.

DAD: Sí, un poco.

DOCTOR: So, the egg is fertilized by the sperm and they form the first complete cell, or library. Each of you contributed half the information, or half the 23 pairs of books. That's why children look like their parents, just like your daughter looks like you both, right? She received genetic instructions for development from each of you. That's what determines her eye color, hair color, which cells will become the heart, the toenails, etc. Do you understand?

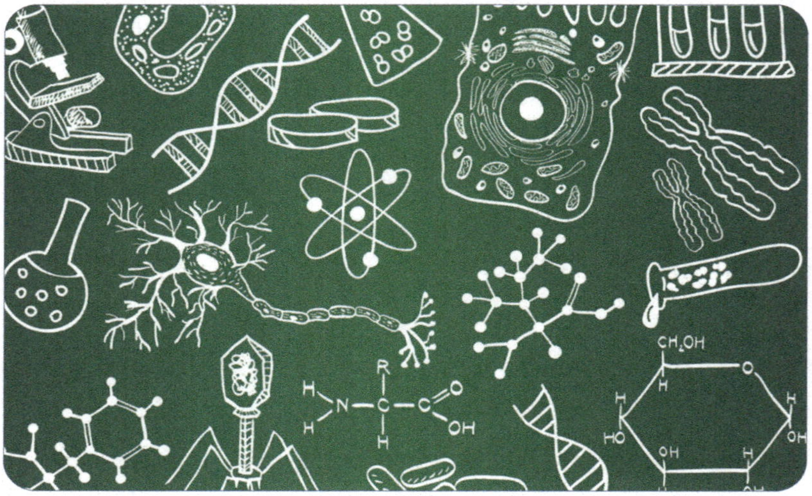

MOM: Sí.

DOCTOR: So that first fertilized egg had a complete set of genetic instructions, and then it started to divide and copy itself, over and over, with all the details and all the mistakes.

DAD: ¿Entonces hubo un error?

DOCTOR: In a way, or just a change. Imagine there are two copies of each book, and these pairs of books are the chromosomes. Imagine if you open a book and see lots of chapters with pages, lots of lines with sentences, words, all made up of letters. Those lines are like hundreds of instructions for development, which are what we call genes.

DAD: Sí, ya entiendo un poco más.

DOCTOR: Now, imagine if one of the lines on a page, or one of the pages, is missing from a book. That could cause big changes in the outcome. Usually, if there is a mistake on one of the lines, there's another set of instructions from the identical volume that formed the pair of books, and we can compensate.

MOM AND DAD: Sí.

DOCTOR: Or you could think of it like a cake recipe with changes in the amount of sugar or salt. The cake would come out differently.

DAD: Sí, sí.

DOCTOR: ¿Comprendo? *(Doctor uses wrong verb form.)*

MOM: No, es que sí, digo, ya me estoy acordando. Pero si es así, ¿por qué dicen que no tenemos la culpa, si es que todo lo que tiene ella es de nosotros?

DOCTOR: Well, good question. *(to interpreter)* It shows they understand. *(to parents)* This is nature, or God, or however you see the world. Sometimes things happen that are completely out of our control. We can't control it or cause it. There are several ways this can happen. Sometimes, well, remember the example of the library?

MOM AND DAD: Sí.

DOCTOR: Well, one way a thing like this can happen is at the time of conception, when half the books from the ovum get together with the other books from the sperm. That's a lot of detail and a lot of moving around. Sometimes for example, let's say, a phrase on line 638 from page 232 from chapter six, in volume one, of pair 17, gets mixed up and when the two halves of information get together, that phrase is moving around and then attaches itself to a different volume. That can cause a change. Or a change can happen if both parents have a page ripped out of the same chapter of the same book. When the child receives that chromosome with the missing page, or gene, from both parents, then there is no way to compensate for that. It can also cause a change. If one of the volumes isn't missing the page, then usually things are OK because there's always another copy of the genetic information. Does that seem reasonable?

MOM AND DAD: Sí, sí.

DOCTOR: Other times, maybe the egg or the sperm has *extra* information, so for example, instead of giving one volume of a pair to the forming embryo, it gives two. I'm sure you've seen children with Down syndrome. Those babies have an extra copy of one of the volumes, or in other words, three copies of a book instead of a pair of books.

MOM: ¿Es por eso que nos dijeron que no lo pueden remediar, no hay medicinas ni cirugías ni nada?

DOCTOR: Exactly. We can treat the symptoms, for example, do surgery on a defective heart, but in Jessica's case, the change is throughout the whole body because of how cells copy and reproduce themselves.

MOM: Oh, sí, yo entiendo.

DOCTOR: So back to Jessica and her case. Jessica has the condition I mentioned, partial androgen insensitivity syndrome. It isn't as uncommon as you might think. I believe about two to five of every 100,000 people are born this way.

MOM: ¿Y entonces por qué nos dijeron al comienzo que no sabían qué tenía o si era niña o niño?

DOCTOR: Well, I believe that in the beginning, after they did the prenatal testing, they were concerned that they didn't get a cell sample from more than one place. You see, remember when we talked about the first cell dividing and being duplicated with all its chromosomal arrangements?

MOM AND DAD: Sí.

DOCTOR: Well, sometimes this change or rearrangement doesn't take place at conception. Maybe it takes place after two or four or eight divisions, and only some cells are affected. This is what is sometimes referred to as a mosaic condition. Your baby was born with what appeared to be a large clitoris, but the doctors were concerned that it was a penis. There were vaginal labia, but also scrotal tissue. They wanted to get genetic samples from different tissues in the body before going forward with definitive information. Some children exhibit the appearance of one gender externally, while genetically they are the other gender. The last of the 23 pairs of chromosomes are either XX or XY, and that is a lot of what determines whether a baby is a girl or a boy. Though researchers are discovering new things all the time, and some scientists think that gender is something much more complicated and determined in multiple places at multiple times during fetal development. Some people go through most of their lives and don't find this out until much later, when they try to have children and have trouble with pregnancy, for example.

DAD: Bueno, ¿y qué opina usted? ¿Estamos haciendo lo correcto?

DOCTOR: You know, first of all, I want you to know that I think you are doing an excellent job. I think this is one of the hardest things for parents to go through. I think you are doing a wonderful job. I know it isn't easy, especially when you aren't sure who you can share this with or how people may react.

MOM: Pues, sí. Todavía no le hemos dicho nada a nadie. Solamente a mi hermana, y eso fue hace apenas cuatro o cinco meses.

DOCTOR: Well, you are wonderful parents, and Jessica seems like a happy, healthy girl.

MOM: Entonces, ¿cuándo podríamos hacer la cirugía?

DOCTOR: I think that you are talking with Jessica and the psychologist, and that's the right place to start. I have a note here from the psychologist. She says that you've discussed the fact that about 80 percent of children respond to testosterone at puberty. Now, what does that mean for a child like Jessica? It means that many children hit puberty, and suddenly after being raised their whole childhood as a girl, they realize they feel more like a boy. That is why the most recent recommendation is to wait until that time to do any kind of a permanent surgery.

MOM: Entonces, ¿tenemos que esperar?

DOCTOR: Yes, I know it's hard, but I know you probably also want what's best for your child. We will need to do regular ultrasounds on her to check the status of the gonads in her abdomen.

DAD: ¿Qué es eso?

DOCTOR: Well, they are the egg cells, they would have become testicles, but in Jessica's case they will never develop and sometimes they can become cancerous. So we will just have to watch them and at a certain point we should probably remove them, but I think we need to hold off on any other kind of surgery until she's a little older. It will be important for her to keep working with the psychologist to make sure she is really ready and comfortable with her choice when the time comes. Does that sound OK?

MOM AND DAD: Sí.

DOCTOR: OK, then, should we call Jessica back in to do a physical exam?

(Jessica is called back into the room.)

DOCTOR: Jessica, I just need to do a quick exam down below like last time. Is that OK with you?

PATIENT: Yes.

DOCTOR: OK, Jessica. I'm just going to measure you here; everything looks just fine. *(to parents)* I'm

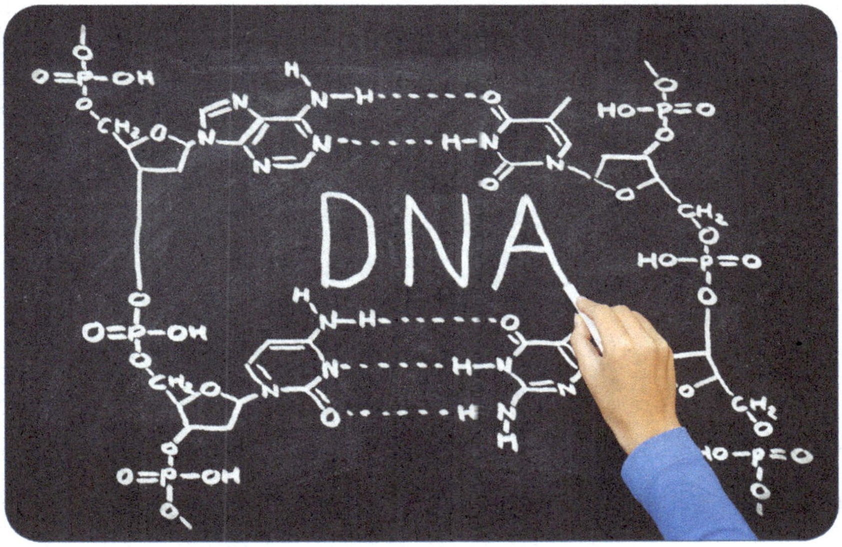

just measuring the size of her clitoris to see if there has been much growth. She looks fine. I don't see much change. *(to patient)* OK, Jess, that's all. You can sit up now. Do you have any questions for me?

PATIENT: No.

DOCTOR: OK. Well, then, we'll see you in about six months. I'll get my assistant to give you a call and we'll set up your next appointment. You'll come early and go to ultrasound first, and then we'll see you up here.

MOM AND DAD: Gracias, doctor.

DOCTOR: You're welcome. It was great to see you, you're doing a wonderful job and Jessica looks great. We'll see you again in November.

Pediatric urology and genetics—gender identity role play (English only)

DOCTOR: *(to interpreter)* Great, you're here. *(to the parents)* I do understand quite a bit of your language but I can't speak it. Hi, I'm Dr. Pavignani, how are you?

MOM: Well, we're fine.

DOCTOR: And how has Jessica been?

MOM: Good.

DOCTOR: You're just here for a regular checkup, right?

MOM: Yes.

DOCTOR: So how's she doing? Have there been any problems or changes since the last time we saw you?

MOM: No. Everything's the same.

DOCTOR: Have you noticed any change in the size of her clitoris? Does it seem to be growing?

MOM: Yes, it does seem to have grown a little.

DOCTOR: Has she noticed it? Does she know she's different? Has anyone at school noticed?

MOM: Uh...I believe so. She was very young before, but yes, she's starting to ask us about it. We've started talking with a psychologist as well.

DOCTOR: Well, that's good. We have a lot to talk about today then. Do you have any specific questions to start with?

MOM: Not really. The questions we have are the same ones we always have, and we always get the same answers.

DOCTOR: Oh, well, what are the questions you have? But before we start, would Jessica like to wait out in the waiting room, or would you rather have her stay here while we talk?

DAD AND MOM: It would be better if she stays in the waiting room. Jessie, do you want to go wait out where the television is?

DOCTOR: Jessica, how about if I talk to your mom and dad a little while, and then one of us will come get you and talk? *(Jessica leaves the room.)*

MOM: Well, the questions we always have are...Why did this happen, what exactly does she have and what can we expect?

DOCTOR: All right. *(silence)*

MOM: We always ask ourselves if we've done the right thing. The doctors told us that according to their experience, we should bring her up as a girl, and that's what we've done, but we wind up asking ourselves if this is what we should be doing. It's just that we saw a program on the television, and what if later on she wants to be a man?

DOCTOR: Well, first of all, if the other doctors you've seen haven't made it clear to both of you yet, this has nothing to do with anything you could or couldn't have done. Your child was born with a condition that was determined before you probably even knew you were pregnant. It's a chromosomal condition, a condition called partial androgen receptor insensitivity. Did the genetics doctors explain all of this to you?

DAD: Well, mostly they just confused us.

DOCTOR: Did they explain about the genetic condition?

DAD: Well, something.

MOM: But like my husband said, we were so crushed and with so many things going on, they got us all confused.

DOCTOR: Well, I'm not a geneticist, but let me see. In every cell in our bodies we have what we call genetic instructions, like a blueprint for development.

DAD: Yes, yes. We're all made up of cells, I remember something about that in a science class.

DOCTOR: And each cell has 46 chromosomes. Chromosomes are strings of instructions. If something is different about them, then it causes a change, so for example, if your blueprint called for 6-inch steel bolts and someone were to use 4-inch steel bolts, or mix the cement wrong, the building might not be as strong.

DAD: *(Both parents turn to the interpreter, looking more puzzled and anxious.)* I'm totally lost with all that stuff about blueprints and cement and bolts.

DOCTOR: I'm sorry. Let's start with the pregnancy. I imagine you know that it starts with conception when the sperm and egg get together.

MOM AND DAD: Right, right.

DOCTOR: Let's say we start out with this fertilized egg, which is like a library. There are millions and millions of cells in the body and they are all copies of that first one. So, let's say that each cell has a library, and in the library there are two copies of each of 23 volumes. So that's 46 books, or 23 pairs of books. Do you understand? Every cell has the library.

MOM AND DAD: Yes.

DOCTOR: Well, the sex cells, the ovum and sperm are different. They have only half the set of instructions each, or one of the two volumes in each pair. They each have half the necessary information for development. Does that sound familiar?

MOM: Yes, yes.

DAD: Yes, a little.

DOCTOR: So, the egg is fertilized by the sperm and they form the first complete cell, or library. Each of you contributed half the information, or half the 23 pairs of books. That's why children look like their parents, just like your daughter looks like you both, right? She received genetic instructions for development from each of you. That's what determines her eye color, hair color, which cells will become the heart, the toenails, etc. Do you understand?

MOM: Yes.

DOCTOR: So that first fertilized egg had a complete set of genetic instructions, and then it started to divide and copy itself, over and over, with all the details, and all the mistakes.

DAD: So then there was a mistake?

DOCTOR: In a way, or just a change. Imagine there are two copies of each book, and these pairs of books are the chromosomes. Imagine if you open up a book and see lots of chapters with pages, lots of lines with sentences, words, all made up of letters. Those lines are like hundreds of instructions for development, which are what we call genes.

DAD: OK, I'm understanding a little better now.

DOCTOR: Now, imagine if one of the lines on a page, or one of the pages, are missing from a book. That could cause big changes in the outcome. Usually, if there is a mistake on one of the lines, there's another set of instructions from the identical volume that formed the pair of books, and we can compensate.

MOM AND DAD: Yes.

DOCTOR: Or you could think of it like a cake recipe with changes in the amount of sugar or salt. The cake would come out differently.

DAD: OK, I get it.

DOCTOR: *(with grammatical mistakes in patient's language)* I understand?

MOM: No, well, yes, I mean, now I'm remembering. But if it's like you say, why do they tell us that it isn't our fault, if everything she is comes from us?

DOCTOR: Well, good question. *(to interpreter)* It shows they understand. *(to parents)* This is nature, or God, or however you see the world. Sometimes things happen that are completely out of our control. We can't control it or cause it. There are several ways this can happen. Sometimes, well, remember the example of the library?

MOM AND DAD: Yes.

DOCTOR: Well, one way a thing like this can happen is at the time of conception, when half the books from the ovum get together with the other books from the sperm. That's a lot of detail and a lot of moving around. Sometimes for example, let's say, a phrase on line 638 from page 232 from chapter six, in volume one, of pair 17, gets mixed up and when the two halves of information get together, that phrase is moving around and then attaches itself to a different volume. That can cause a change. Or a change can happen if both parents have a page ripped out of the same chapter of the same book. When the child receives that chromosome with the missing page, or gene, from both parents, then there is no way to compensate for that. It can also cause a change. If one of the volumes isn't missing the page, then usually things are OK because there's always another copy of the genetic information. Does that seem reasonable?

MOM AND DAD: Yes, yes.

DOCTOR: Other times, maybe the egg or the sperm has *extra* information, so for example, instead of giving one volume of a pair to the forming embryo, it gives two. I'm sure you've seen children with Down syndrome. Those babies have an extra copy of one of the volumes, or in other words, three copies of a book, instead of two books.

MOM: Is that why they told us that there's no cure, no medicine or surgeries or anything?

DOCTOR: Exactly. We can treat the symptoms, for example, do surgery on a defective heart, but in Jessica's case, the change is throughout the whole body because of how cells copy and reproduce themselves.

MOM: Oh, I understand.

DOCTOR: So back to Jessica and her case. Jessica has the condition I mentioned, partial androgen insensitivity syndrome. It isn't as uncommon as you might think. I believe about two to five of every 100,000 people are born this way.

MOM: So then why did they tell us at the beginning that they didn't know what was wrong with her, or if she was a girl or a boy?

DOCTOR: Well, I believe that in the beginning, after they did the prenatal testing, they were concerned that they didn't get a cell sample from more than one place. You see, remember when we talked about the first cell dividing and being duplicated with all its chromosomal arrangements?

MOM AND DAD: Yes.

DOCTOR: Well, sometimes this change or rearrangement doesn't take place at conception. Maybe it takes place after two or four or eight divisions, and only some cells are affected. This is what is sometimes referred to as a mosaic condition. Your baby was born with what appeared to be a large clitoris, but the doctors were concerned that it was a penis. There were vaginal labia, but also scrotal tissue. They wanted to get genetic samples from different tissues in the body before going forward with definitive information. Some children exhibit the appearance of one sex externally, while genetically they are the other. The last of the 23 pairs of chromosomes are either XX or XY, and that is a lot of what determines whether a baby is a girl or a boy. Though researchers are discovering new things all the time, and some scientists think that gender is something much more complicated and determined in multiple places at multiple times during fetal development. Some people go through most of their lives and don't find this out until much later, when they try to have children and have trouble with pregnancy, for example.

DAD: Well, what do you think? Are we doing the right thing?

DOCTOR: You know, first of all, I want you to know that I think you are doing an excellent job. I think this is one of the hardest things for parents to go through. I think you are doing a wonderful job. I know it isn't easy, especially when you aren't sure who you can share this with or how people may react.

MOM: Yes. We still haven't said anything to anybody. Just to my sister, and that was only four or five months ago.

DOCTOR: Well, you are wonderful parents, and Jessica seems like a happy, healthy girl.

MOM: So when do you think we might do the surgery?

DOCTOR: I think that you are talking with Jessica and the psychologist, and that's the right place to start. I have a note here from the psychologist. She says that you've discussed the fact that about 80 percent of children respond to testosterone at puberty. Now, what does that mean for a child like Jessica? It means that many children hit puberty, and suddenly after being raised their whole childhood as a girl, they realize they feel more like a boy. That is why the most recent recommendation is to wait until that time to do any kind of a permanent surgery.

MOM: So we have to wait?

DOCTOR: Yes, I know it's hard, but I know you probably also want what's best for your child. We will need to do regular ultrasounds on her to check the status of the gonads in her abdomen.

DAD: What's that?

DOCTOR: Well, they are the egg cells, they would have become testicles, but in Jessica's case they will never develop and sometimes they can become cancerous. So we will just have to watch them and at a certain point we should probably remove them, but I think we need to hold off on any other kind of surgery until she's a little older. It will be important for her to keep working with the psychologist to make sure she is really ready and comfortable with her choice when the time comes. Does that sound OK?

MOM AND DAD: Yes.

DOCTOR: OK, then, should we call Jessica back in to do a physical exam?

(Jessica is called back into the room.)

DOCTOR: Jessica, I just need to do a quick exam down below like last time. Is that OK with you?

PATIENT: Yes.

DOCTOR: OK, Jessica. I'm just going to measure you here; everything looks just fine. *(to parents)* I'm just measuring the size of her clitoris to see if there has been much growth. She looks fine. I don't see much change. *(to patient)* OK, Jess, that's all. You can sit up now. Do you have any questions for me?

PATIENT: No.

DOCTOR: OK. Well, then we'll see you in about six months. I'll get my assistant to give you a call and we'll set up your next appointment. You'll come early and go to ultrasound first, and then we'll see you up here.

MOM AND DAD: Thank you, doctor.

DOCTOR: You're welcome. It was great to see you, you're doing a wonderful job and Jessica looks great. We'll see you again in November.

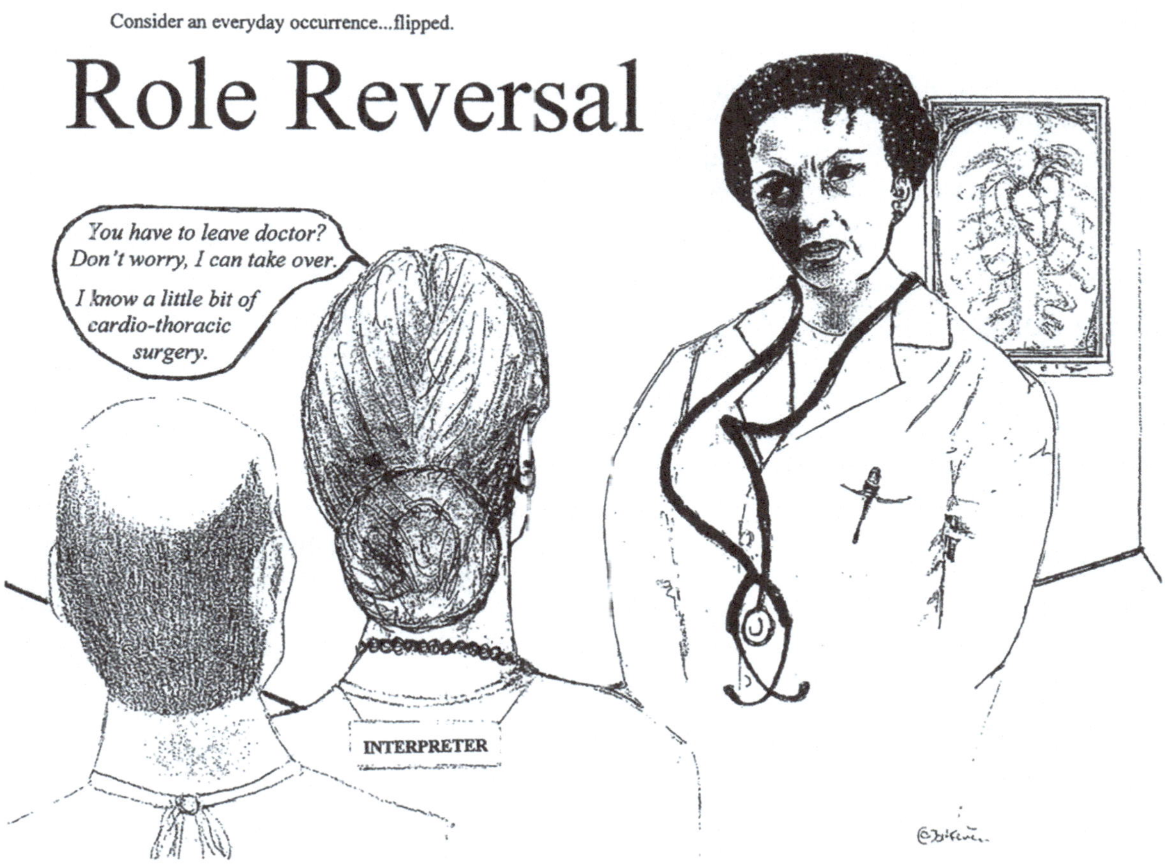

What's important to know about this chapter?

Suggested reading

If you would like to know more about gender identity through reading a work of fiction, you might enjoy a novel called *Middlesex*, a Pulitzer Prize-winning work of fiction by Jeffrey Eugenides published in 2002. In this book you can pick up historical, medical and scientific information about aspects of gender identity. The book itself is entertaining, realistic and often moving. The plot addresses genetics, gender confusion, Greek-Turkish immigrants and race relations in the 1960s in the United States (among other subjects).

Terminology

The following vocabulary is of special importance. Please read it closely and carefully. These definitions are from the website of GLAAD (formerly the Gay & Lesbian Alliance Against Defamation), a U.S. nongovernmental media monitoring organization founded by lesbian/gay/bisexual/transgender (LGBT) people in the media. The GLAAD website is www.glaad.org. You will find glossaries and other educational material and information on the website.

Sex: The classification of people as male or female. At birth infants are assigned a sex, usually based on the appearance of their external anatomy. (This is what is written on the birth certificate.) However, a person's sex is actually a combination of bodily characteristics including: chromosomes, hormones, internal and external reproductive organs and secondary sex characteristics.

Gender Identity: One's internal, deeply held sense of one's gender. For transgender people, their own internal gender identity does not match the sex they were assigned at birth. Most people have a gender identity of man or woman (or boy or girl). For some people, their gender identity does not fit neatly into one of those two choices. Unlike gender expression (see below) gender identity is not visible to others.

Gender Expression: External manifestations of gender, expressed through one's name, pronouns, clothing, haircut, behavior, voice, or body characteristics. Society identifies these cues as masculine and feminine, although what is considered masculine and feminine changes over time and varies by culture. Typically, transgender people seek to make their gender expression align with their gender identity, rather than the sex they were assigned at birth.

Sexual Orientation: Describes an individual's enduring physical, romantic and/or emotional attraction to another person. Gender identity and sexual orientation are not the same. Transgender people may be straight, lesbian, gay or bisexual. For example, a person who transitions from male to female and is attracted solely to men would identify as a straight woman.

Interpreter and social gender identity attitudes

What attitudes do we each have toward children with undetermined (the genitalia of an infant or child does not clearly suggest a gender), unassigned (health providers and/or parents may choose not to declare a child's gender), or nonconforming (a person appears and/or behaves like someone of a gender that does not match the gender assigned at birth), gender identity and expression? Do those attitudes change with regard to adults?

Urology

This specialty involves the bladder, kidneys and conduits, such as the ureter and urethra. Obviously, it will involve a lot of discussion of urination. There are many ways to talk about urination both formally and informally, with children and adults—for example, *urinate*, *pee*, *piss* and *number one*. Can you think of others? What about similar terms in your other working language(s)? Follow the lead of the speakers and try to maintain the register.

It may come as a surprise when you interpret in urology, but there may also be a lot of discussion about bowel movements, also known as *pooping*. It turns out that constipation in children often has a lot to do with bladder infections. While these systems are separate, constipation can keep people from completely emptying their bladders, where urine can remain and become infected. Regarding bowel movements, be prepared both psychologically and in terms of your vocabulary in your working languages to talk about texture, color, form, shape and frequency. Be sure that your face and body language do not reflect your own feelings but those of the speakers.

Urology also involves the genitals. You may interpret information about conditions such as hypospadias, difficulty with intercourse or circumcision. Review the graphic and corresponding vocabulary that accompanies this dialogue.

Child patient and parents

The interpreter is present for everyone, to facilitate clear communication. The age of the child may change how you interpret. When children are young, interpreting to them in first person can be confusing. If you try to speak in first person and the child gets confused, switch to third person, for example, "The doctor wants to listen to your heart now." When children grow older and develop more abstract thinking, often after the age of eight or so, you can interpret for them as you usually would. As much as possible, follow the doctor's and guardian's lead and see how well the child appears to understand.

Formal or informal—adolescents

If you are interpreting in a language that has formal and informal pronouns and corresponding grammar, which should you use when speaking with an adolescent or young adult? There is no distinction in English, so you will have to gauge the effects if your other language requires that you make a choice. If you use the informal with an adolescent, you may make them feel like a child, which can be demeaning or a relief for them. If you speak to them in a formal adult manner, you may be empowering them and establishing rapport and respect, or unduly burdening or confusing them. Use your best judgment.

Direct or indirect—elders and children or caretakers

A situation where you are interpreting for a provider and an elder in the presence of a grown child or

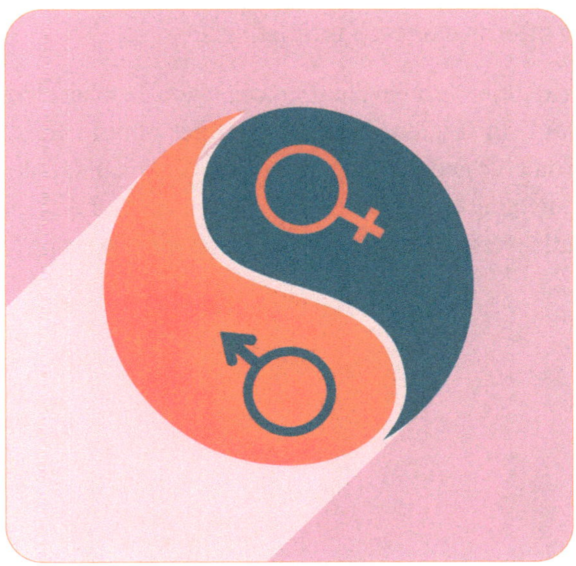

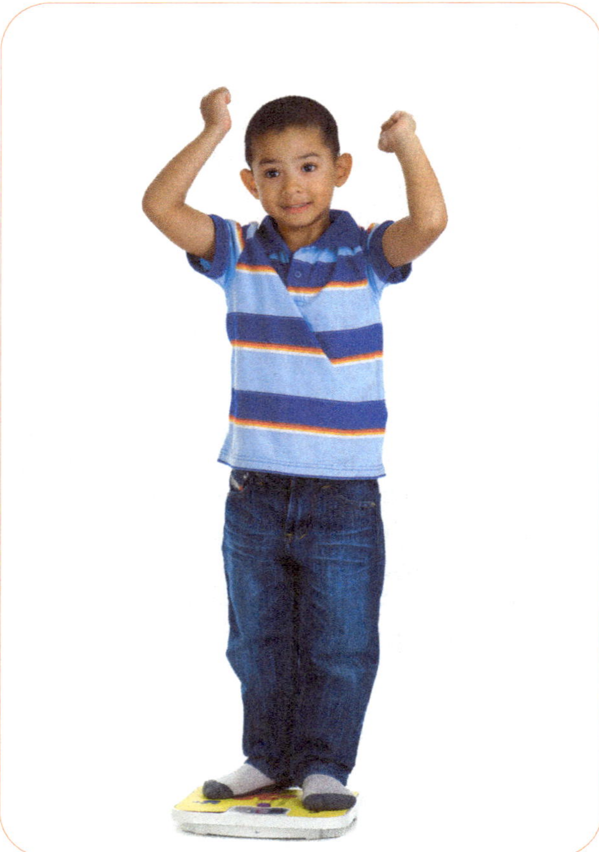

caretaker can lead to questions for interpreters. For example, when a patient is an older adult, some doctors may ignore them and have a conversation with the grown child or caretaker about the patient. If the elder is mentally competent and aware, this can be offensive or even infuriating.

In addition, grown children can override what elders want. In this case, the interpreter should follow protocols and interpret as she usually would, unless something compels her to do otherwise. Is the elderly patient attempting to speak but no one is hearing? Is the grown child contradicting the patient, who is not being heard? These are situations that might lead an interpreter to consider advocacy, which is discussed in the "Guide to Advocacy" introductory section in this book.

Gender identity

In the same way that some languages require you to speak formally or informally, other languages require you to specify gender. Beyond pronouns, some languages require you to speak to males and females in different ways—and you have to use one or the other. If this is your situation, how would you speak to a transgender or nongender-conforming person? Other languages have only one third-person pronoun and it is genderless, not *he* or *she*. In this dialogue, the parents have a child with undetermined gender, but they have chosen to raise her as a girl, with a girl's name. Here the interpreter does not have to make a split-second decision.

How can you tell if someone should be addressed as male, female or transgender, and what does that mean for your second language? If you work with a patient whose gender you cannot tell (because the patient has both "feminine" and "masculine" features and mannerisms), you might possibly get help from the patient name. However, some names are used for both males and females (e.g., Terry, Kim, Jamie). You may also see a conflict in names on different records, identifications (IDs) or the electronic records; a patient may be "Justin" on one record and "Justina" on another. Ask a provider, if you can. You can also introduce yourself to the patient and say, "Hello, I am _____, your interpreter. What may I call you?" or ask in some other polite way how the patient would like to be addressed.

Ethics and standards: Reflect and practice

Goal 7: Professionalism

Translation and paraphrasing

1. Look at the eight NCIHC standards of practice related to professionalism (Standards 19-26, NCIHC, 2005, p. 10). Working individually, *paraphrase* the objective, its related ethical principle and the six standards.
2. Working individually, *translate* the original text of these standards into your other working language(s) or interpret it into sign language.
3. Find a partner or partners. Compare, discuss and modify your translations and paraphrasing until you are satisfied with your final products as a group.
4. If you can, pick a group representative and discuss your final versions with any other groups that share your working languages. Compare and discuss your differences.

Suggested reading

Roat, C. E. (2010). *Healthcare Interpreting in Small Bites: 50 Nourishing Selections from the "Pacific Interpreters Newsletter," 2002-2010.* Victoria, British Columbia: Trafford, pp. 89-93.

Consider and discuss

1. Write your own definition of the word *professional* in the context of medical interpreters and interpreting. What does this word mean to you?
2. **Standard 19** What are some of the purposes of interpreter credentials? What are the purposes of any type of credential? Discuss the benefits of a standard measure of competency, for example, among lawyers or nurses. How would a standard national measure of interpreter competency benefit the interpreting profession? How might it help and hurt interpreters?
3. **Standard 20** What are some resources for enhancing your medical terminology? Where might you be able to practice medical interpretation outside of a clinical appointment?
4. **Standard 21** An interpreter is assigned with advance notice to a genetics appointment. When

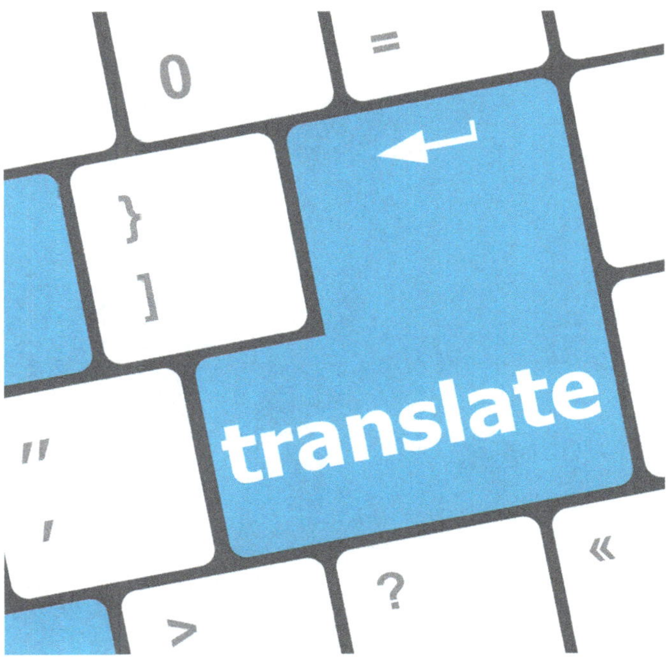

he comes across the term *deoxyribonucleic acid (DNA)* in the assignment, should he know how to interpret the term, should he know what it means, or both? Why or why not? What is deoxyribonucleic acid (DNA)?

5. **Standard 21** An interpreter finds herself in an assignment with complicated terminology regarding physiology at the cellular level (mitochondrial DNA, amino acid deficiencies, metabolic conditions, different functions of specific immune cells, etc.) that she is unfamiliar with: she is lost. What should she do?
6. **Standard 22** What are some of the problems associated with the sight translations of long, complex, legally binding standard forms that are vital? What are the obligations of an institution in the United States receiving federal funds (such as Medicaid payments, grants, used equipment) with regard to written translation of standard "vital forms" when those forms are needed by a significant percentage of a patient population? What are some examples of vital forms? (Try searching for this information at www.lep.gov and other government websites.)
7. **Standard 23** This standard states that as the interpreter you are accountable for your own performance. Do you agree or disagree? Why?
8. **Standard 24** How might fatigue compromise interpreter performance? Do a search online (using the quotation marks) for the document, "Remote interpreting: Assessment of human factors and performance parameters" (Moser-Mercer, 2003). Read the abstract section. What happens to interpreter performance after 30 minutes of remote interpreting?
9. **Standard 24** How could you convince an employer to pay for continuing education for interpreters, interpreter participation in professional conferences and to prepare for or sit for national or other certifications? Give at least two reasons why this investment would benefit the interpreter's employer.
10. **Standard 25** Healthcare providers sometimes complain to an interpreter about the performance or behavior of another interpreter—who is perhaps the interpreter's colleague. Some of the complaints are valid. How should a professional interpreter handle these remarks?

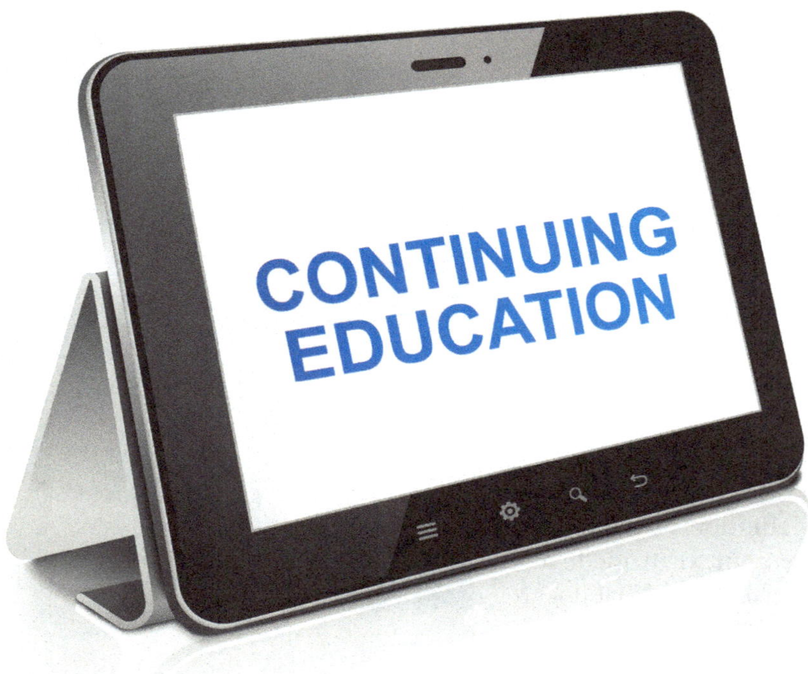

Occupational therapy for interpreters

EXERCISES FOR THE TONGUE, HEART AND MIND

You will now revisit part of the original role play dialogue in this chapter. In this version, the interpreter takes action. Each time the interpreter speaks or acts, decide if you agree with what the interpreter did by answering the questions that follow each excerpt.

Then read the commentary that follows the eight excerpts and see if you want to change any of your answers.

> *Interpreter alert! Where does this interpreter's conduct fall in the range between impartial interpreter and patient advocate, or is it entirely unprofessional? Under what circumstances, if any, should an interpreter engage in the interventions described below?*

PART 1

INTERPRETER: *(observes that the parents look somewhat bewildered)* Dr. Pavignani, as the interpreter, I need to clarify something, I think they might need some clarification. *(to parents)* Has anyone ever explained to you the meaning of the words *chromosomes* and *genes*? Do you know what he's referring to when he talks about a genetic condition?

DAD: Well, a little bit.

MOM: But like my husband said, we were so upset dealing with so many things, more than anything we just got confused.

Do you agree that the interpreter here did the right thing? Circle your answer.

YES NO MAYBE

Why did you agree or disagree with the interpreter's intervention?

PART 2

INTERPRETER: *(to doctor)* They definitely need more information and there is confusion. Can you go back and start with an explanation of what genes and chromosomes are? *(to parents)* I'm telling the doctor that he needs to explain all of this again because it still hasn't been explained to you well.

DOCTOR: *(to interpreter)* Why don't you go ahead?

Do you agree that the interpreter here did the right thing? Circle your answer

YES NO MAYBE

Why did you agree or disagree with the interpreter's intervention?

PART 3

DOCTOR: *(to interpreter)* Why don't you go ahead?

INTERPRETER: I don't know; I'm not really supposed to do that. I mean, you're the doctor. I'm the interpreter.

DOCTOR: Well, that's true, let me see. I'm not a geneticist, so if you have any questions, please ask me at any time. Now, let me see. In every cell in our bodies we have what we call genetic instructions, like a blueprint for development.

Do you agree that the interpreter here did the right thing? Circle your answer.

YES NO MAYBE

Why did you agree or disagree with the interpreter's intervention?

PART 4

INTERPRETER: *(After interpreting the doctor's statement above, the interpreter asks the parents.)* Dr. Pavignani, the interpreter needs to clarify some terms with the parents. *(to parents)* Do you know what a cell is? Did you have an opportunity to study that in school?

DAD: Yes, yes. We are all made up of cells, I remember something about that in a science class.

INTERPRETER: *(to doctor)* Well, they know what cells are. But I think you need to start with the basics about genes and chromosomes.

Do you agree that the interpreter here did the right thing? Circle your answer.

YES NO MAYBE

Why did you agree or disagree with the interpreter's intervention?

PART 5

DOCTOR: And each cell has 46 chromosomes. Chromosomes are strings of instructions. If something is different about them, then it causes a change, so for example, if your blueprint called for 6-inch steel bolts and someone were to use 4-inch steel bolts, or mix the cement wrong, the building might not be as strong.

DAD: *(Both parents turn to interpreter, looking more puzzled and anxious.)* I'm totally lost with all that stuff about blueprints and cement and bolts.

INTERPRETER: *(to doctor)* They're really lost.

Do you agree that the interpreter here did the right thing? Circle your answer.

YES NO MAYBE

Why did you agree or disagree with the interpreter's intervention?

PART 6

DOCTOR: *(to interpreter)* Can you give it a try? You've probably spent a lot of time in the genetics clinic.[41]

> **INTERPRETER:** Yes, I have, and I actually know this family from lots of other appointments. But it's really not my role.

DOCTOR: Are you sure?

> **INTERPRETER:** It's probably better left to you, but I have a suggestion. I've heard doctors use models of kitchen recipes and file cabinets, but I heard a geneticist here use a library as a model. Two copies of each volume for two copies of each chromosome and pages, lines, words and letters for deleted or rearranged genetic info. That comparison seemed to help.

Do you agree that the interpreter here did the right thing? Circle your answer.

YES NO MAYBE

Why did you agree or disagree with the interpreter's intervention?

PART 7

DOCTOR: Jessica, I just need to do a quick exam down below like last time. Is that OK with you?

PATIENT: Yes.

> **INTERPRETER:** *(to the patient, who speaks English)* Jessica, do you want me to go outside? I can go out until after your exam. Your mom can stay here with you. You know it's OK for the doctor to examine you because your mom is here and she says it's OK. Right?

41 Interpreter alert! Where does this interpreter's conduct fall in the range between neutral party and patient advocate, or is it entirely off the grid? Under what circumstances, if any, should an interpreter do this?

PART 8

PATIENT: You can stay, I don't care.

INTERPRETER: OK, I'll just sit over here with your dad, behind this curtain *(interpreter draws the curtain between chairs and the exam table for patient privacy).*

Do you agree that the interpreter here did the right thing? Circle your answer.

YES NO MAYBE

Why did you agree or disagree with the interpreter's intervention?

Commentaries

Now read the commentaries about each of the eight excerpts and see if you want to change any of your answers.

Commentary on Part 1

INTERPRETER: *(observes that the parents look somewhat bewildered.)* Dr. Pavignani, as the interpreter, I need to clarify something, I think they might need some clarification. *(to parents)* Has anyone ever explained to you the meaning of the words *chromosomes* and *genes*? Do you know what he's referring to when he talks about a genetic condition?

DAD: Well, a little bit.

MOM: But like my husband said, we were so upset dealing with so many things, more than anything we just got confused.

This interpreter has crossed a line. First, the interpreter was not transparent: she did not say the same thing to the parents that she said to the doctor. Why didn't she say, "I just told the doctor I needed to clarify something because I think you might need some clarification"? How might that message sound to the patient?

Also, instead of suggesting to the doctor that there might be a possible misunderstanding about chromosomes, genes or genetic conditions, and then allowing the doctor to check for understanding, the interpreter checked for understanding herself, but doing so, as discussed in the previous chapter, is the provider's job.

Say *you* check for the patient's understanding. Now the doctor doesn't realize that he needs to be checking for understanding—instead, this looks like a task that is better to leave to the interpreter. The doctor is missing an opportunity to realize the importance of improving his communication skills.

Look at it this way. Nagging your children or spouse to do more house chores is work. It's often easier just to do it yourself, right? Actually, no. It might feel easier in the short term to do the work yourself, but in the long run it's more work for you, taking time from your schedule—and then your family members are not learning their own responsibilities and duties.

In this medical case, the doctor probably has the same communication problems with other patients but not all interpreters might be as alert to misunderstandings as you are. The doctor needs to start changing and perhaps simplifying the way he communicates. In short, help the *provider* to check for understanding. Don't do it yourself.

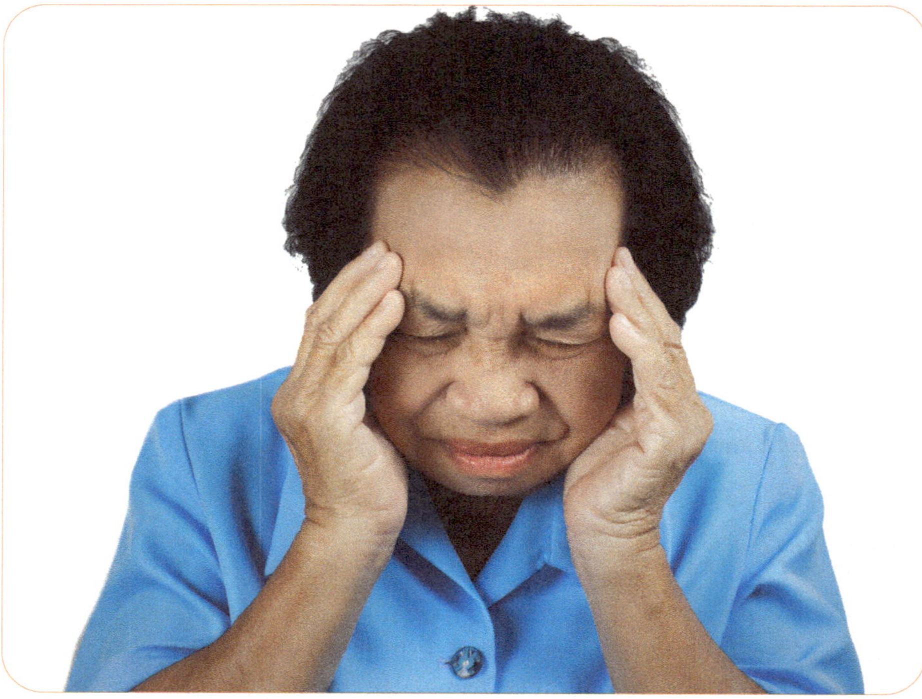

Commentary on Part 2

> **INTERPRETER:** *(to doctor)* They definitely need more information and there is confusion. Can you go back and start with an explanation of what genes and chromosomes are? *(to parents)* I'm telling the doctor that he needs to explain all of this again because it still hasn't been explained to you well.

DOCTOR: *(to interpreter)* Why don't you go ahead?

Oh-oh! Once again, this interpreter is not transparent. Why not? Imagine telling the doctor, "I just informed the parents you need to explain all this again because it still hasn't been explained to them well." Or imagine telling the parents that you told the doctor what to say and also told him how to say it.

This interpreter might not have been transparent because unconsciously she knew how being transparent might sound—in this case, perhaps unprofessional, inappropriate or domineering (depending partly on the tone of voice and body language). Also, telling the doctor how to do the job is really not *your* job. Your job in this case is to make sure the doctor finds out what the parents didn't understand so that the doctor can explain it more clearly.

Commentary on Part 3

DOCTOR: *(to interpreter)* Why don't you go ahead?

> **INTERPRETER:** I don't know; I'm not really supposed to do that. I mean, you're the doctor. I'm the interpreter.

DOCTOR: Well, that's true, let me see. I'm not a geneticist, so if you have any questions, please ask me at any time. Now, let me see. In every cell in our bodies we have what we call genetic instructions, like a blueprint for development.

Ah! So now the interpreter realizes she stepped out of role! But what an awkward moment. How professional does the interpreter sound in this part? Acting on her own advice ("I'm not really supposed to do that") could have avoided this awkward situation.

Commentary on Part 4

Interpreter: *(After interpreting the doctor's statement above, the interpreter asks the parents.)* Dr. Pavignani, the interpreter needs to clarify some terms with the parents. *(to parents)* Do you know what a cell is? Did you have an opportunity to study that in school?

> **DAD:** Yes, yes. We are all made up of cells, I remember something about that in a science class.

> **INTERPRETER:** *(to doctor)* Well, they know what cells are. But I think you need to start with the basics about genes and chromosomes.

Once again, the interpreter is telling the doctor what to do and taking over the doctor's role, asking the parents questions, making decisions about how much the parents do or do not understand based on their medical knowledge. This is the doctor's decision. Help the doctor to take the right action to find out how much the parents do or don't know.

Commentary on Part 5

DOCTOR: And each cell has 46 chromosomes. Chromosomes are strings of instructions. If something is different about them, then it causes a change, so for example, if your blueprint called for 6-inch steel bolts and someone were to use 4-inch steel bolts, or mix the cement wrong, the building might not be as strong.

> **DAD:** *(Both parents turn to interpreter, looking more puzzled and anxious.)* I'm totally lost with all that stuff about blueprints and cement and bolts.

INTERPRETER: *(to doctor)* They're really lost.

The interpreter here needs to interpret what the father said, not summarize it. The information that the interpreter omitted (perhaps to avoid offending the doctor) could really help the doctor to understand the problem better.

Commentary on Part 6

DOCTOR: *(to interpreter)* Can you give it a try? You've probably spent a lot of time in the genetics clinic.

INTERPRETER: Yes, I have, and I actually know this family from lots of other appointments. But it's really not my role.

DOCTOR: Are you sure?

INTERPRETER: It's probably better left to you, but I have a suggestion. I've heard doctors use models of kitchen recipes and file cabinets, but I heard a geneticist here use a library as a model. Two copies of each volume for two copies of each chromosome and pages, lines, words and letters for deleted or rearranged genetic info. That comparison seemed to help.

When the doctor asks the interpreter, "Can you give it a try? You've probably spent a lot of time in the genetics clinic." (*Can you just take over and practice medicine for me?*) Under what circumstances, if any, should an interpreter do what the doctor suggests? The answer is simple: The interpreter should not be providing medical information or medical explanations of any kind to patients or families, *even if healthcare providers ask them to do so.*

Such requests are not unusual, by the way. Be ready to know what to say. For example, "I'd be happy to interpret anything you suggest, or I could interpret for a health educator if you'd like to bring one in. As the interpreter, I'm not ethically permitted to provide health information for reasons of liability, professional ethics and lack of training." (The fact is that you are also not permitted to practice medicine.) Whatever you say, be sure to report it to the other party.

Commentary on Part 7

DOCTOR: Jessica, I just need to do a quick exam down below like last time. Is that OK with you?

PATIENT: Yes.

INTERPRETER: *(to the patient, who speaks English)* Jessica, do you want me to go outside? I can go out until after your exam. Your mom can stay here with you. You know it's OK for the doctor to examine you because your mom is here and she says it's OK. Right?

The interpreter in this dialogue made a decision here to add something that was not spoken by anyone present. In short, the interpreter (again) stepped out of role. Say that she makes a conscious, personal choice to breach interpreting ethical guidelines. What might the motives be? What could the consequences be? What would *you* do?

In general, such action would be considered *advocacy* and there does not appear to be any justification for advocacy in this situation. See the introductory section of this book, "Guide to Advocacy," which addresses advocacy, for details.

Commentary on Part 8

PATIENT: You can stay, I don't care.

INTERPRETER: OK, I'll just sit over here with your dad, behind this curtain *(interpreter draws the curtain between chairs and the exam table for patient privacy).*

In this case, the interpreter is not transparent with the parents while she spoke to the child in English, which is absolutely necessary, but otherwise the interpreter is acting in role. The interpreter should not leave, since the parents might have questions, but the interpreter should still respect privacy. As long as there is no reason for the interpreter *not* to be behind the curtain with the father, the interpreter's decision and conduct here (except for the lack of transparency) is perfectly appropriate.

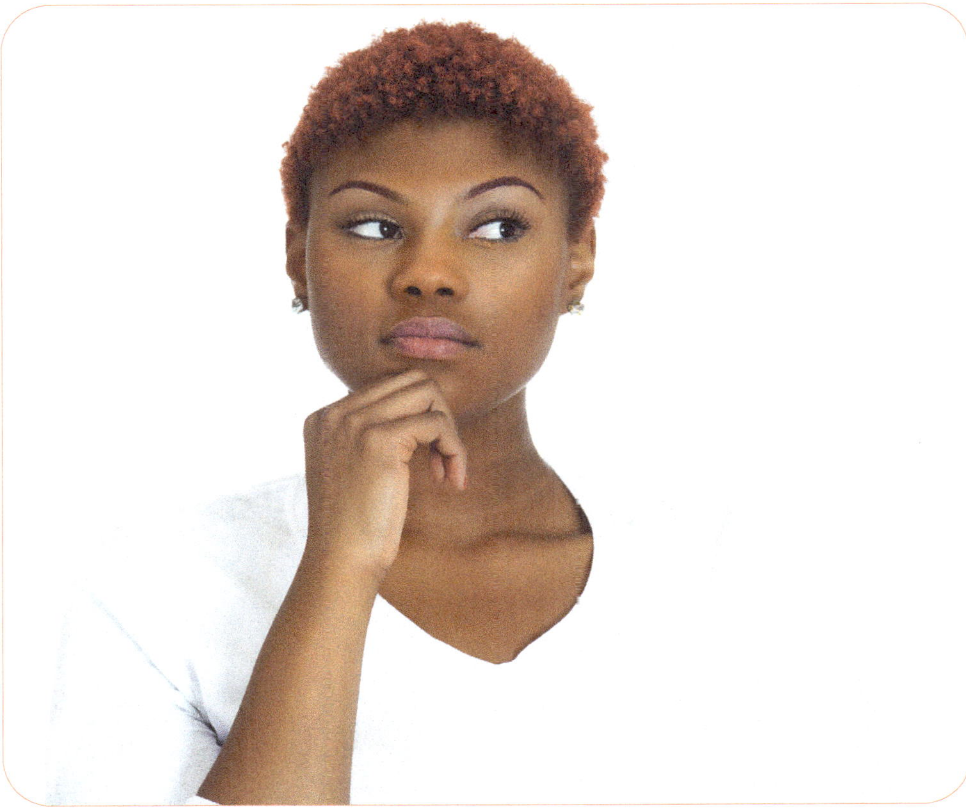

Medical terminology: The male and the female genitourinary systems

Below you will find anatomical drawings relevant to the content of this chapter. Follow the instructions found at the end of Chapter 1 to study the terminology in this section.

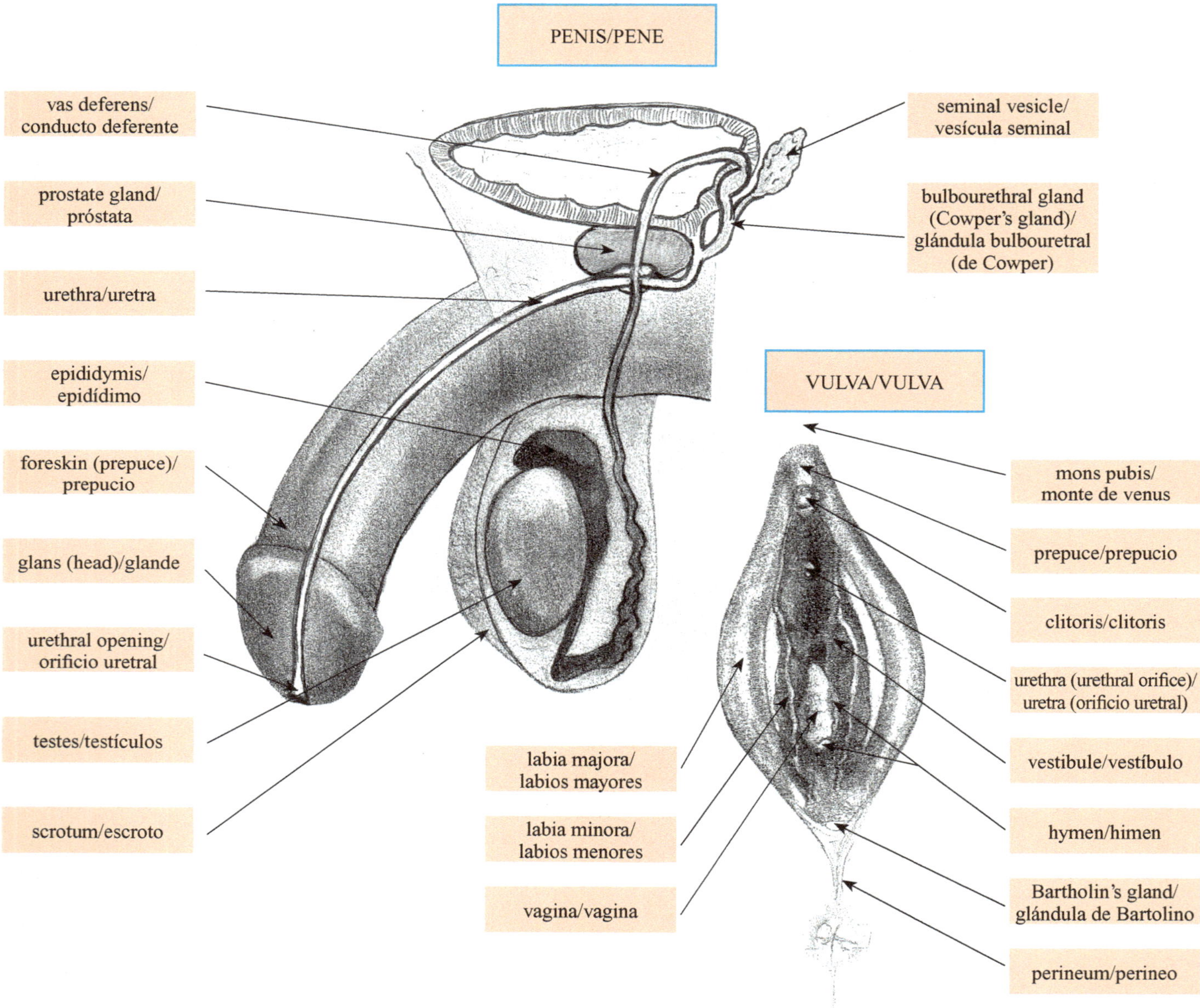

Figure 7-A: The male and the female genitourinary systems (English and Spanish)

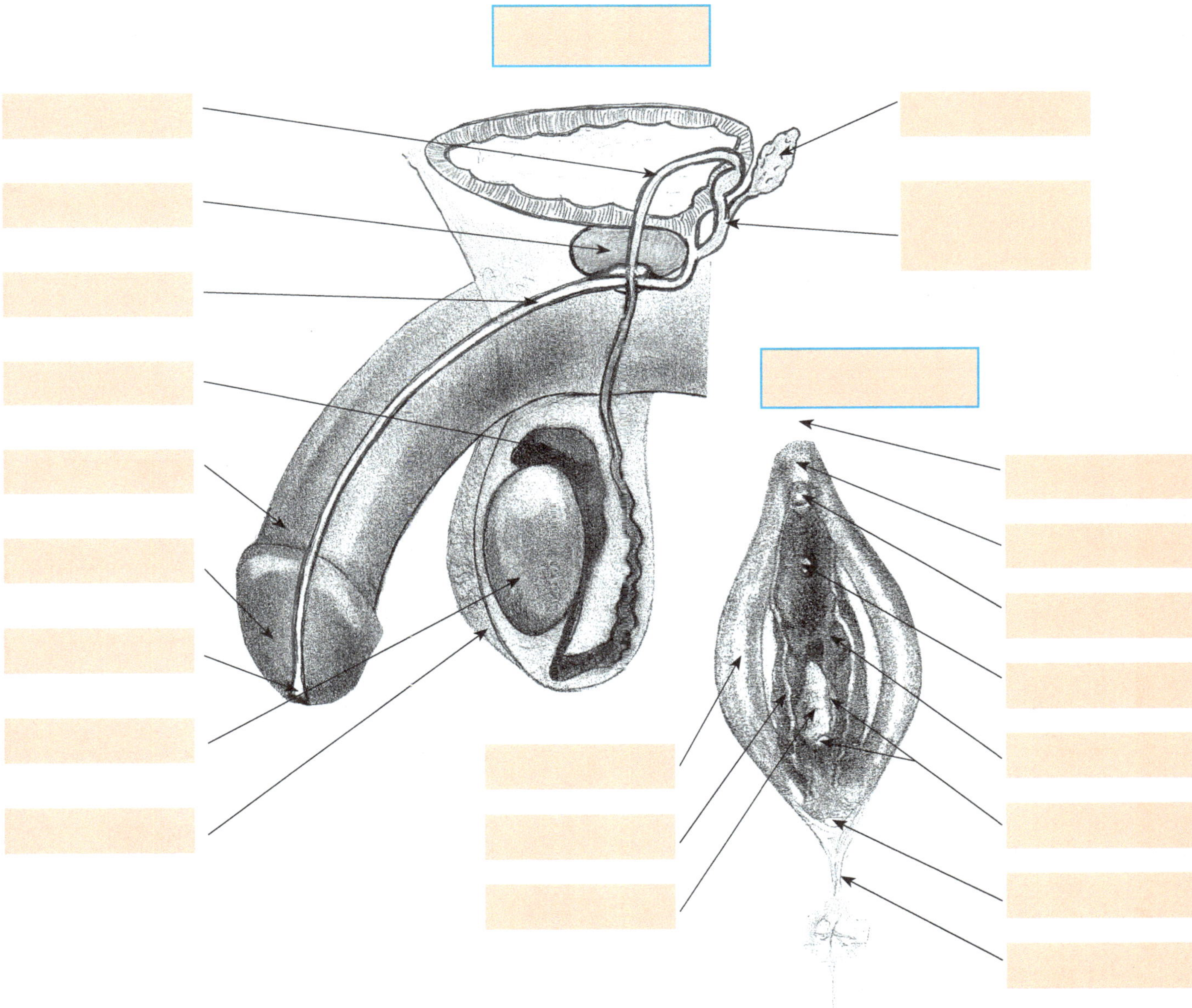

Figure 7-B: The male and the female genitourinary systems (blank labels)

Medical terminology list

The male and the female genitourinary systems

VOCABULARY FOR GRAPHIC–IN ENGLISH	VOCABULARY FOR GRAPHIC–IN SPANISH	ANY OTHER LANGUAGE
FEMININE	FEMENINO	
Bartholin's gland	glándula de Bartolino	
clitoris	clítoris	
hymen	himen	
labia	labios	
labia majora	labios mayores	
labia minora	labios menores	
mons pubis	monte de venus	
ovarian ligament	ligamento ovárico	
perineum	perineo	
prepuce	prepucio	
urethra (urethral orifice)	uretra (orificio uretral)	
vagina	vagina	
vestibule	vestíbulo	
vulva	vulva	
MASCULINE	MASCULINO	
bulbourethral gland (Cowper's gland)	glándula bulbouretral (de Cowper)	
ejaculatory duct	conducto eyaculatorio	
epididymis	epidídimo	
foreskin (prepuce)	prepucio	
glans (head)	glande	
penis	pene	
prostate gland	próstata	
scrotum	escroto	
seminal vesicle	vesícula seminal	
testes	testículos	
urethra	uretra	
urethral opening	orificio uretral	
vas deferens	conducto deferente	

Gynecology 8

Advisory

This chapter involves some material about gynecology, cancer and gynecological procedures.

This patient is a 58-year-old woman who has come in for a checkup with her primary care women's health practitioner. She has lived through a war. She is a patient with a long history of coming to her appointments complaining of many symptoms and complaints, including stomach pain and depression. It appears that her healthcare providers have not explored the possibility that her wartime experiences have had a deep psychological impact that might affect her physical health and/or her perception of her own health.

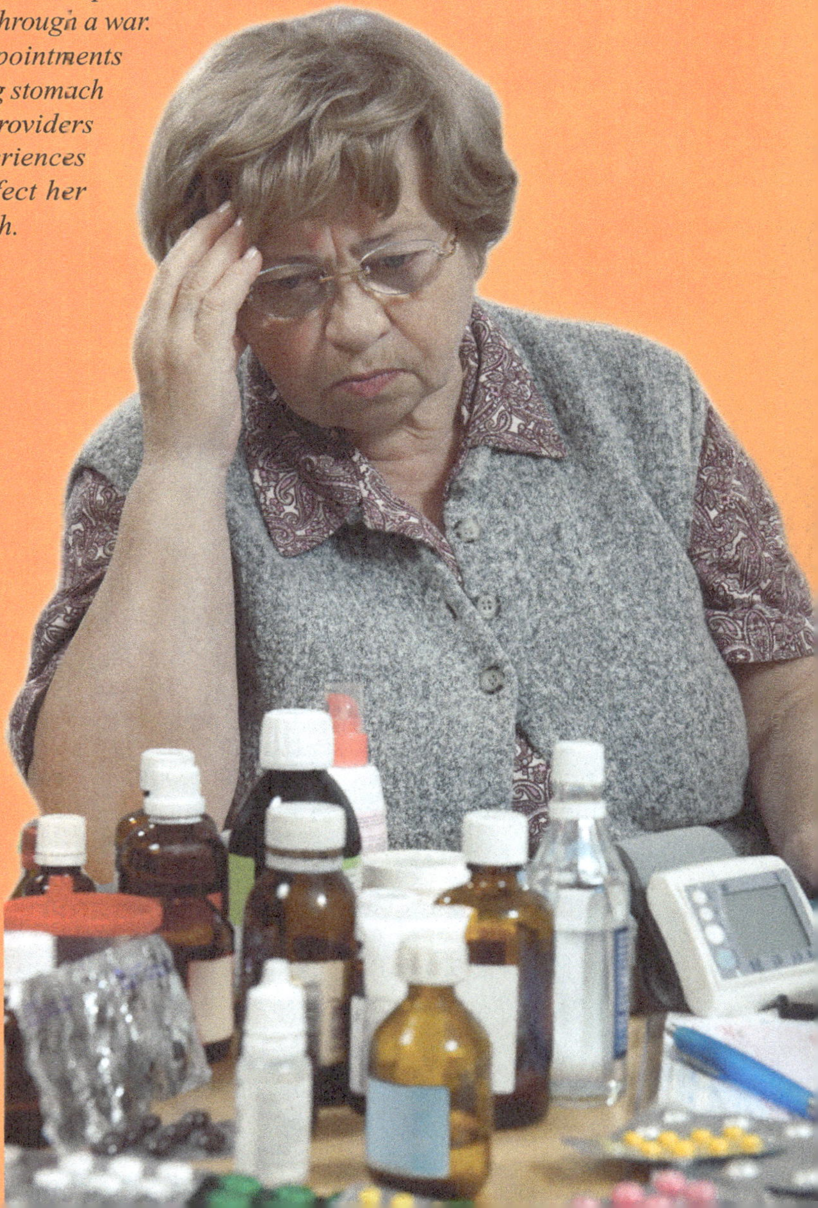

Gynecology role play (English-Spanish)

NURSE PRACTITIONER: Good morning, Mrs. Fuentes. How can I help you today?

PATIENT: Pues, creo que tengo una infección en la orina. También quiero que me haga un examen de la matriz. Mi mamá se murió de cáncer de la matriz y quiero que me haga un examen, una biopsia.

NURSE PRACTITIONER: All right. Now what makes you think you have a bladder infection?

PATIENT: Cuando orino, me arde mucho.

NURSE PRACTITIONER: Well, let's see. My assistant just came back with your urine sample. It doesn't show any bacteria, so I don't think you have a bladder infection or a urinary tract infection. Do you think it might be the outside, your labia, when you urinate?

PATIENT: Pues, puede ser, sí.

NURSE PRACTITIONER: Well, I think there may be some chafing or some atrophy. Let's take a look. Maybe you need some kind of hormone cream. Let me look at your chart.

PATIENT: También me arde todo mi cuerpo. A veces siento que me estoy quemando.

NURSE PRACTITIONER: First of all, didn't you have an endometrial biopsy not too long ago? If I remember correctly, it was very difficult for you. Now we don't want to repeat that if it's not necessary. Ah, here it is, yes, we did a biopsy in June, the results are here and everything is fine. Now is there a reason why you want that done again? Has something changed?

PATIENT: Pues, quiero que me diga si tengo cáncer. También quiero que me haga un examen de Papanicolau, no me lo han hecho en tres años.

NURSE PRACTITIONER: Well, let's see. You've been coming here for about that long. And I've been seeing you. I can't believe that it's been all that time and nobody ever did a Pap smear, especially if they did an endometrial biopsy. Oh, it looks like you're right, it has been that long. Wow. Well, I guess you've just been coming here for acute problems and we've been dealing with those.

PATIENT: Sí.

NURSE PRACTITIONER: Now, the Pap smear is just a scraping of cells from the cervix, not from the uterine lining, so we won't have to insert the tube.

PATIENT: Sí. Mire, doctora, también necesito un mamograma. Tengo mucho cáncer en mi familia. A mi hermana le tuvieron que quitar un pecho.

NURSE PRACTITIONER: Right, now let's see. It looks like you had one six months ago. Why did you go over to the cancer center?

PATIENT: Usted me dijo que fuera porque me encontré una bolita en el pecho.

NURSE PRACTITIONER: Oh, yes, well, it looks like you went and the doctors said everything is fine, but you are due for a follow-up exam and a mammogram. It looks like they wanted you to come back in six months.

PATIENT: Sí. Tengo una cita para el veintiuno, pero necesito que usted me dé la orden. Siempre que llego para hacerme el mamograma, me dicen que me falta algún papel.

NURSE PRACTITIONER: Actually, I don't think you should have any problem with that since the cancer center already recommended the follow-up appointment, but I'll take care of it before you go. Now let's get back to your original complaint. You said you're having hot flashes?

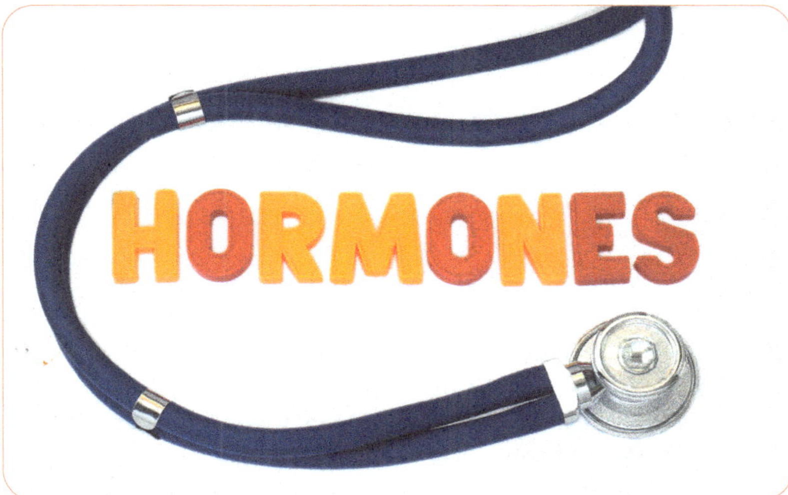

PATIENT: Sí.

NURSE PRACTITIONER: Are you still taking the hormones?

PATIENT: No, tengo tres meses de no tomarlas.

NURSE PRACTITIONER: Why is that?

PATIENT: Usted me dijo que las suspendiera.

NURSE PRACTITIONER: I think it's just a question of finding a balance. You know if you take them, we can regulate your bleeding and alleviate your hot flashes, but you may have breast tenderness again. If the hot flashes are really bothering you, I think we should try hormones again. We can try a different dose. There are many kinds we can try.

PATIENT: Está bien, pero yo no quiero esas que tomé la vez pasada. Creo que el problema fue que en la farmacia me dieron estas hormonas que son genéticamente modificadas.

NURSE PRACTITIONER: Genetically modified? Do you mean—generic medications?

> **PATIENT:** Pues sí, algo así, pero yo no quiero esta medicina. Quiero medicina verdadera y no esa que tiene la genérica o genética como usted dice.

NURSE PRACTITIONER: Mrs. Fuentes, "generic" just means that what I prescribed was the same medicine, but made by a different company. The pharmacy was probably giving it to you because it's not covered by your health plan and the generic medicine is much less expensive, but it's not genetically modified. That's a completely different thing.

> **PATIENT:** Pues, yo no quiero esas cosas genéricas o genéticas, yo les tengo miedo.

NURSE PRACTITIONER: OK. We'll write you a new prescription and you can get the original medication, not a generic brand. But I don't think that was the problem. I think maybe we just need to do a different dose. Would you like to try that? Hopefully you won't have the breast tenderness.

> **PATIENT:** Sí, está bien.

NURSE PRACTITIONER: Great. Right now, I'd like to do your Pap smear and a breast exam. We really don't need to do another biopsy because you had one relatively recently. It sounds like you're set up for your next mammogram, which I'll give you a referral for. And I'll write you a new prescription for hormones. Now, let's talk about the burning.

> **PATIENT:** Está bien.

NURSE PRACTITIONER: I'm also going to give you some samples of this hormone cream for the burning. Now, I only want you to use this cream for a few weeks. Just put a little bit on your fingertips and rub it on the outside, on the labia, not inside the vagina. Once you're taking the hormones it should get better. All right? I think the burning sensation is caused by dry tissues from a drop in hormonal levels. When the urine hits those dry tissues it can feel like burning. I really think that's what's going on.

> **PATIENT:** Sí, entonces ¿no la pongo allí dentro de mi parte?

NURSE PRACTITIONER: Not inside, only outside, where you have the burning, on the labia. Now, I think we can get through the rest of the appointment without the interpreter. Do you have any questions for me before we do the exam?

> **PATIENT:** *(to interpreter)* Oh, ¿usted se va?

(LET THE INTERPRETER RESPOND.)

> **PATIENT:** No tengo más preguntas. Pero oiga, dígame algo. Ella es judía, ¿no? Parece que todos los doctores aquí son judíos. ¿Ella es judía? Siempre son judíos. Pues mejor que si fuera negra. O musulmana. ¿Es judía?

(LET THE INTERPRETER RESPOND.)

NURSE PRACTITIONER: What did she just say?

Gynecology role play (English only)

NURSE PRACTITIONER: Good morning, Mrs. Fuentes. How can I help you today?

PATIENT: Well, I think I have a urine infection. I also want you to do an exam on my uterus. My mother died of cancer of the uterus, and I want you to check me, to do a biopsy.

NURSE PRACTITIONER: All right. Now what makes you think you have a bladder infection?

PATIENT: When I urinate, it burns a lot.

NURSE PRACTITIONER: Well, let's see. My assistant just came back with your urine sample. It doesn't show any bacteria, so I don't think you have a bladder infection or a urinary tract infection. Do you think it might be the outside, your labia, when you urinate?

PATIENT: Well, it could be, yes.

NURSE PRACTITIONER: Well, I think there may be some chafing or some atrophy. Let's take a look. Maybe you need some kind of hormone cream. Let me look at your chart.

PATIENT: My whole body burns too. Sometimes I feel like I'm burning up.

NURSE PRACTITIONER: First of all, didn't you have an endometrial biopsy not too long ago? If I remember correctly, it was very difficult for you. Now we don't want to repeat that if it's not necessary. Ah, here it is, yes, we did a biopsy in June, the results are here and everything is fine. Now is there a reason why you want that done again? Has something changed?

PATIENT: Well, I want you to tell me if I have cancer. I also want you to do a Pap smear; I haven't had one in three years.

NURSE PRACTITIONER: Well, let's see. You've been coming here for about that long. And I've been seeing you. I can't believe that it's been all that time and nobody ever did a Pap smear, especially if they did an endometrial biopsy. Oh, it looks like you're right, it has been that long. Wow. Well, I guess you've just been coming here for acute problems and we've been dealing with those.

PATIENT: Yes.

NURSE PRACTITIONER: Now, the Pap smear is just a scraping of cells from the cervix, not from the uterine lining, so we won't have to insert the tube.

PATIENT: Yes. Look, doctor, I also need a mammogram. There's a lot of cancer in my family. My sister had to have a breast removed.

NURSE PRACTITIONER: Right, now let's see. It looks like you had one six months ago. Why did you go over to the cancer center?

PATIENT: You told me to go there because I found a lump in my breast.

NURSE PRACTITIONER: Oh yes, well, it looks like you went and the doctors said everything is fine, but you are due for a follow-up exam and a mammogram. It looks like they wanted you to come back in six months.

PATIENT: Yes. I have an appointment for the twenty-first, but first I need you to give me a paper. Every time I go over there for a mammogram, they tell me I need some paper.

NURSE PRACTITIONER: Actually, I don't think you should have any problem with that since the cancer center already recommended the follow-up appointment, but I'll take care of it before you go. Now let's get back to your original complaint. You said you're having hot flashes?

PATIENT: Yes.

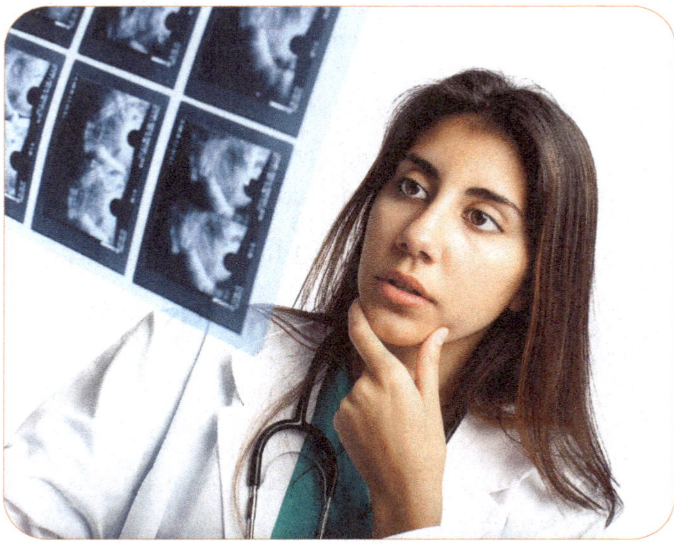

NURSE PRACTITIONER: Are you still taking the hormones?

PATIENT: No, I haven't taken them for three months.

NURSE PRACTITIONER: Why is that?

PATIENT: You told me I should stop.

NURSE PRACTITIONER: I think it's just a question of finding a balance. You know if you take them, we can regulate your bleeding and alleviate your hot flashes, but you may have breast tenderness again. If the hot flashes are really bothering you, I think we should try hormones again. We can try a different dose. There are many kinds we can try.

PATIENT: All right, but I don't want the ones I took last time. I think the problem was that the pharmacy gave me hormones that are genetically modified.

NURSE PRACTITIONER: Genetically modified? Do you mean—generic medications?

PATIENT: Yes, something like that. But I don't want that medicine. I want real medicine and not that kind that has the generic or genetic or whatever that is you are saying.

NURSE PRACTITIONER: Oh, "generic" just means that it's the same medicine, but made by a different company. The pharmacy was probably giving it to you because it's not covered by your health plan and the generic medicine is much less expensive, but it's not genetically modified. That's a completely different thing.

PATIENT: Well, I don't want those generic or genetic things, I'm afraid of those.

NURSE PRACTITIONER: OK. We'll write you a new prescription and you can get the original medication, not a generic brand. But I don't think that was the problem. I think maybe we just need to do a different dose. Would you like to try that? Hopefully you won't have the breast tenderness.

PATIENT: Yes, all right.

NURSE PRACTITIONER: Great. Right now, I'd like to do your Pap smear and a breast exam. We really don't need to do another biopsy because you had one relatively recently. It sounds like you're set up for your next mammogram, which I'll give you a referral for. And I'll write you a new prescription for hormones. Now, let's talk about the burning.

PATIENT: It's fine.

NURSE PRACTITIONER: I'm also going to give you some samples of this hormone cream for the burning. Now, I only want you to use this cream for a few weeks. Just put a little bit on your fingertips and rub it on the outside, on the labia, not inside the vagina. Once you're taking the hormones it should get better. All right? I think the burning sensation is caused by dry tissues from a drop in hormonal levels. When the urine hits those dry tissues it can feel like burning. I really think that's what's going on.

PATIENT: All right, so then I shouldn't put it there, inside my private part?

NURSE PRACTITIONER: Not inside, only outside, where you have the burning, on the labia. Now, I think we can get through the rest of the appointment without the interpreter. Do you have any questions for me before we do the exam?

PATIENT: *(to interpreter)* Oh, are you leaving?

(LET THE INTERPRETER RESPOND.)

PATIENT: No. I don't have any more questions. *(turns to the interpreter and speaks into the interpreter's ear.)* Hey, tell me something, she's Jewish, right? It seems like all the doctors are Jewish. Is she a Jew? They're always Jewish. Well, better than if she were a Muslim. Or Black. Is she Jewish?

(LET THE INTERPRETER RESPOND.)

NURSE PRACTITIONER: What did she just say?

What's important to know about this chapter?

Trauma history and its impact on health

The patient in this dialogue has seen war. She suffered from mental illness when political upheaval in her country turned to violent civil war. She fled before the worst happened, but the turmoil left no one there unscathed. Now she comes to see the doctor often, and some providers and staff regard her as a "difficult patient" with a list of chronic complaints. Healthcare providers have a hard time figuring out what to focus on because she has so many symptoms and health concerns.

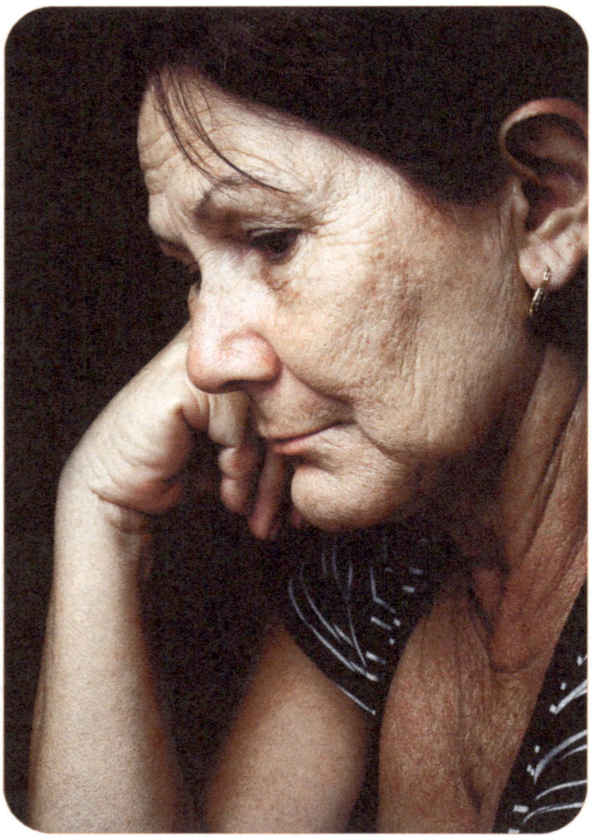

Every person is unique, and so is the adaption to trauma, but there are common patterns. Some patients who suffer frequently from many chronic conditions, such as stomach pain, headache, depression or other symptoms, might be living with trauma. Often, that suffering is never recognized or treated. Reread the dialogue with this knowledge. Does the patient sound any different to you now?

Patients who know some English

This patient speaks just enough English to get confused in medical appointments. She confuses the terms and ideas behind words like "genetic," "genetically modified" and "generic" (as they refer to medication). Such confusion of terms and concepts often happens when interpreters do not intervene because practitioners or patients think they understand each other but often they do not. Such problems can lead to an appreciation of the phrase, "Don't believe everything you think."

Vocabulary

Interpreters who work in gynecology, urology, women's health, women's clinics, reproductive health and also general medicine need to be prepared with the corresponding vocabulary. You need to know the anatomical vocabulary (male and female) in both languages and be familiar with some of the euphemisms that are used to refer to intimate body parts. In addition to medical vocabulary for this chapter, make a list of euphemisms in your other working language for sexual organs (e.g., "down there," "private part(s)," etc.).

Cultural orientation

It's important to be or become familiar with common cultural beliefs about urinary tract infections and conditions of the uterus and the ovaries. In some places, women are taught that sitting on a cold surface (such as a cement bench) can cause ovarian cysts or cause a "cold" in the ovaries. In some places where women swim in the sea, women never stay in a wet bathing suit, for fear of yeast infections. Instead, even to sunbathe, they change into a dry bathing suit. There are also many remedies for bladder or urinary tract infections, such as cranberry juice and corn silk tea. A health worker in a Planned Parenthood clinic in New York once described two young women who believed they could prevent pregnancy by douching with 7 Up.

Sensitivity, observation and intuition

It is probable that in the course of an interpreting career you will come across women, girls, men and boys who have suffered trauma, be it emotional, physical, violent, sexual or a combination. Paying attention to body language and the contextual cues is a serious matter. While you are not a licensed health practitioner, language and body language often reveal things that the interpreter notices and others miss. Such missed information can have serious implications for a diagnosis or treatment plan, and it's often important that the issue be brought to the attention of the provider. Here are a few examples.

Urology

A woman goes to a clinic for help because of painful intercourse with her husband. As she describes her discomfort, the interpreter notices a nervousness, a lowered gaze, sadness, depression or shame. The interpreter (when she accompanies the doctor as he leaves the room to fetch a printout of a prescription) tells the doctor what she senses in the patient's communication style. The doctor then goes back and asks the patient if someone has hurt her. Tears trickle down—and the patient discloses her rape as a young woman before she married. She has never spoken to anyone about it before. As a result, this sensitive provider proceeds to gently assure the patient that she has nothing to be ashamed of, but that the perpetrator does. The patient receives additional support services. The interpreter made a difference.

General medicine

A patient visits her doctor every few months with a list of chronic ailments: headache, stomach ache, inflammation, pain. She also seems downcast, and while the provider listens to the patient, focused on the computer screen where he enters data, the interpreter observes tears welling in the patient's eyes. The interpreter, with transparency and delicacy, conveys to the provider the need to return to the patient. The doctor turns, sees and inquires. The patient is being battered and verbally abused by her alcoholic husband on a regular basis. Now aware, the doctor attends to his patient with sympathy, and treats her physical ailments in addition to referring her to appropriate social, psychological and legal services. The interpreter made a difference.

Transplant donor workup

A doctor describes the gynecological exam she is about to perform on a prospective organ donor, a woman in her thirties. The interpreter notices the patient's change in demeanor; she is nervous, tense and quiet. Outside the room, the interpreter alerts the provider, who then comes back and carefully asks about the patient's sexual history. She has never had sexual relations, a pelvic exam or a Pap smear. The doctor decides she can forgo this part of the workup. The interpreter made a difference.

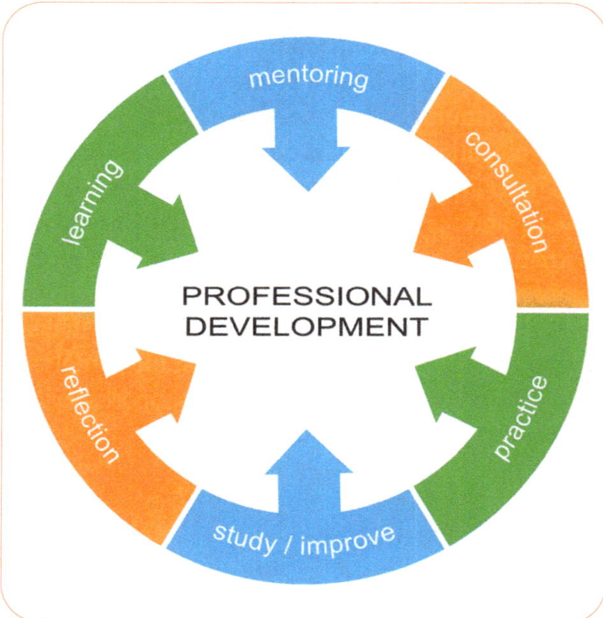

Culturally sensitive exams

The patient is at the clinic for a pelvic exam and a Pap smear. The interpreter enters the room to find the patient in a gown. In the course of the doctor's introduction, it becomes apparent that the patient is unfamiliar with the procedure and the medical terminology being used. She says she was advised by an aunt not to have the exam and asks if it will "change anything," or if she will "be different afterward." The doctor's response is, "No! It's a relatively noninvasive procedure." (Relative to what? What is the doctor's point of reference?) The interpreter is female and finds the comment somewhat astounding but focuses on her composure and alerts the doctor that she senses some miscommunication that needs to be clarified. By the end of the appointment, the patient, who has never had sex and comes from a culture where an intact hymen upon marriage is extremely important, gets a lesson in human anatomy and basic gynecological exams and opts out of the pelvic exam and Pap smear. Again, the interpreter made a difference.

Teen clinic

An uncle of a monolingual teenage girl hovers a bit too close to her and insists on doing all the interpreting, answering many questions for the girl. He is reluctant to leave the room so that the provider can talk privately with the adolescent as is customary. The teenager is clearly nervous. Something isn't right. Outside the room, the interpreter conveys what she senses from the uncle and patient's communication styles to the provider. As a result, the provider and a social worker speak to the girl without the "uncle." The teenager turns out to be a victim of human trafficking. The interpreter made a huge difference.

An interpreter is sometimes faced with decisions about whether or not to share certain things he or she notices and how to do so in a professional manner. This issue will be discussed again later in this chapter.

Do I really have to interpret that?

The interpreter in this dialogue is familiar with the patient's national history, including the many wars, mass rape, genocide and suffering. It may seem hard to imagine that the patient believes some of the same ideology that has caused her own suffering, but she does criticize whole groups of people based on their religion. As a result, some of the patient's comments make the interpreter uncomfortable. She might be tempted to omit them or change those messages. She might ask herself, "Do I really have to interpret that?" But the answer is yes. She does have to interpret everything that is said or signed, as unpleasant as it may be.

Interpret as accurately as you can. The person who speaks will have to bear the responsibility and consequences, not you.

Ethics and standards: Reflect and practice

Goal 8: Professional development

Translation and paraphrasing

1. Look at the four NCIHC standards of practice related to professional development (Standards 27-30, NCIHC, 2005, p. 10). Working individually, *paraphrase* the objective, its related ethical principle and the two standards.
2. Working individually, *translate* the original text of these standards into your other working language(s) or interpret it into sign language.
3. Find a partner or partners. Compare, discuss and modify your translations and paraphrasing until you are satisfied with your final products as a group.
4. If you can, pick a group representative and discuss your final versions with any other groups that share your working languages. Compare and discuss your differences.

Suggested reading

Roat, C. E. (2010). *Healthcare Interpreting in Small Bites: 50 Nourishing Selections from the "Pacific Interpreters Newsletter," 2002-2010.* Victoria, British Columbia: Trafford, pp. 161-163.

Consider and discuss

1. **Standard 27** List three ways that you can develop your medical terminology and regional varieties.
2. **Standard 27** Define and discuss "shadowing" for interpreter skill development.
3. **Standard 28** How can an interpreter and coworkers (e.g., other staff interpreters or bilingual employees who interpret) confer and consult regularly about challenging assignments? How might a freelance interpreter without regular coworkers engage in this kind of professional development?
4. **Standard 29** How can mentor interpreters support novice interpreters? What could mentor interpreters gain from such activities? What are the most important things that novice interpreters might learn from being mentored?

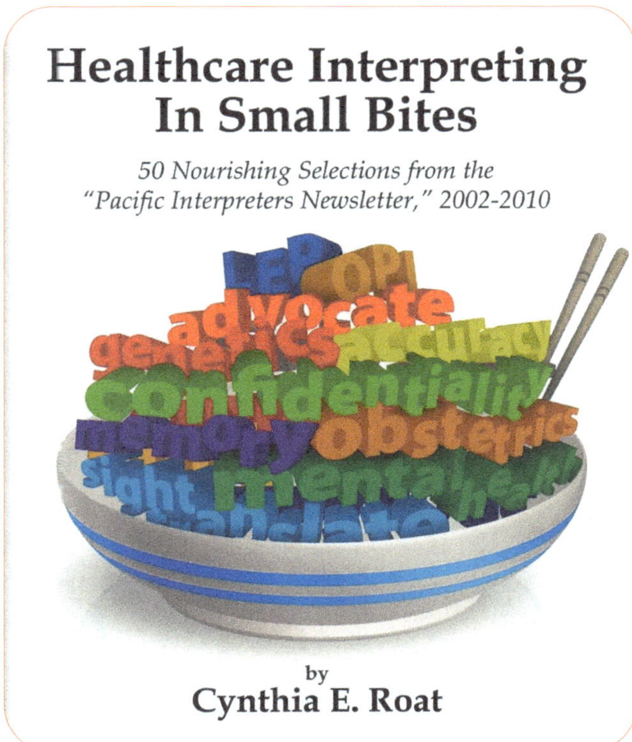

5. **Standard 29** One of the most valuable ways you can support your own professional development and that of other interpreters is to join a professional association, such as American Translators Association, or ATA (www.atanet.org) in the United States, which also supports interpreters. But what is a professional association? Is NCIHC a professional association? Why or why not? (To find out, go to the website www.ncihc.org.) Is IMIA a professional association? (See www.imiaweb.org.) Give examples of associations that might be good for you to join. You can check the list of professional associations under the resources tab of www.ncihc.org for ideas.
6. **Standard 30** List three organizations that you might join to support your own professional development as an interpreter. Seek information about local, state, national and international organizations online and share the most relevant information and your recommendations with interpreters in your study group.
7. **Standard 30** Identify two professional conferences that you might attend in the near future. Review the programs. Attending a conference can be one of the most stimulating and rewarding activities you can do for professional development. Choose wisely. In general, the larger the conference you can afford to attend, the more opportunities you will find to learn. However, local or nearby conferences have the advantage that they often focus on issues relevant to your geographic area and circumstances. (They are also less expensive to attend!)

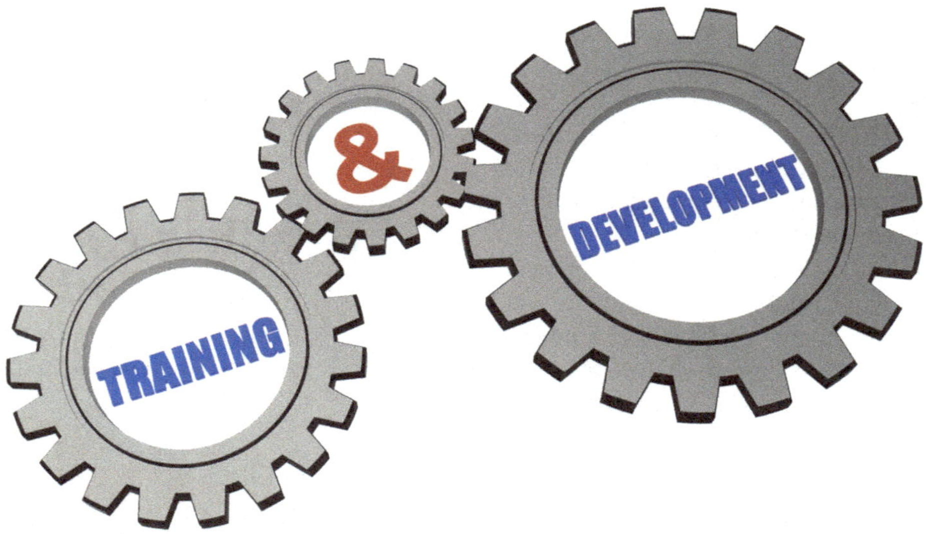

Occupational therapy for interpreters

EXERCISES FOR THE TONGUE, HEART AND MIND

You will now revisit part of the original role play dialogue in this chapter. In this version, the interpreter takes action. Each time the interpreter speaks or acts, decide if you agree with what the interpreter does by answering the questions that follow each excerpt.

Then read the commentary that follows the excerpts and see if you want to change any of your answers.

PART 1

NURSE PRACTITIONER: Genetically modified? Do you mean—generic medications?

> **PATIENT:** Yes, something like that. But I don't want that medicine.

NURSE PRACTITIONER: *(turns to interpreter)* Wait, I'm not sure what she means.

> **INTERPRETER:** *(to doctor)* May the interpreter clarify? The interpreter thinks she means "generic" and she's mixed up about the terms. May the interpreter clarify that with her?

NURSE PRACTITIONER: Oh, sure.

Interpreter: Do you mean the label on the medicine says it's "generic"?

> **PATIENT:** Yes, something like that. But I don't want that medicine. I want real medicine and not that kind that has the generic or genetic or whatever that is you are saying.

> **INTERPRETER:** OK, I understand. *(to doctor)* Yes, she's mixed up about the terms. The pharmacy gave her a generic brand, and she's getting that mixed up with the term "genetically modified." She wants nongeneric and nongenetically modified medicine.

Do you agree with the interpreter's actions here? Circle your answer.

YES NO MAYBE

Why did you agree or disagree with the interpreter's intervention?

PART 2

NURSE PRACTITIONER: Now, I think we can get through the rest of the appointment without the interpreter. Do you have any questions for me before we do the exam?

PATIENT: *(to interpreter)* Oh, are you leaving?

INTERPRETER: *(to patient)* Yes. The doctor says she can go ahead without the interpreter. Is that OK with you? *(repeats in English for the doctor)*

Do you agree with the interpreter's actions here? Circle your answer.

YES NO MAYBE

Why did you agree or disagree with the interpreter's intervention?

PART 3

PATIENT: No. I don't have any more questions. *(turns to the interpreter and speaks into the interpreter's ear.)* Hey, tell me something, she's Jewish, right? It seems like all the doctors are Jewish. Is she Jewish? They're always Jewish. Well, better than if she were a Muslim. Or Black. Is she Jewish?

INTERPRETER: *(pauses for a moment, uncomfortable, unsure what to do)*

NURSE PRACTITIONER: What did she just say?

INTERPRETER: *(to patient, in the patient's language)* Can I remind you as the interpreter that I have to interpret *everything* you say? *(to the provider)* I just clarified my role with the patient.

Do you agree with the interpreter's actions here? Circle your answer.

YES NO MAYBE

Why did you agree or disagree with the interpreter's intervention?

COMMENTARIES

Now read the commentaries about each of the three excerpts and see if you want to change any of your answers.

Commentary on Part 1

NURSE PRACTITIONER: Genetically modified? Do you mean—generic medications?

> **PATIENT:** Yes, something like that. But I don't want that medicine.

NURSE PRACTITIONER: *(turns to interpreter)* Wait, I'm not sure what she means.

> **INTERPRETER:** *(to doctor)* May the interpreter clarify? The interpreter thinks she means "generic" and that she's mixed up about the terms May the interpreter clarify that with her?

NURSE PRACTITIONER: Oh, sure.

> **INTERPRETER:** Do you mean the label on the medicine says it is "generic"?

> **PATIENT:** Yes, something like that. But I don't want that medicine. I want real medicine and not that kind that has the generic or genetic or whatever that is you are saying.

> **INTERPRETER:** OK, I understand. *(to doctor)* Yes, she's mixed up about the terms. The pharmacy gave her a generic brand, and she's getting that mixed up with the term "genetically modified." She wants nongeneric and nongenetically modified medicine.

As a professional medical interpreter, it is not your job to check for understanding. You are there to facilitate communication in order to support access to the service. By checking for understanding, you are taking over the provider's role.

However, the interpreter's assumption in this case is correct. Therefore, just as you saw in the previous chapter, it would be preferable for the interpreter to *request* clarification from the patient so that the *provider* can ask the right questions and check for understanding.

For example, the interpreter could say, "Excuse me, as the interpreter I sense a possible misunderstanding about the meaning of the term 'generic' versus 'genetic,'" or "The interpreter suggests you ask the patient what she means by 'generic.'" In this way the interpreter can solve the problem without taking over the provider's job, and the provider in the future can be more alert to this type of misunderstanding.

Commentary on Part 2

NURSE PRACTITIONER: Now, I think we can get through the rest of the appointment without the interpreter. Do you have any questions for me before we do the exam?

> **PATIENT:** *(to interpreter)* Oh, are you leaving?

> **INTERPRETER:** *(to patient)* Yes. The doctor says she can go ahead without the interpreter. Is that OK with you? *(repeats in English for the doctor)*

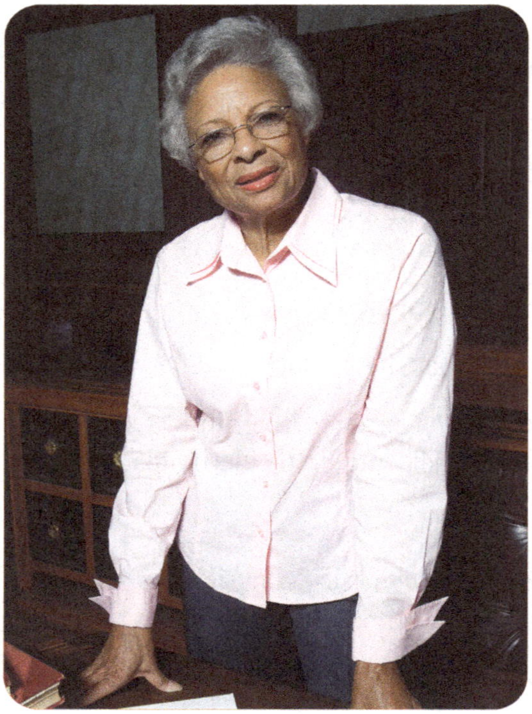

This is a difficult situation! If the hospital's policy is that health professionals can conduct physical exams on patients who need interpreters without an interpreter being present, there might be nothing the interpreter can do except to participate in language access efforts to change such policies, for example, by working with professional associations and groups like NCIHC.

However, it is unlikely that it is a hospital policy to conduct exams on LEP patients without an interpreter. In this case, the situation suggests a need for potential interpreter advocacy because (a) possible discrimination is taking place (patients who speak the language can ask questions and get answers from their health professionals during the exam); (b) there is a potential for misunderstandings, miscommunication and concerns about patient safety; (c) the hospital might be in violation of its obligations under language access laws, such as the federal Title VI of the Civil Rights Act and other relevant federal, state and/or local language access laws; (d) the situation potentially undermines the patient's sense of well-being, safety and human dignity.

On these grounds the interpreter could consider engaging in advocacy if such action is permissible and appropriate. See the introductory section of this book, "Guide for Advocacy," for guidance on how to engage appropriately in advocacy.

Commentary on Part 3

PATIENT: No. I don't have any more questions. *(turns to the interpreter and speaks into the interpreter's ear.)* Hey, tell me something, she's Jewish, right? It seems like all the doctors are Jewish. Is she Jewish? They're always Jewish. Well, better than if she were a Muslim. Or Black. Is she Jewish?

INTERPRETER: *(pauses for a second, uncomfortable, unsure how to start)*

NURSE PRACTITIONER: What did she just say?

INTERPRETER: *(to patient, in the patient's language)* Can I remind you as the interpreter that I have to interpret *everything* you say? *(to the provider)* I just clarified my role with the patient.

This is another tricky situation!

a. First, yes, the question is offensive. But if it were your doctor, wouldn't you want to know if your provider was bigoted against certain groups—perhaps your group? Similarly, the provider has a right to know what the patient feels.

b. Second, the professional interpreter is ethically obligated to interpret everything. So it is better—far better—to emphasize in your introduction that you will interpret *everything* than to find yourself in this position. Many interpreters now add a statement like this to their introduction to both or all parties: *Please don't say anything that you don't want me to interpret, as I am ethically obligated to interpret EVERYTHING.*
c. Also, many providers speak some words in other languages—and many patients understand more English than they speak. If the provider (or patient) realizes you are not interpreting what was said because he or she understands some statements in the other language, how does that omission make you look? Could it anger the provider? Lead to a complaint against you? Consider the consequences of every decision you make!
d. By making the decision to sometimes omit information, you are taking on the role of deciding what is important to interpret and what is not. That is not really your decision to make. Yes, it can be tough to interpret everything. Yes, there can be extreme exceptions to this ethical requirement, including emergencies, psychotic patients, dangerous situations and more. But as a general policy, walk in with the firm intention to interpret everything stated during the session and then do so. That habit and reflex will provide a solid foundation for your interpreting!

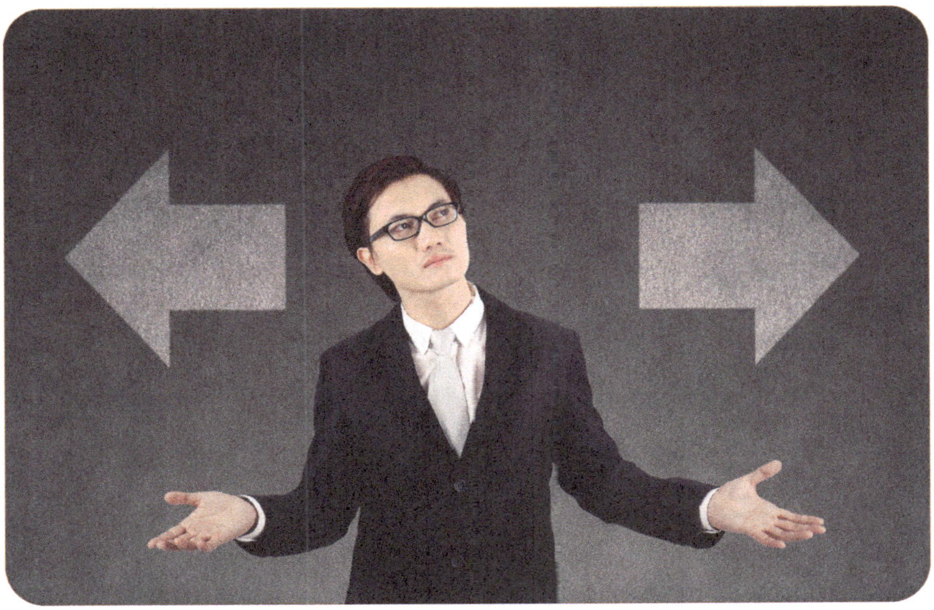

Medical terminology: The uterus

Below you will find anatomical drawings relevant to the content of this chapter. Follow the instructions found at the end of Chapter 1 to study the terminology in this section.

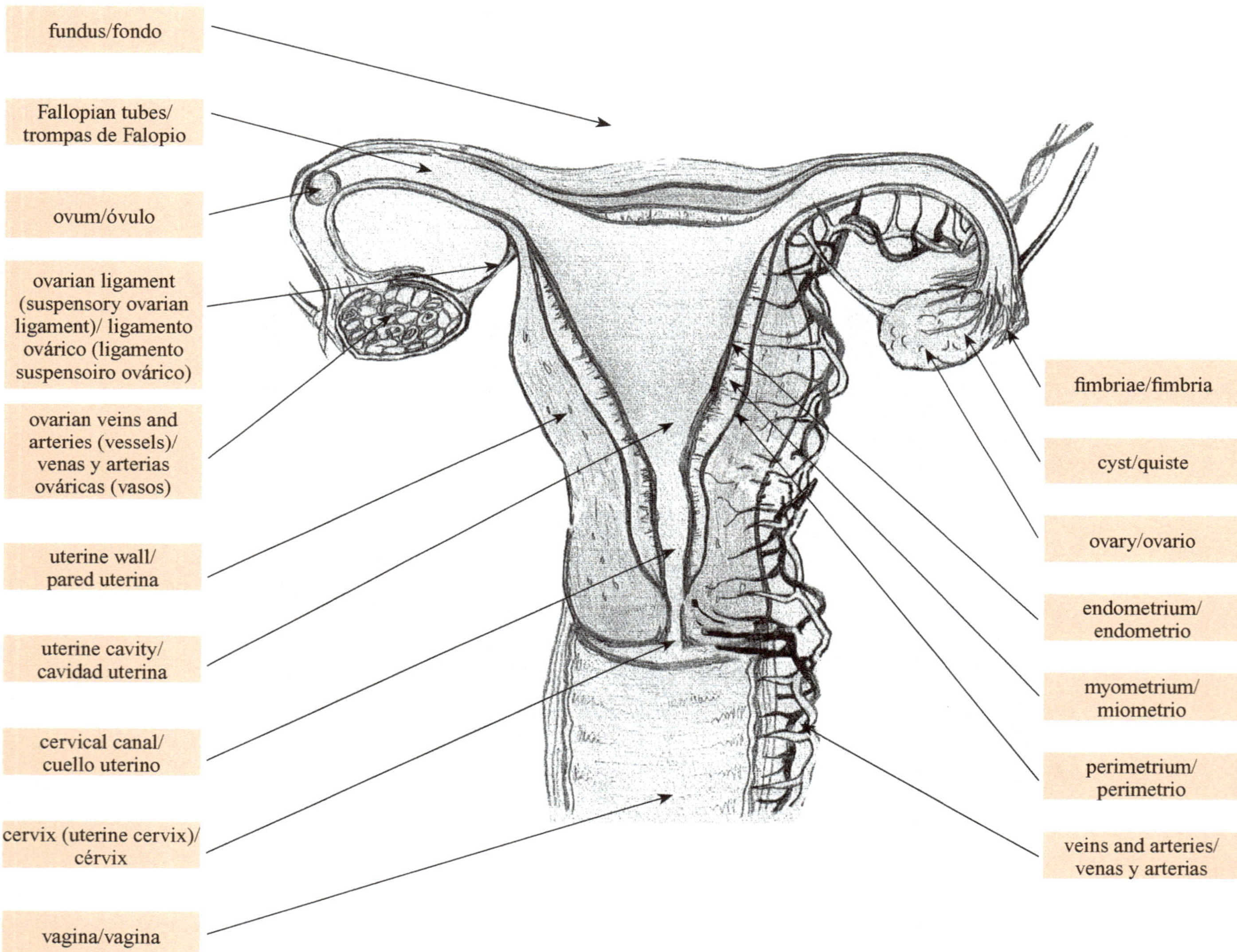

Figure 8-A: The uterus (English and Spanish)

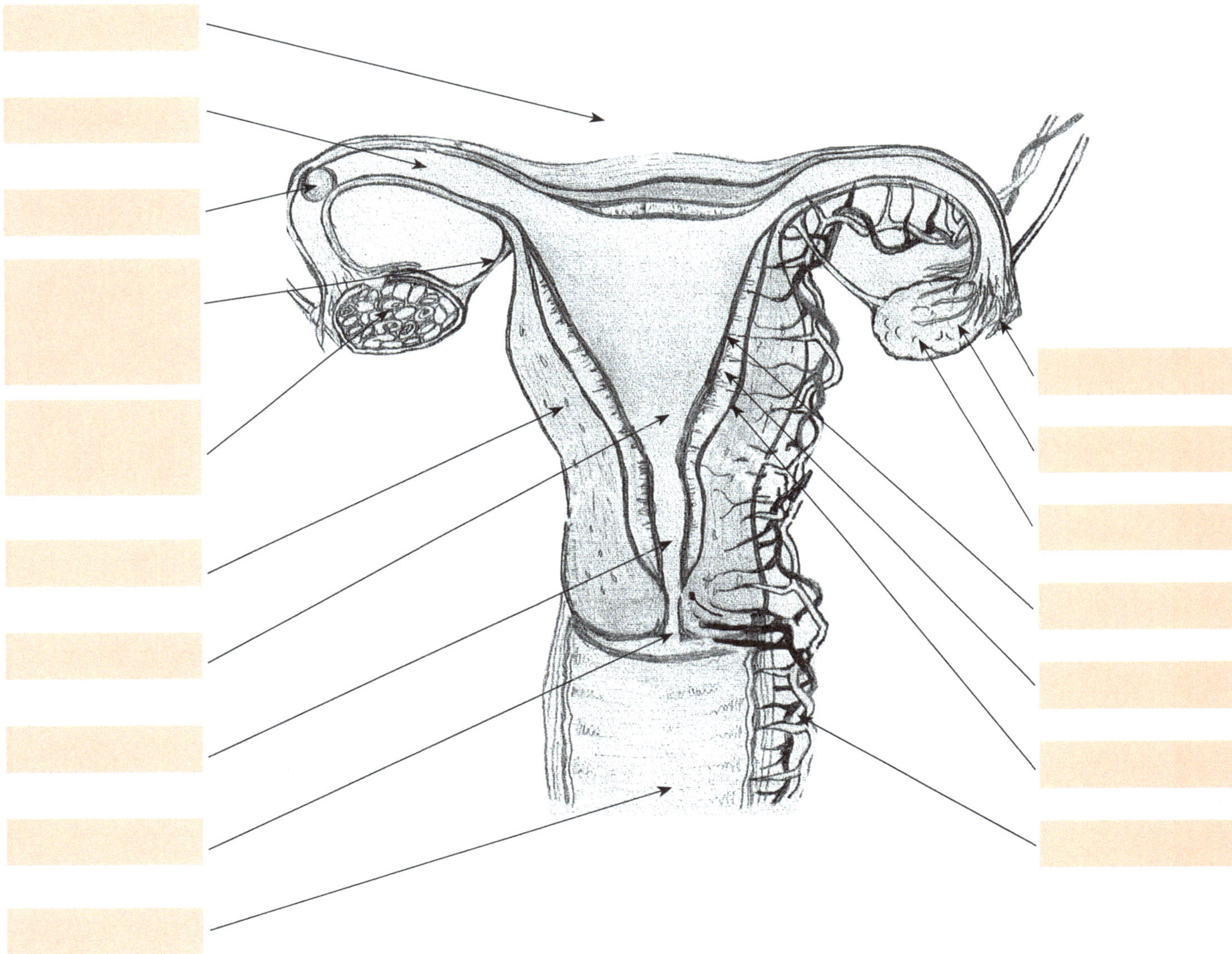

Figure 8-B: The uterus (blank labels)

Medical terminology list

The uterus

VOCABULARY FOR GRAPHIC—IN ENGLISH	VOCABULARY FOR GRAPHIC—IN SPANISH	ANY OTHER LANGUAGE
cervical canal	cuello uterino	
cervix (uterine cervix)	cérvix	
cyst	quiste	
endometrium	endometrio	
Fallopian tubes	trompas de Falopio	
fibroid	fibroide	
fimbriae	fimbria	
fundus	fondo	
myometrium	miometrio	
ovarian ligament (suspensory ovarian ligament)	ligamento ovárico (ligamento suspensoiro ovárico)	
ovarian veins and arteries (vessels)	venas y arterias ováricas (vasos)	
ovary	ovario	
ovum	óvulo	
perimetrium	perimetrio	
uterine body	cuerpo uterino	
uterine cavity	cavidad uterina	
uterine wall	pared uterina	
uterus	útero (matriz)	
vagina	vagina	

Rheumatology 9

Advisory

This chapter involves material about autoimmune conditions and arthritis. It includes some colorful vocabulary and uninhibited sexual innuendo.

This patient is a 45-year-old woman of Mexican descent (for the Spanish-English dialogue only) with arthritis and a great sense of humor. The interpreter has been in the waiting room and is called in with the patient. Patient and provider know each other well and enjoy working together.

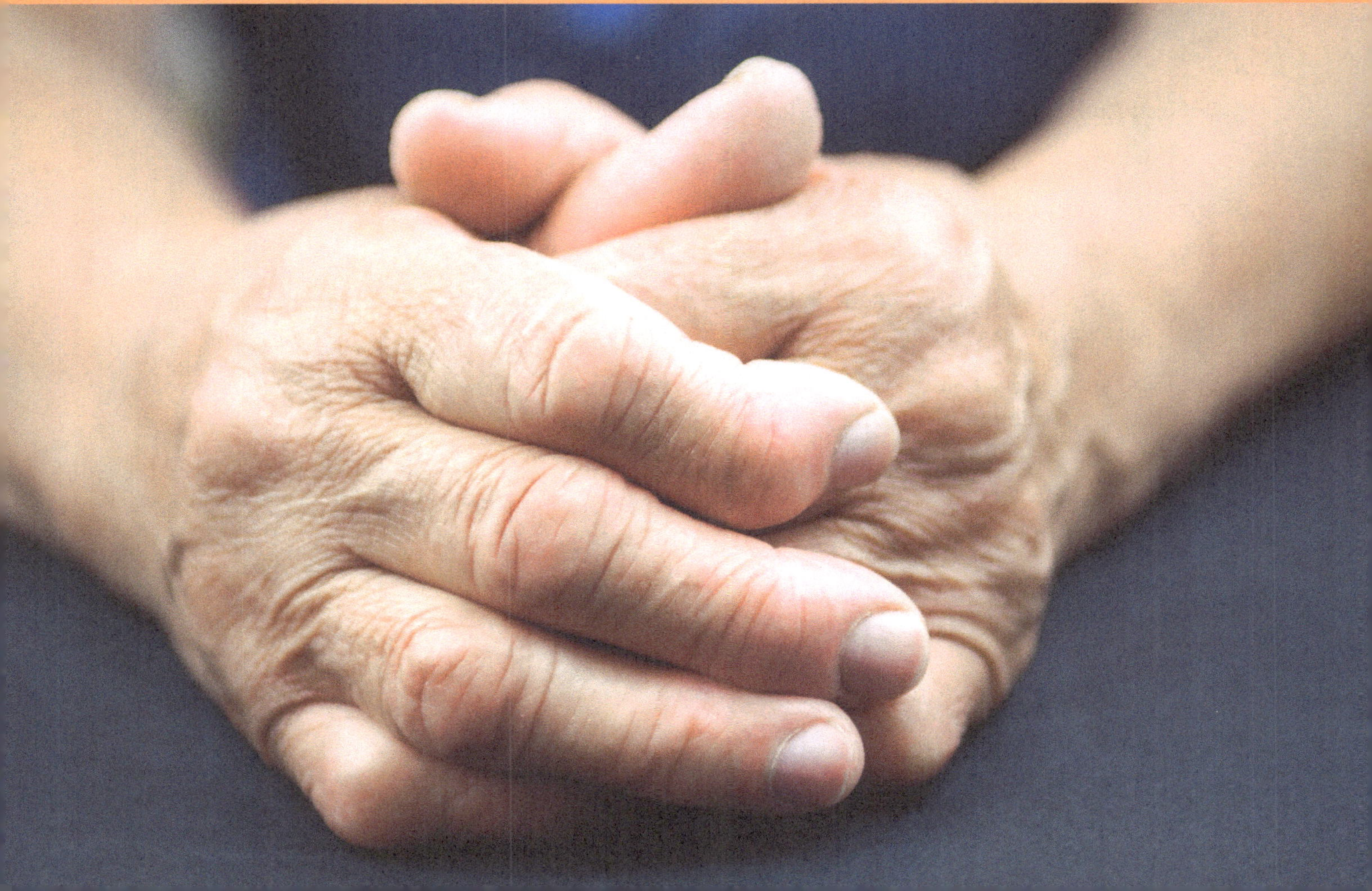

Adult arthritis clinic role play (English-Spanish)

DOCTOR: Good morning, Esme, right this way. How are you?

PATIENT: Bien, bien, doctorcito. ¿Cómo está usted?

DOCTOR: I'm fine. But we're here to take care of you today. So, how can I help you? How are the knees?

PATIENT: Pos doctorcito, esta que me inyectó la vez pasada está más o menos, pero la otra, pos está remal.[42]

DOCTOR: Let's see, and your other joints? *(Doctor begins to examine the patient, starting with the shoulder joints.)* How are you here in the shoulders?

PATIENT: ¡Ay, ay, ay!

DOCTOR: Does that hurt?

PATIENT: ¡Ay, cabrón!

DOCTOR: Oh, sorry. And here?

PATIENT: ¡Si! Ay, ay, allí es donde duele mucho.

DOCTOR: And the medicine I gave you last time, did it help at all?

PATIENT: ¡Pos no hizo ni, pos ni madres!

DOCTOR: Oh, I'm sorry to hear that, Esme. We're going to have to do something about that. Why didn't you call and make an appointment to see me sooner instead of waiting two months?

PATIENT: Es que sabía que le iba a ver ahora y seguramente no me hubieran dado una cita más temprano. ¿Pa' qué entonces?

DOCTOR: I'm so sorry you've been in so much pain all this time. How long has it been taking you to start moving around in the morning?

PATIENT: Pos, depende de lo que estoy haciendo antes de levantarme, ¿ei? Pero pos me encuentro mal cuando me despierto, con mis dedos de pie tiesos, pero me baño y a la media hora estoy mejor. Pero no es como antes doctor, antes estaba pero remal.

DOCTOR: I'm really very sorry, Esme. We'll have to see about getting you in more quickly next time.

PATIENT: Qué bueno que es usted, mi doctorcito. *(to interpreter)* Es que yo quiero mucho a mi doctorcito. Ay, si yo fuera más joven. Yo me caso con él, calvito y todo. *(Patient winks at interpreter.)*

42 What is "pos" in other parts of México? What is the function of the suffix "re" in México? In English?

DOCTOR: Gracias, Esme. I'm flattered. Now back to the knees. Can I see your knees?

PATIENT: Pos claro que sí doctorci— ¡ay! Allí, allí, allí es donde estoy pero madreada, ¿ei? ¿No me va a inyectar otra vez, doctor?

DOCTOR: Esme, I want you to lie down and let me rotate your knees. Relax your muscles and let me move them.

PATIENT: Ay, ay, eso sí duele, pero refeo.

DOCTOR: Well, I think we could go ahead and do that in this knee. The other one still seems to be OK. I think I also want to prescribe something a little stronger for your shoulders. You're still taking the other medicine regularly, the Naprosyn, right? And the Zantac for your stomach?

PATIENT: Sí, doctor.

DOCTOR: And how are your hips? Are they OK? And your neck?

PATIENT: Más o menos, doctor, echándole ganas.

DOCTOR: All right. I want you to keep taking those, and then in addition, I'd like you to try this new one. Try taking one of these for pain and see how you do. If you need more, you can take one up to every four hours.

PATIENT: Como usted mande, doctorcito.

DOCTOR: Now be sure to call me if you don't get some relief from this, all right?

PATIENT: Pos, claro que sí.

DOCTOR: I'm going to consult with my attending and come right back with the injection for that leg. Do you need a refill for your other medications?

PATIENT: Sí doctor, pero es que, pos, es que el mes que entra voy pa' México, y voy a estar un buen rato. Así que *(to interpreter)* dígale al doctorcito que me de una receta, pero con huevos, ¿ei?

DOCTOR: OK, Esme, I'll do my best. Is there anything else, because I think we can let the interpreter go. I'll just give you the injection, the prescription for stronger medicine and a prescription for refills.

PATIENT: No, doctorcito, creo que vamos a estar bien.

DOCTOR: And I want you to come back and see me when you get back from your vacation, all right?

PATIENT: Lo que usted diga, doctorcito. *(to the interpreter)* Gracias señorita, muy amable.

Adult arthritis clinic role play (English only)

DOCTOR: Good morning, Esme, right this way. How are you?

PATIENT: Well, well, dearie. How are you?

DOCTOR: I'm fine. But we're here to take care of you today. So, how can I help you? How are the knees?

PATIENT: Well, honey, this one here, the one they injected last time is so-so, but the other one, well, it's real bad; it's throwing me for a loop.

DOCTOR: Let's see, and your other joints? *(Doctor begins to examine the patient, starting with the shoulder joints.)* How are you here in the shoulders?

PATIENT: Oh, oh, oh!

DOCTOR: Does that hurt?

PATIENT: Ouch, damn!

DOCTOR: Oh, sorry. And here?

PATIENT: Yes! Oh, oh, that's where it hurts a bunch.

DOCTOR: And the medicine I gave you last time, did it help at all?

PATIENT: Well, it didn't really, it didn't do shit!

DOCTOR: Oh, I'm sorry to hear that, Esme. We're going to have to do something about that. Why didn't you call and make an appointment to see me sooner instead of waiting two months?

PATIENT: Well, I knew I was going to see you today and I'm sure they wouldn't have given me an appointment any sooner. So why bother?

DOCTOR: I'm so sorry you've been in so much pain all this time. How long has it been taking you to start moving around in the morning?

PATIENT: It depends on what I'm doing before I get up, eh? But, it's bad when I wake up; my toes are stiff, but I bathe and then half hour later I'm better. But it's not like before, doc, I was bad, but *really* bad before.

DOCTOR: I'm really very sorry, Esme. We'll have to see about getting you in more quickly next time.

PATIENT: Doctor, honey, you are so good. *(to interpreter)* I just love my little doctor. My, if I were younger I'd marry him, bald as he is! *(Patient winks at interpreter.)*

DOCTOR: Thanks, Esme. I'm flattered. Now back to the knees. Can I see your knees?

PATIENT: Well, of course, doctor hon—ouch! There, there, there, that's where I'm really fucked up, eh? Aren't you gonna inject me again, doctor?

DOCTOR: Esme, I want you to lie down and let me rotate your knees. Relax your muscles and let me move them.

PATIENT: Oh, oh, that hurts real, real bad.

DOCTOR: Well, I think we could go ahead and do that in this knee. The other one still seems to be OK I think I also want to prescribe something a little stronger for your shoulders. You're still taking the other medicine regularly, the Naprosyn, right? And the Zantac for your stomach?

PATIENT: Yes, doctor.

DOCTOR: And how are your hips? Are they OK? And your neck?

PATIENT: So-so, doctor, it's all I can do.

DOCTOR: All right. I want you to keep taking those, and then in addition, I'd like you to try this new one. Try taking one of these for pain, and see how you do. If you need more, you can take one up to every four hours.

PATIENT: Whatever you say, doctor honey.

DOCTOR: Now be sure to call me if you don't get some relief from this, all right?

PATIENT: I sure will.

DOCTOR: I'm going to consult with my attending, and come right back with the injection for that leg. Do you need a refill for your other medications?

PATIENT: Yes, doctor, but next month I'm going to my country, and I'll be gone for a good while. So *(to interpreter)* tell my sweetheart doctor to give me a prescription, but one with balls, eh?

DOCTOR: OK, Esme, I'll do my best. Is there anything else, because I think we can let the interpreter go. I'll just give you the injection, the prescription for stronger medicine and a prescription for refills.

PATIENT: No, doctor honey, I think we'll be fine.

DOCTOR: And I want you to come back and see me when you get back from your vacation, all right?

PATIENT: Whatever you say, sweetheart. *(to the interpreter)* Thank you, miss, you've been very nice.

What's important to know about this chapter?

Terminology

For this specialty, you will need to become familiar with terms for arthritis, anatomy of joints and autoimmune conditions.

Interpreting "inappropriate" remarks

The patient in this chapter is good-natured and gregarious. She is harmlessly flirting but says things that can make the interpreter and/or the physician uncomfortable. Some of the comments would be considered inappropriate, but in this case the physician doesn't seem to be bothered. The doctor and patient know each other fairly well, and this type of conversation is part of their working rapport. It doesn't seem to impede care.

All that said, an interpreter needs to be accurate, complete, impartial and professional. Sometimes this kind of conversation is not easy to interpret. Some of the comments may be inappropriate and may not be well-received. A provider may also say things that the patient or interpreter finds inappropriate or offensive.

Barring the rare exception, the interpreter needs to interpret it all. Other actions may need to be taken (such as addressing inappropriate language during the appointment with all parties present, addressing it outside the appointment with the provider or healthcare staff, or reporting the situation to the appropriate authority). It is helpful to think about these situations in advance so that, if they happen to you, you are prepared.

As the interpreter, you need to capture this type of language in all its nuances. An accurate reflection of the patient's speech is an indicator of many things that may be important for diagnosis. The interpreter does not have to determine that diagnosis, the practitioner does. Remember, the interpreter is not responsible for what is said by the other parties; she is responsible for interpreting it.

Idioms

What are some of the many ways you could interpret, "It didn't do shit"? How can you say it in different registers from the more formal to the less formal?

Variations

In English, regional varieties allow for emphasis on a word in different ways. *Very bad* can be stated as *super bad, real bad, hella bad, totally bad, hideously bad,* or in more "colorful" or crude expressions such as *fucking bad, really fucking bad* or expressions that imply "bad" without using the word itself such as *hellacious,* etc. What are some of the ways you can play with to add on to a word like *bad* in your working languages?

Suggested presentation

For a hilarious yet informative presentation, try to attend a conference session on how to interpret profanity, in particular (if you can) one like the presentation by Alvaro Vergara-Mery, PhD, CMI, of the Nevada Interpreters & Translators Association and interpreter and trainer at University Medical Center in Las Vegas, Nevada. His presentation, "Interpreting Profanity In Healthcare: Nurse, I Want My F-ing Pills Now!"[43] has been given at several conferences. Attending it might be the most educational fun you will ever have at a conference!

43 Retrieved from www.nitaonline.org/interpreting-profanity-in-healthcare-nurse-i-want-my-f-ing-pills-now/

Ethics and standards: Reflect and practice

Goal 9: Advocacy

Translation and paraphrasing

1. Look at the last two NCIHC standards of practice, which are related to advocacy (Standards 31 and 32, NCIHC, 2005, p. 10). Working individually, *paraphrase* the objective, its related ethical principle and the two standards.
2. Working individually, *translate* the original text of these standards into your other working language(s) or interpret it into sign language.
3. Find a partner or partners. Compare, discuss and modify your translations and paraphrasing until you are satisfied with your final products as a group.
4. If you can, pick a group representative and discuss your final versions with any other groups that share your working languages. Compare and discuss your differences.

Suggested reading

Roat, C. E. (2010). *Healthcare Interpreting in Small Bites: 50 Nourishing Selections from the "Pacific Interpreters Newsletter," 2002-2010.* Victoria, British Columbia: Trafford, pp. 47-51 and 129-132.

Consider and discuss

1. **Standard 31** According to the National Code of Ethics for Interpreters in Health Care, advocacy is defined as follows.

   Objective: *To prevent harm to parties that the interpreter serves.*

   Glossary definition: *Advocacy is understood as an action taken on behalf of an individual that goes beyond facilitating communication, with the intention of supporting good health outcomes. In general, advocacy means that a third party (in this case, the interpreter) speaks for or pleads the cause of another party, thereby departing from an impartial role.*

   How do the objective and the definition contradict or support each other?

2. **Standard 31** What is the difference between impartiality and indifference?
3. **Standard 31** In a posttransplant clinic, an interpreter works with a patient who has a central intravenous line in her neck. She is having pain, trouble unbending her neck and difficulty swallowing. She is losing weight. It is agreed that this situation is fairly serious and will be reassessed in two weeks. There may be adhesions that require a surgery.

   Three weeks later, the interpreter is working over the phone with the same clinic. The patient asks, "Will I be able to move my neck again?" The clinical nurse practitioner (CNP) answers, "Yes. When the line comes out." The interpreter suddenly remembers the previous scenario, and the importance of reassessing the neck for possible required surgery over a week ago as stated by the previous provider. She identifies herself as the interpreter and asks if this might be the same patient. The CNP says she doesn't know and moves on. Concerned, the interpreter again identifies herself as the interpreter and recounts the previous visit, including the plan to reassess the neck at this time and asks again if it might be the same patient. The CNP says she doesn't know and goes on. Finally, the interpreter

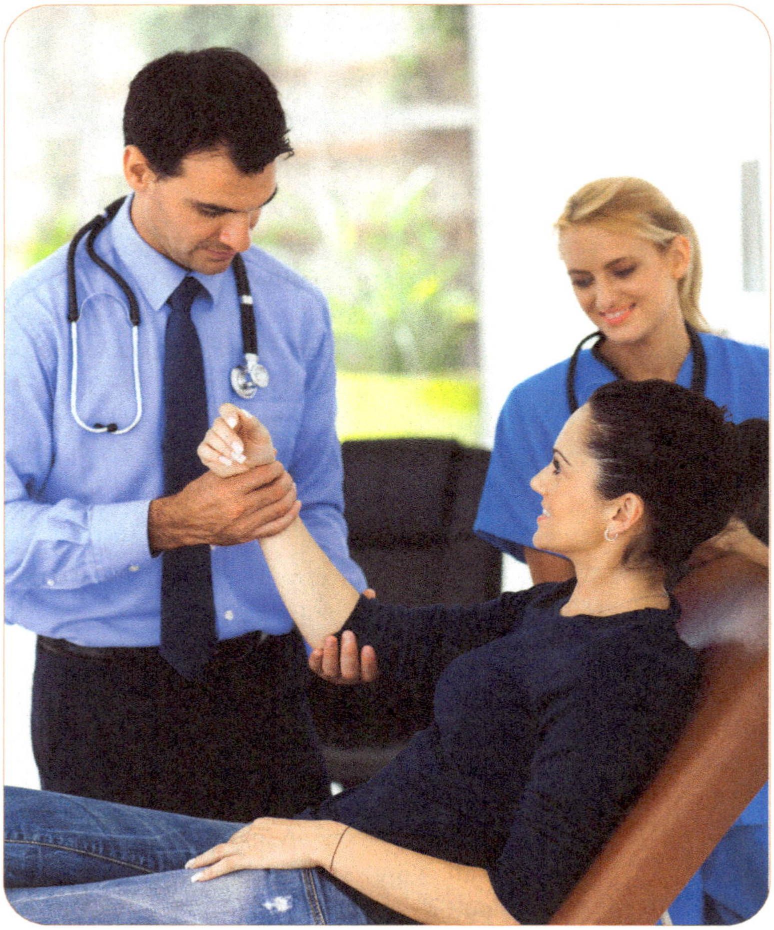

asks the CNP permission to clarify. It is in fact the same patient. Is this an intervention? Is it crossing a professional boundary? Is it doing harm? Is it harmful to stay silent? Critique the interpreter's behavior according to Standard 31.

4. **Standard 32** In a pediatric intensive care unit, a mother is distressed and anxious about the cause and treatment for her child's severe abdominal pain. A physician comes to talk to her and insists on speaking to her directly without an interpreter, but his Spanish is limited and difficult to understand. The mother tells the physician that she cannot understand, yet he keeps speaking to her in incomprehensible Spanish. Mom turns to the interpreter and says, "I don't understand anything he says." The interpreter tells the doctor, "She doesn't understand you." He ignores her and continues in his incomprehensible Spanish to explain a complicated procedure and the risks of anesthesia involved. The mother is more and more distressed. What should the interpreter do? To whom can she appeal?
5. **Standard 32** An orthopedist is sending a patient for a leg x-ray and asks if the patient could be pregnant. The patient looks at her husband and answers, "Well, not that I *know* of." The doctor says it's probably fine. Just before the patient leaves for the x-ray, she asks the doctor if he can help her with contraceptives. Is there a reason for advocacy here?
6. **Standard 32** Consider two complementary types of advocacy: ***Language access* advocacy and *patient* advocacy.** Language access advocacy is something that any interpreter can support, for example, by joining NCIHC, sitting on language advocacy boards or groups, presenting on language access at a conference or educating providers and administrators about the benefits of complying with federal guidelines for language access. Patient advocacy is what you might choose to do, for example, if you see patient safety at risk due to providers or healthcare staff who fail to provide an interpreter when one is needed.

Now look at the table about these two types of advocacy. Discuss any unfamiliar terms or concepts you find with other interpreters. Circle one heading at the top of each column to indicate which list or column refers to ***language access* advocacy** and which is more focused on ***patient* advocacy**.

	Language Access Advocacy or Patient Advocacy?	Language Access Advocacy or Patient Advocacy?
1	Specific, acute, "downstream"	Broad, chronic, "upstream"
2	Occurs at the individual health encounter	Occurs outside the individual health encounter
3	On behalf of a specific patient	On behalf of groups
4	Occurs at the interpersonal level	Occurs at institutional, community, group levels
5	More controversial for interpreter	May be controversial or threatening to stakeholders, questioning factors that contribute to systemic, institutional language access issues
6	Potentially influences perceptions of interpreter's neutrality, confidence in accurate communication, trust in the interpreter	Addresses behaviors, policies and systems
7	Addresses actions in a specific encounter	Draws focus to legal, ethical obligations, levels of compliance and allocation of resources across multiple encounters
8	Can be patronizing or empowering	Can be stressful and empowering

7. **Standards 31 and 32** Select one of the following quotes about advocacy or find another one and translate it.

"The hottest places in hell are reserved for those who, in times of great moral crisis, maintain their neutrality."

—Dante Alighieri, *Inferno*

"Washing one's hands of the conflict between the powerful and the powerless means to side with the powerful, not to be neutral."

—Paulo Freire

"If you are neutral in situations of injustice, you have chosen the side of the oppressor. If an elephant has its foot on the tail of a mouse and you say that you are neutral, the mouse will not appreciate your neutrality."

—Bishop Desmond Tutu

"In the end, we will remember not the words of our enemies, but the silence of our friends."

—Martin Luther King Jr.

Occupational therapy for interpreters

EXERCISES FOR THE TONGUE, HEART AND MIND

Learning how to read the research literature

Some studies, of greater or less quality, have been conducted on various aspects of medical interpreting. As an example, some studies focus on the differences between remote (telephone or video) and in-person interpreting, and sometimes these studies are cited to support a particular mode (in-person, video remote interpreting or VRI, telephone). Other studies focus on a particular kind of interpreter (qualified medical interpreter, bilingual employee who was never trained to interpret, or ad hoc interpreter such as family members, friends or children of the patient). Other studies might compare the results of utilizing trained versus untrained interpreters.

Interested parties are called stakeholders. Stakeholders who care about the results of such research could be interpreters themselves, patients, clinicians, administrators, sales representatives, government agencies, policymakers or advocates for patient safety, to name only a few.

All these stakeholders could have different opinions, agendas and goals. They may see the world through different lenses. Often they might mention certain studies to support a particular position (for example, "Telephone interpreters are all we need in hospitals"). However, if you carefully read such studies you may find that in fact the conclusions are often not clear or simple, and don't lend claimed support for a position.

As an interpreter or language access advocate, you can find such studies useful and important to read. It is important to understand what is really being assessed. With rapid changes in technology, studies will probably be used to make claims about the benefits or negative impacts of technological innovation for interpretation. For example, remote interpreting might affect the terms, conditions and compensation for your work. It could have an impact on the required training, skill or certifications of interpreters. It might affect the quality of service offered to patients of a particular national origin or ethnicity, and ultimately, their health. It may narrow or widen the gap in health disparities.

Here are a few examples of the kinds of points you might want to keep in mind as you read studies about medical interpreting.

Consider and discuss

Resource

> Nápoles, A.M. et al. (2010). Clinician ratings of interpreter mediated visits in underserved primary care settings with ad hoc, in-person professional and video conferencing modes. *Journal of Healthcare for the Poor and Underserved, 21*(1), pp. 301-317.

The abstract for this article presents important concepts such as "quality of interpretation and communication," "degree of patient engagement" or "cultural competence." It is clear that "clinician ratings"—the first two words in the title—are a high priority. But below are some essential questions to explore to help you assess the validity and strength of the article.

1. What skills and capabilities are needed in order to rate interpreting?

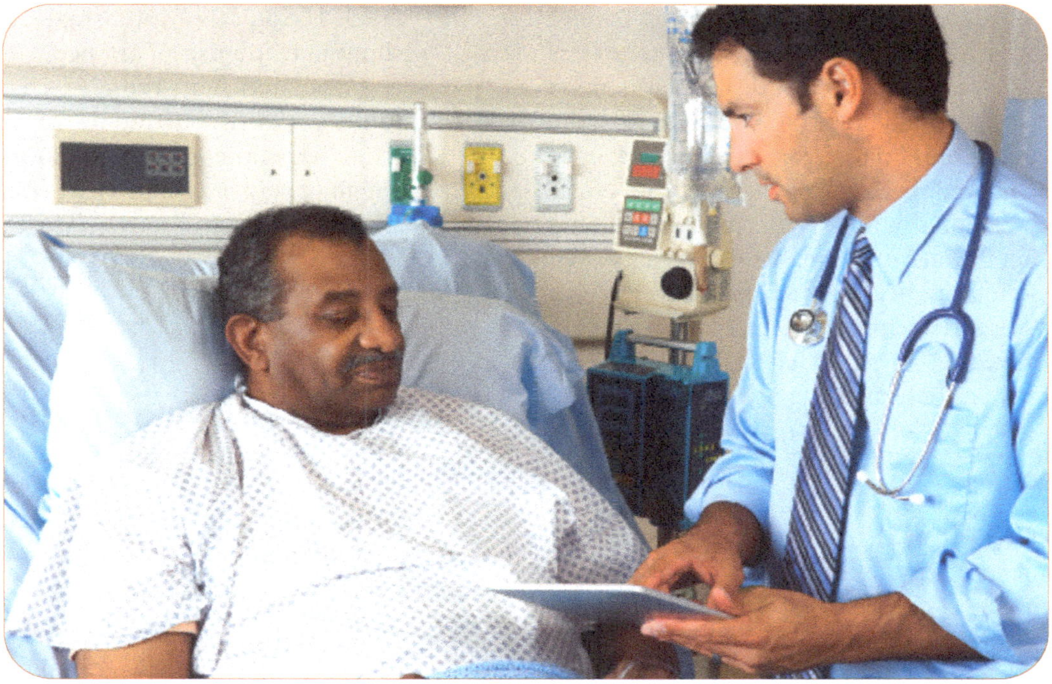

2. Do the clinicians who rated the visits possess these skills or capabilities?
3. What credentials or measures of competencies were required of raters?
4. Does the presence or absence of these credentials and measures affect the validity of the study?
5. What makes an assessment of interpreters by clinicians subjective or objective?
6. Do the assessments in this article appear to be subjective or objective? Why?

Resource

> Kuo, D., and Fagan, M. (1991). Satisfaction with methods of Spanish interpretation in an ambulatory care clinic. *Journal of General and Internal Medicine*, *14*, pp. 547-550.

The focus of this study was physicians' and their Spanish-speaking patients' satisfaction with different methods of interpreting. Both physicians and patients concurred that specific characteristics they considered highly important in an interpreter were availability, accuracy and confidentiality. Where they diverged was patients' appreciation for personal familiarity, gender concordance and the ability of the interpreter to assist after the visit in contrast with clinicians' appreciation for availability and understanding of customs and beliefs.

1. What skills or competencies must one possess in order to assess whether an interpreter is accurate? If these assessment capabilities are not addressed, does that affect the validity of the study?

   Below is a description of the clinicians and the patient participants. From the description, is it possible to tell if any of the participants have the required skills for interpreter assessment?

   > "All 149 patients who participated in our study (response rate, 94%) were native speakers of Spanish, with 92.5% originating from the Dominican Republic, Puerto Rico and Guatemala. The patients were predominantly female, with mean age of 52.6 years and on average had resided in the United States for 14 years.
   >
   > Fifty-one medical residents (69%) responded to our survey. None of them assessed themselves to be fluent in Spanish; fewer than 16% felt they were moderately proficient."

2. Helpful discussion of topics such as patient comfort levels with family-member interpreters and costs are included in the "discussion" section of the study. Yet accuracy (additions, censorship, omissions, opinions, error) does not seem to be considered. If a patient and practitioner are highly satisfied with an interpreter-mediated visit, but the interpreter makes significant errors with serious clinical consequences, is that visit a good or satisfactory encounter?
3. Can measures of satisfaction be considered subjective or objective?

Resource

> Flores, G. et al., (2003). Errors in medical interpretation and their potential clinical consequences in pediatric encounters. *Pediatrics, 111*(1), 6-14.

This is an example of a study in which interpreter error was measured. Audio recordings were analyzed post-visit. Interpreter error was described by degree of seriousness in terms of consequence and type of interpreter was defined in greater depth (professional, ad hoc, heritage speaker nurse, etc.).

Conclusions are based on systematically gathered data by thorough, reliable methodologies, performed by researchers with the appropriate skills. This study clearly illuminates the health impacts of the varying quality of interpreting provided to patients:

> "Errors in medical interpretation are common, averaging 31 per clinical encounter and omissions are the most frequent type. Most errors have potential clinical consequences and those committed by ad hoc interpreters are significantly more likely to have potential clinical consequences than those committed by hospital interpreters" (Reiss-Končar, 2010).

> "Aside from the social costs, inequities in healthcare are expensive. Errors in understanding may increase the cost of healthcare because of unnecessary testing, medical error, lack of compliance with treatments, return visits and liability (Dower 2003; Hardt, 1999). Alternatively, studies show that the use of trained interpreters is associated with reduced costs in ED [emergency department] return rates, increased clinic utilization, no increase in length of stay or cost of visit" (Bernstein et al., 2002, p. 4).

1. Briefly, what main points did the authors of this report make about the studies they considered?

Consider the following information

Multiple sources document that LEP patients have lower health outcomes (Jacobs et al., 2003) and less access to a regular source of care, fewer physician visits, lower rates of preventive service (Fox & Stein, 1991; Kirkman-Liff & Mondragón, 1991; Woloshin et al., 1997; Fiscella et al., 2002) and typically longer hospital stays than English proficient patients with the same conditions (John-Baptiste et al., 2004). A lack of regular, systemic interpretation and translation services are a problem (Jacobs et al., 2003). In cases where LEP patients are able to access care, they have poorer adherence to treatment and follow-up for chronic illnesses, increased medication complications, decreased understanding of diagnoses and treatment after emergency department (ED) visits and lower rates of satisfaction with care (Manson, 1988; Crane, 1997; Carrasquillo et al., 1999; Gandhi et al., 2000). One study found that some degree of detectable physical harm occurred in adverse events reported in 49.1% of LEP cases, as opposed to 29.5% of those cases of English-speaking patients and that language barriers appear to increase the risks to patient safety (Divi et al., 2007, p. 61).

2. In the multiple studies cited above, what are the two populations being compared?

3. Which set of comparisons interests you most? Why?

Other studies to consider reading

Review the following abstracts for the articles listed. Do you find these articles relevant for medical interpreters to read and understand? Why or why not? (Specify the reasons for each article.)

Abstract

Schiaffino, M.K., Nara, A., and Mao, L. (2016). Language services in hospitals vary by ownership and location. *Health Affairs*, *35*(8), pp. 1399-1403.

> *Twenty-four million people in the United States have limited English proficiency. They experience barriers to healthcare because of their inability to communicate effectively with providers. Hospitals are required to provide language services that reflect the needs of people in their communities, but these services are not available systematically.*

Abstract

Eneriz-Wiemer, M., Sanders, L.M., Barr, D.A., and Mendoza, F.S. (2014). Parental limited English proficiency and health outcomes for children with special healthcare needs: A systematic review. *Academic Pediatrics, 14*(2), pp. 128-136.

> ***BACKGROUND:*** *One in 10 US adults of childbearing age has limited English proficiency (LEP). Parental LEP is associated with worse health outcomes among healthy children. The relationship of parental LEP to health outcomes for children with special healthcare needs (CSHCN) has not been systematically reviewed.*
>
> ***OBJECTIVE:*** *To conduct a systematic review of peer-reviewed literature examining relationships between parental LEP and health outcomes for CSHCN...*
>
> ***ELIGIBILITY CRITERIA:*** *US studies published between 1964 and 2012 were*

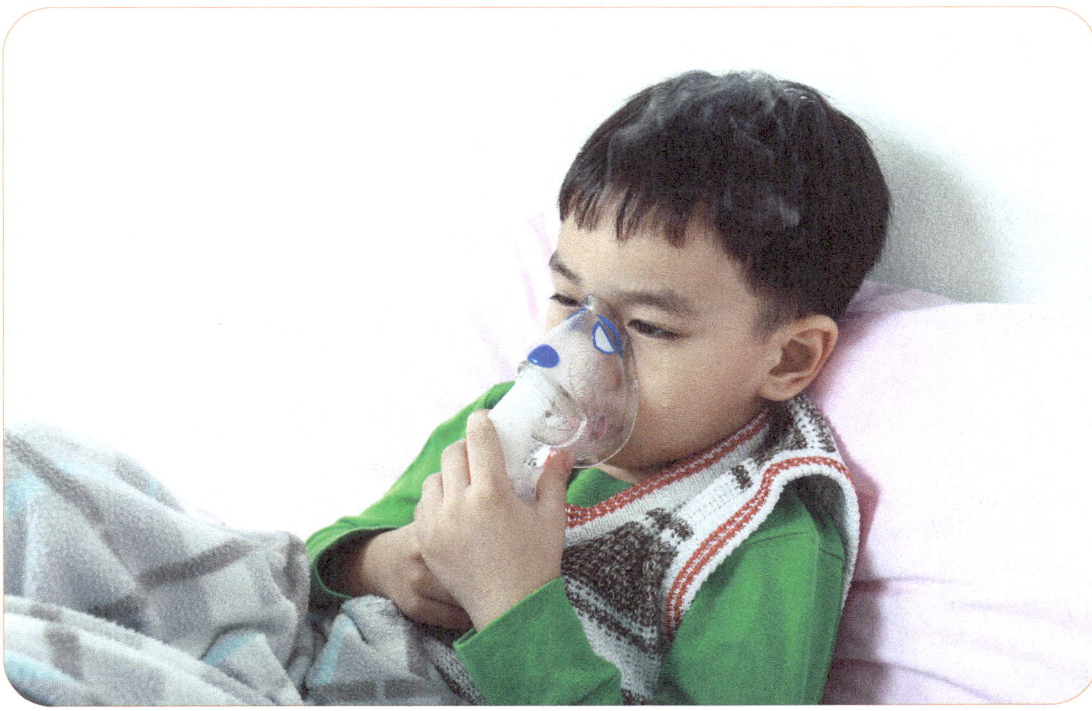

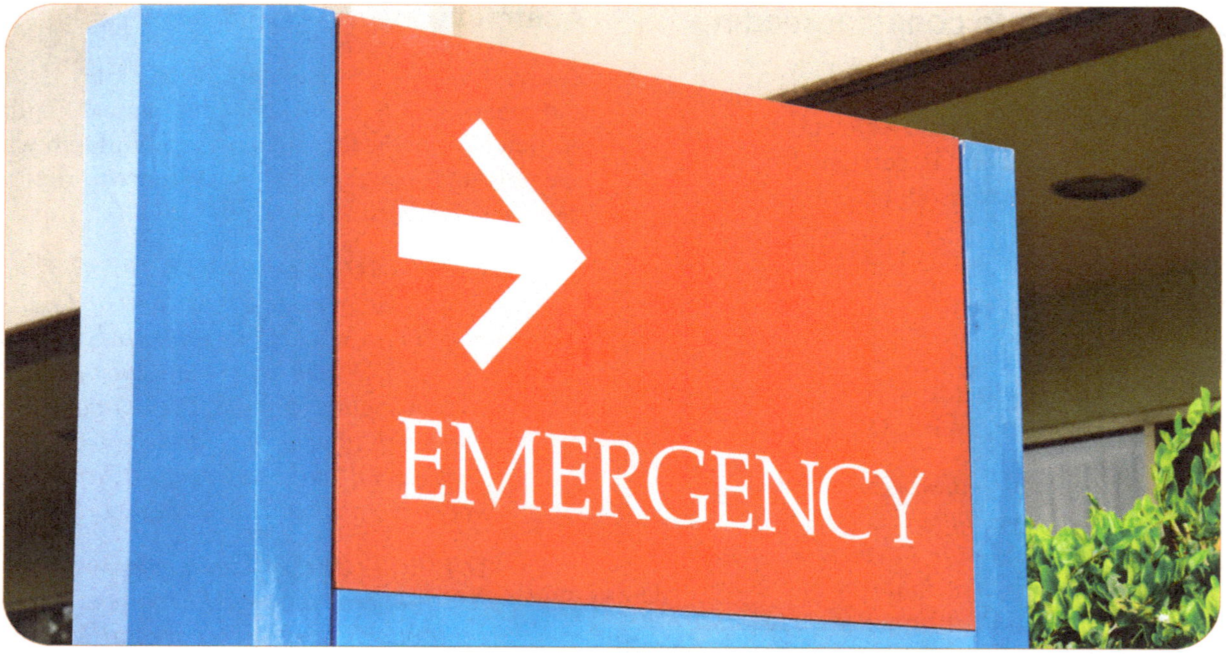

included if: 1) subjects were CSHCN; 2) studies included some measure of parental LEP; 3) at least 1 outcome measure of child health status, access, utilization, costs, or quality; and 4) primary or secondary data analysis.

METHODS: *Three trained reviewers independently screened studies and extracted data. Two separate reviewers appraised studies for methodological rigor and quality.*

RESULTS: *From 2765 titles and abstracts, 31 studies met eligibility criteria. Five studies assessed child health status, 12 assessed access, 8 assessed utilization, 2 assessed costs, and 14 assessed quality. Nearly all (29 of 31) studies used only parent- or child-reported outcome measures, rather than objective measures. LEP parents were substantially more likely than English-proficient parents to report that their CSHCN were uninsured and had no usual source of care or medical home. LEP parents were also less likely to report family-centered care and satisfaction with care. Disparities persisted for children with LEP parents after adjustment for ethnicity and socioeconomic status.*

CONCLUSIONS AND IMPLICATIONS: *Parental LEP is independently associated with worse healthcare access and quality for CSHCN. Healthcare providers should recognize LEP as an independent risk factor for poor health outcomes among CSHCN. Emerging models of chronic disease care should integrate and evaluate interventions that target access and quality disparities for LEP families.*

Abstract

Njeru, J.W. et al., (2015). Emergency department and inpatient healthcare utilization among patients who require interpreter services. *BMC Health Services Research, 15*:214.

BACKGROUND: *Limited English proficiency is associated with health disparities and suboptimal health outcomes. Although Limited English proficiency is a barrier to effective healthcare, its association with inpatient healthcare utilization is unclear. The aim of this study was to examine the association between patients with limited English proficiency, and emergency department visits and hospital admissions.*

METHODS: We compared emergency department visits and hospitalizations in 2012 between patients requiring interpreter services and age-matched English-proficient patients (who did not require interpreters), in a retrospective cohort study of adult patients actively empanelled to a large primary healthcare network in a medium-sized United States city (n = 3,784).

RESULTS: Patients who required interpreter services had significantly more Emergency Department visits (841 vs 620; P≤.001) and hospitalizations (408 vs 343; P≤.001) than patients who did not require interpreter services. On regression analysis the risk of a first Emergency Department visit was 60 percent higher for patients requiring interpreter services than those who did not...

CONCLUSIONS: Patients who required interpreter services had higher rates of inpatient healthcare utilization compared with patients who did not require an interpreter. Further research is required to understand factors associated with this utilization and to develop sociolinguistically tailored interventions to facilitate appropriate healthcare provision for this population.

Abstract

Juckett, G., and Unger, K. (2014). Appropriate use of medical interpreters. *American Family Physician, 90*(7), pp. 476-480.

More than 25 million Americans speak English "less than very well," according to the U.S. Census Bureau. This population is less able to access healthcare and is at higher risk of adverse outcomes such as drug complications and decreased patient satisfaction. Title VI of the Civil Rights Act mandates that interpreter services be provided for patients with limited English proficiency who need this service, despite the lack of reimbursement in most states. Professional interpreters are superior to the usual practice of using ad hoc interpreters (i.e., family, friends, or untrained staff). Untrained interpreters are more likely to make errors, violate confidentiality, and increase the risk of poor outcomes. Children should never be used as interpreters except in emergencies. When using an interpreter, the clinician should address the patient directly and seat the interpreter next to or slightly behind the patient. Statements should be short, and the discussion should be limited to three major points. In addition to acting as a conduit for the discussion, the interpreter may serve as a cultural liaison between the physician and patient. When a bilingual clinician or a professional interpreter is not available, phone interpretation services or trained bilingual staff members are reasonable alternatives. The use of professional interpreters (in person or via telephone) increases patient satisfaction, improves adherence and outcomes, and reduces adverse events, thus limiting malpractice risk.

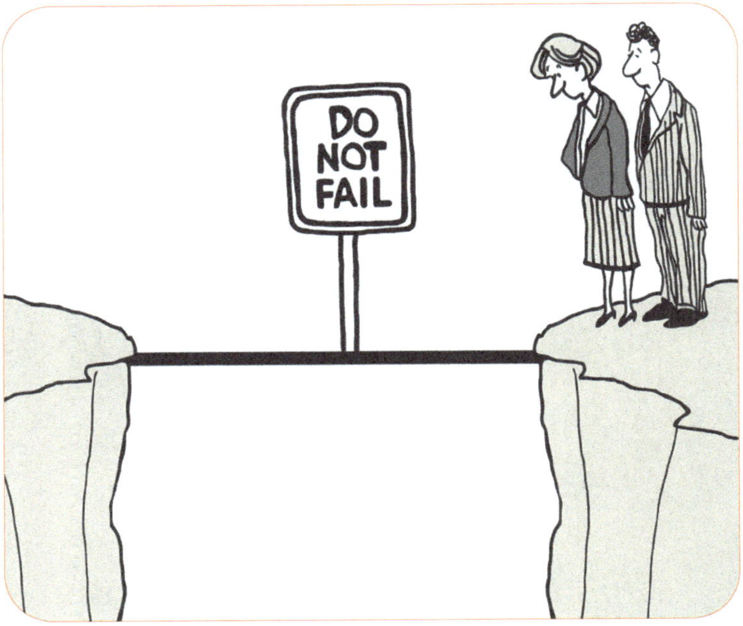

Medical terminology: Bones and joints

Below you will find anatomical drawings relevant to the content of this chapter. Follow the instructions found at the end of Chapter 1 to study the terminology in this section.

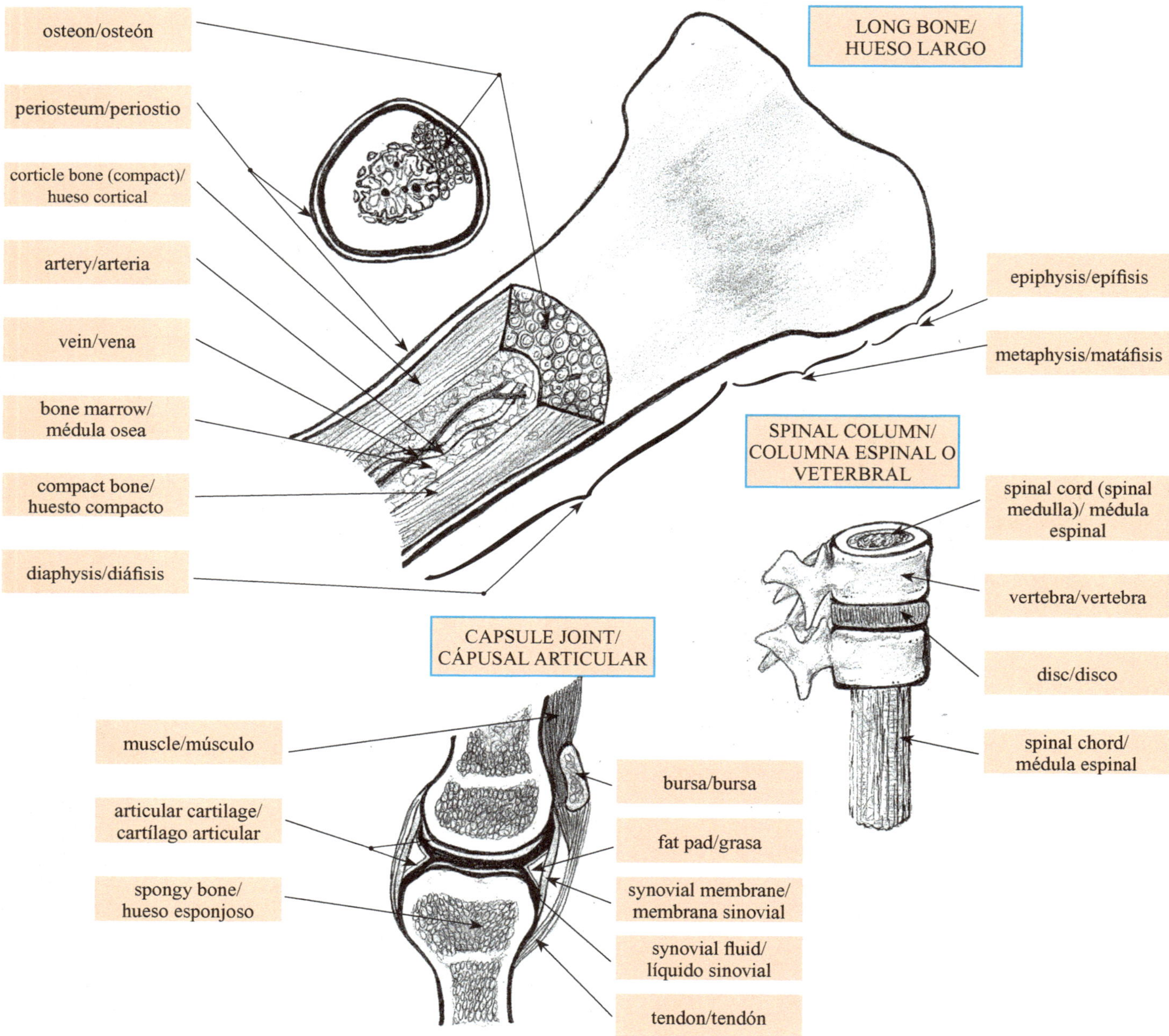

Figure 9-A: Bones and joints (English and Spanish)

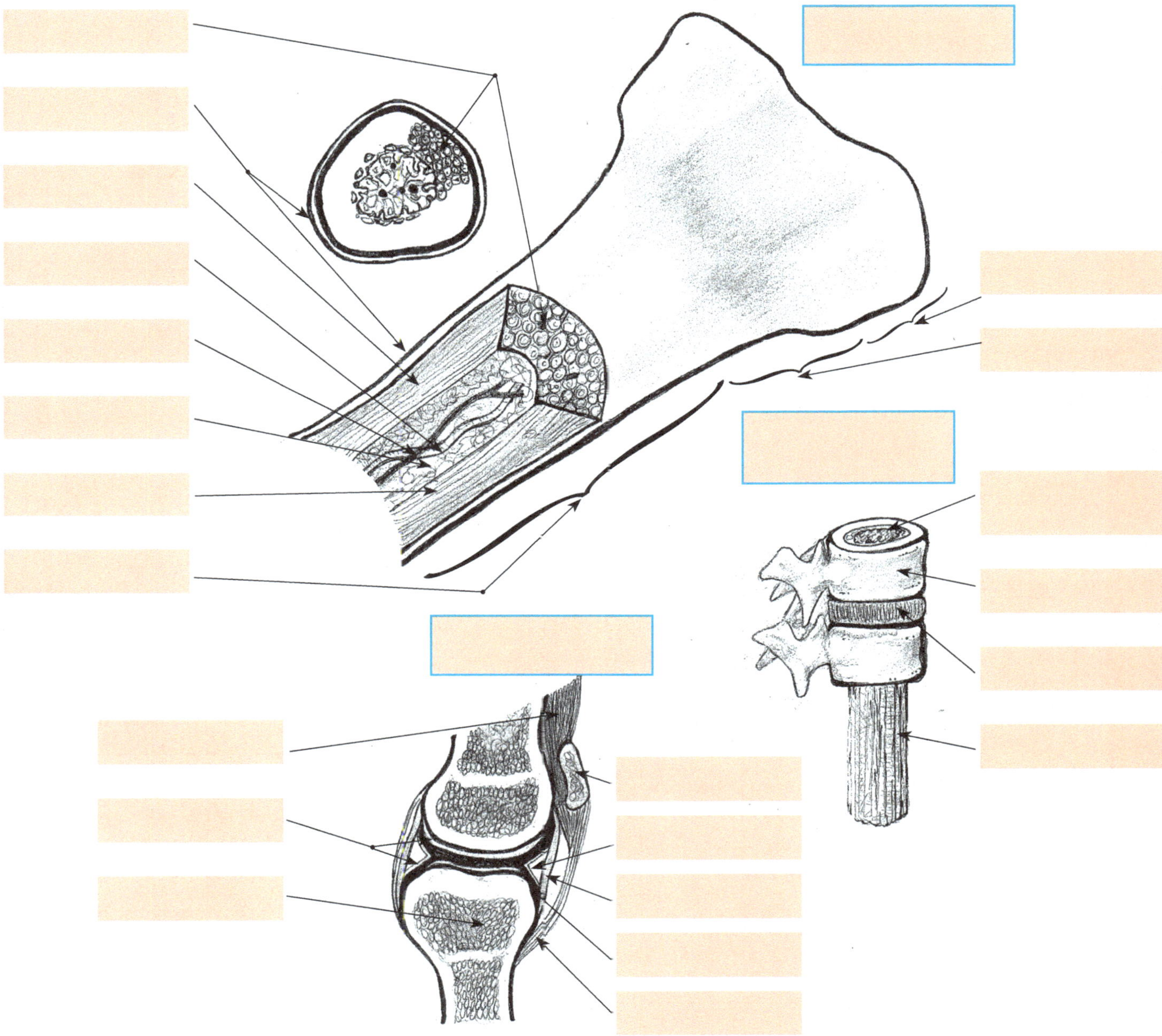

Figure 9-B: Bones and joints (English only)

Medical terminology list

Bones and joints

VOCABULARY FOR GRAPHIC–IN ENGLISH	VOCABULARY FOR GRAPHIC–IN SPANISH	ANY OTHER LANGUAGE
artery	arteria	
articular cartilage	cartílago articular	
bone marrow	médula osea	
bones	hueso	
bursa	bursa	
capsule joint	cápusal articular	
cartilage	cartílago	
compact bone	huesto compacto	
corticle bone (compact)	hueso cortical	
diaphysis	diáfisis	
ellipsoid joint	articulación elipsoidal	
epiphysis	epífisis	
flat bones	huesos planos	
gliding joint	articulación deslizante	
growth plate (epiphyseal line)	cartílago de crecimiento (placa epifisaria, cartílago e[ifisario)	
hinge joint	articulación en bisagra	
irregular bones	huesos irregulares	
joint	articulación, coyuntura	
long bone	hueso largo	
medullary cavity	cavidad medular	
metaphysis	matáfisis	
muscle	músculo	
osteon	osteón	
periosteum	periostio	
pivot joint	articulación en pivote	
saddle joint	articulación en silla de montar	
short bones	huesos cortos	
spheroidal joint	articulación esférica	
spinal column	columna espinal o veterbral	
spinal cord (spinal medulla)	médula espinal	
spongy bone	hueso esponjoso	
synovial fluid	líquido sinovial	
synovial joint	articulación sinovial	
synovial membrane	membrana sinovial	
tendon	tendon	
vein	vena	
vertebra	vertebra	

Pharmacology and Referrals 10

Advisory

This chapter addresses pediatric hospitalizations, interpreting protocols regarding minors and developmental delay in children.

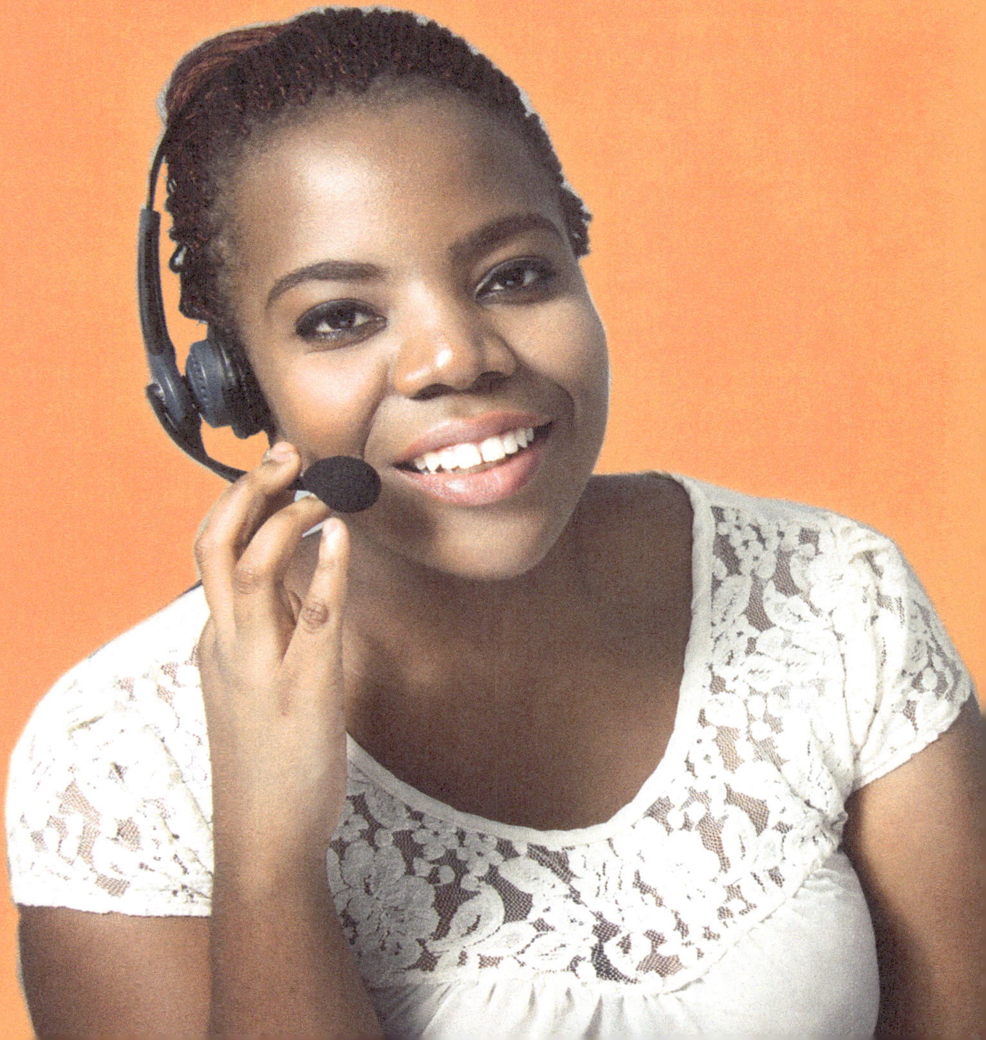

Remote interpreting role play dialogue I—pediatric inpatient pharmacology (English-Spanish)

Note: In these two dialogues, the interpreter is part of the script. Do not act out this dialogue as a regular role play (where the interpreter should not read the dialogue but only interpret it). Instead, this time allow the interpreter to see the script as you act it out. After doing so, discuss the interpreter's decisions for each dialogue and whether or not you agree with those decisions.

This telephone dialogue is between a patient and a pharmacist on a pediatric hospital ward. The patient is a 16-year-old boy. The parent or guardian is not present and the pharmacist would like to get some background information, or medical history, from the patient. The pharmacist is in the patient room and the interpreter is in a different location on the telephone. The interpreter has no specific information about this patient regarding why he is being hospitalized. This conversation takes place over the phone.

PHARMACIST: Hello, this is Bridget from pediatric pharmacy. I was told you could help me speak to a patient in Spanish.

INTERPRETER: Sure. Can I get the name of the patient and the location?

PHARMACIST: Yes, let's see, the patient's name is Alejandro Castillo. He's 16 years old, and I just want to get some background information from him.

INTERPRETER: Will we be speaking with a parent or guardian?

PHARMACIST: No, the mom isn't here right now, but it's pretty basic information. I'm here in the room with the patient.

INTERPRETER: OK. And you said your name is Bridget? From the pediatric pharmacy on which floor of the hospital?

PHARMACIST: Yes, we're on the eighth floor. We're using a dual-set-interpreter telephone so we won't have to pass the telephone back and forth. I'll hand him his line now. *(gives patient his telephone)* Now, could you ask the patient, let's see, Alejandro, if he's had a flu shot this year?

INTERPRETER: Alejandro, ¿te pusieron una vacuna contra la gripe?

PATIENT: ¿Mm? Ah.

INTERPRETER: Alejandro, ¿te pusieron una vacuna para la gripe? Did you get a flu shot this year, Alejandro?

PATIENT: *(silence, breathing)*

INTERPRETER: Alejandro. Yo soy Irma. Soy tu intérprete. ¿Te han puesto la vacuna para la gripe?

PATIENT: *(silence, breathing)*

INTERPRETER: Alejandro, ¿me oyes?

PATIENT: Sí. *(muffled)*

INTERPRETER: Alejandro, ¿te han puesto una vacuna para la gripe este año? ¿Te han puesto una inyección en contra del flu?

PATIENT: No...hm...sé. *(Patient sounds as if he is either groggy or developmentally delayed.)*

INTERPRETER: He doesn't know if he's had the flu shot or not.

PHARMACIST: Can you ask him if they gave him any shots recently?

INTERPRETER: Sure, though as the interpreter, may I clarify with you, you're in the hospital with him, right? I imagine he might be receiving shots or needle sticks every day. So I'll go ahead and ask him, but I'm not sure he will be able to understand your question. I'll ask him. Alejandro, ¿te han inyectado recientemente?

PATIENT: Mm.

INTERPRETER: ¿Sabes qué quiere decir cuando digo inyección o vacuna? ¿Te han picado recientemente?

PATIENT: Sí.

INTERPRETER: ¿Sabes para qué fue?

PATIENT: No sé.

INTERPRETER: *(to the pharmacist)* As the interpreter, Bridget, I'm not really sure he's understanding. He can just tell me he's been injected, or stuck with needles recently, but he's been to the doctor a lot and he is now in the hospital. It could be anything, including blood draws or IVs or blood sugar sticks in the finger.

PHARMACIST: Can you ask him if he's up to date on his vaccines?

INTERPRETER: Alejandro, ¿sabes si te han puesto todas tus vacunas de niño?

PATIENT: No.

INTERPRETER: ¿Crees que no te han puesto las vacunas, o no sabes si te las han puesto?

PATIENT: No sé.

INTERPRETER: *(to pharmacist)* You know, Bridget, speaking as the interpreter, he sounds a little out of it or confused. He's having trouble understanding or answering really basic questions. I can't see his face, but is there any kind of a problem? He really doesn't seem to be responding normally.

PHARMACIST: No, I think maybe he's just shy. Can you just ask him one more thing? I think we're going to go ahead and give him a flu shot, but can you find out if he's allergic to eggs?

INTERPRETER: ¿Alejandro, tienes alergia a los huevos?

PATIENT: No.

INTERPRETER: ¿Tú puedes comer huevos? ¿Comes huevos en casa?

PATIENT: Sí.

INTERPRETER: As the interpreter, I need to clarify a little bit. He says he's not allergic to eggs and he eats them at home, but I need to let you know I'm really uncomfortable with this. I sense there is something going on and it's definitely more than just shyness. There's something else going on here. He's a minor. I would be really hesitant to count on any of this information without talking to a parent.

PHARMACIST: Well, we really need to give him a flu shot, I think it'll be OK.

INTERPRETER: Well, it's your decision, I just have to tell you what I'm picking up, and I really believe there is something going on here. Something's not quite right with his responses, and he is a minor.

PHARMACIST: OK, well, thank you.

INTERPRETER: You're welcome. Bye.

Epilogue: *On a subsequent day, the interpreter worked with this patient's mother and a social worker for a routine visit. In reviewing services that the child was receiving in school and at home, it turned out that the 16 year old had been assessed as being at the developmental stage of a 4 year old. He was enrolled in the special education program with a yearly individual education plan (IEP) through the school district.*

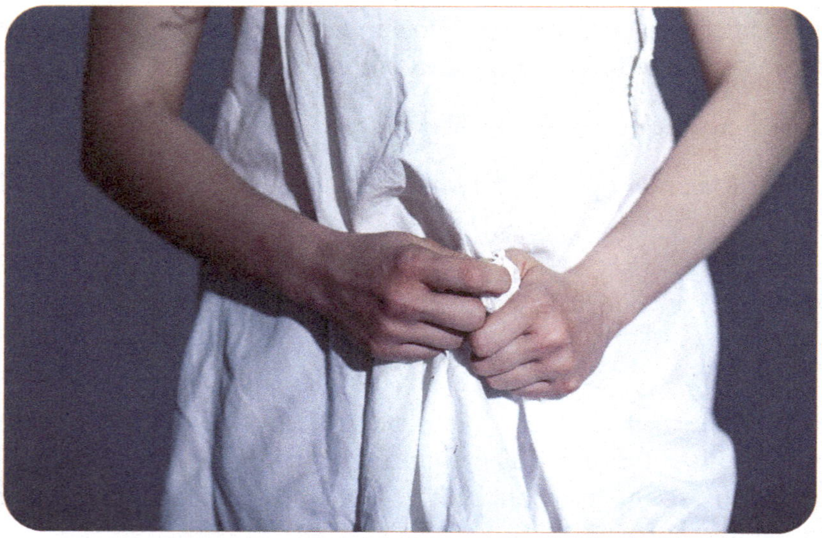

Remote interpreting role play dialogue I—pediatric inpatient pharmacology (English only)

PHARMACIST: Hello, this is Bridget from pediatric pharmacy. I was told you could help me speak to a patient in his language.

INTERPRETER: Sure. Can I get the name of the patient and the location?

PHARMACIST: Yes, let's see, the patient's name is Bilal Hamed. He's 16 years old, and I just want to get some background information from him.

INTERPRETER: Will we be speaking with a parent or guardian?

PHARMACIST: No, the mom isn't here right now, but it's pretty basic information. I'm here in the room with the patient.

INTERPRETER: OK. And you said your name is Bridget? From the pediatric pharmacy on which floor of the hospital?

PHARMACIST: Yes, we're on the eighth floor. We're using a dual-set-interpreter telephone so we won't have to pass the telephone back and forth. I'll hand him his line now. *(gives patient his telephone)* Now, could you ask the patient, let's see, Bilal, if he's had a flu shot this year?

INTERPRETER: Bilal, did you get a flu shot this year?

PATIENT: ¿Mm?

INTERPRETER: Bilal, did you get a flu shot this year? *(tries in English.)* Did you get a flu shot this year, Bilal?

PATIENT: *(silence, breathing)*

INTERPRETER: *(switches back to the patient's language)* Bilal, I am Wafa. I am your interpreter. Did you get a flu shot this year?

PATIENT: *(silence, breathing)*

INTERPRETER: Bilal, can you hear me?

PATIENT: (*speaking his own language*) Yes. *(muffled)*

INTERPRETER: Bilal, did you get a flu shot this year? Did they give you a shot so you won't get the flu?

PATIENT: I don't know. *(Patient sounds as if he is either groggy or developmentally delayed.)*

INTERPRETER: *(switches to English.)* He doesn't know if he's had the flu shot or not.

PHARMACIST: Can you ask him if they gave him any shots recently?

INTERPRETER: Sure, though as the interpreter, may I clarify with you, you're in the hospital with him, right? I imagine he might be receiving shots or needle sticks every day. So I'll go ahead ask him, but I want you to know I'm not sure he will be able to understand your question. I'll ask him. *(switches back to the patient's language.)* Bilal, did you get a shot recently?

PATIENT: Mm.

INTERPRETER: Do you know what I mean when I say shot or injection? Do you know what vaccination is? Did they stick you with a needle or give you a shot recently?

PATIENT: Yes.

INTERPRETER: Do you know what it was for?

PATIENT: No.

INTERPRETER: *(switches to English, speaking to the pharmacist)* As the interpreter, Bridget, I'm not really sure he's understanding. He can just tell me he's been injected, or stuck with needles recently, but he's been to the doctor a lot, and he is now in the hospital. It could be anything, including blood draws or IVs or blood sugar sticks in the finger.

PHARMACIST: Can you ask him if he's up to date on his vaccines?

INTERPRETER: *(switches back to the patient's language.)* Bilal, are you up to date on your vaccines?

PATIENT: No.

INTERPRETER: Do you think they haven't given you your vaccinations, or you don't know if they've given you your vaccinations?

PATIENT: Dunno.

INTERPRETER: *(switches to English, speaking to the pharmacist.)* You know, Bridget, speaking as the interpreter, he sounds a little out of it or confused. He's having trouble understanding or answering really basic questions. I can't see his face, but is there any kind of a problem? He really doesn't seem to be responding normally.

PHARMACIST: No, I think maybe he's just shy. Can you just ask him one more thing? I think we're going to go ahead and give him a flu shot, but can you find out if he's allergic to eggs?

INTERPRETER: *(switches back to the patient's language.)* Bilal, are you allergic to eggs?

PATIENT: *(switches back to the patient's language.)* No.

INTERPRETER: *(switches back to the patient's language.)* Can you eat eggs? Do you eat eggs at home?

PATIENT: *(switches back to the patient's language.)* Yes.

INTERPRETER: As the interpreter, I need to clarify a little bit. He says he's not allergic to eggs and he eats them at home, but I need to let you know I'm really uncomfortable with this. I sense there is something going on and it's definitely more than just shyness. There's something else going on here. He's a minor. I would be really hesitant to count on any of this information without talking to a patient.

PHARMACIST: Well, we really need to give him a flu shot, I think it'll be OK.

INTERPRETER: Well, it's your decision, I just have to tell you what I'm picking up, and I really believe there is something going on here. Something's not quite right with his responses, and he's a minor.

PHARMACIST: OK, well, thank you.

INTERPRETER: You're welcome. Bye.

Epilogue: *On a subsequent day, the interpreter worked with this patient's mother and a social worker for a routine visit. In reviewing services that the child was receiving in school and at home, it turned out that the 16 year old had been assessed as being at the developmental stage of a 4 year old. He was enrolled in the special education program with a yearly individual education plan (IEP) through the school district.*

Remote interpreting role play dialogue II—pediatric referral service and scheduling (English-Spanish)

This telephone dialogue takes place between an operator for a referral service and the patient of a patient. What is the role of the interpreter? How does she manage her role? How might her actions influence patient outcomes and health?

The operator has already given relevant information about the call to the interpreter and dials the patient.

PATIENT: ¿Bueno?

OPERATOR: Hello, this is Wanda. I'm calling from the pediatric referral service. Is this Mrs. Reyes?

PATIENT: No. ¿Quién habla?

OPERATOR: Is this where Tonantzín Reyes lives?

PATIENT: Sí. ¿Quién habla?

OPERATOR: My name is Wanda. I'm calling from White Pines Medical Center. May I speak to the patient or guardian of Tonantzín?

PATIENT: Ella habla. Soy la mamá.

OPERATOR: Oh, all right. Then you are Mrs. Reyes?

PATIENT: No, mi apellido es Ayala. Mi hija se apellida Reyes. ¿Qué desea?

OPERATOR: Well, I'm calling because we have a referral here for Tonantzín to see the dermatologist. Can we go ahead and schedule that appointment?

PATIENT: Oh, pues, ya no. No creo que la necesite. Ya no le duelen los huesos.

OPERATOR: All right, then, we won't schedule it.

INTERPRETER: *(after interpreting)* Excuse me, as the interpreter I need to let you know that there may be some miscommunication that you might want to clear up. *(Interpreter repeats in Spanish.)*

OPERATOR: Oh, really, what's that? *(Interpreter interprets.)*

INTERPRETER: *(in English to operator.)* Well, I noticed that you offered Mom an appointment for a dermatology consultation, but Mom said it wasn't necessary because the child's bones aren't hurting anymore. It seems like there is some confusion here. You said dermatology, but she said bones. *(Interpreter tells the patient, in Spanish, what she told the operator.)*

OPERATOR: Oh, right. Well, go ahead.

INTERPRETER: Did you want to clarify? *(Interpreter tells the patient, in Spanish, what she told the operator.)*

OPERATOR: Yes, can you do that please? *(Interpreter tells the patient, in Spanish, what she told the operator.)*

INTERPRETER: Why don't I let you do that and I'll interpret for you. *(Interpreter tells the patient, in Spanish, what she told the operator.)*

OPERATOR: All right, Mrs. Reyes, I mean Mrs. Ayala, did you know that Dr. Petersen, the pediatrician, had sent out a referral to us for Tonantzín to see a dermatologist for the skin, not for the bones?

PATIENT: Pues, yo no sé nada de eso. Ella tuvo problemas con dolor en los huesos.

OPERATOR: So she didn't have any kind of a skin problem?

PATIENT: No, le dolieron los huesos pero ya se le quitó el dolor. Ya no necesita la cita. Nunca tuvo un problema con la piel.

OPERATOR: Would you like me to call her doctor's office and ask what this is about?

PATIENT: Sí, por favor. Gracias.

OPERATOR: Well, all right. And I'll just write a note here that she no longer has pain in her joints.

INTERPRETER: As the interpreter, I'd like to make a correction. The mother said she had pain in her *bones*, rather than joints, but the pain went away. She doesn't need the appointment anymore. She never had problems with her skin.

OPERATOR: All right, I'll put in my note here that she had pain in her bones, but the pain went away and she doesn't want the appointment. And she never had problems with her skin.

PATIENT: Gracias. Entonces, ¿alguien me va a llamar?

OPERATOR: Yes, as soon as I figure out what this is about I'll give you a call to let you know and see if we still need to schedule an appointment.

PATIENT: Bueno, muchas gracias.

OPERATOR: Thank you.

Remote interpreting role play dialogue II—pediatric referral service and scheduling (English only)

PATIENT: Hello?

OPERATOR: Hello, this is Wanda. I'm calling from the pediatric referral service. Is this Mrs. Lao?

PATIENT: No. Who's calling?

OPERATOR: Is this where Shee Lao lives?

PATIENT: Yes. Who's calling?

OPERATOR: My name is Wanda. I'm calling from White Pines Medical Center. May I speak to the patient or guardian of Shee Lao?

PATIENT: She's speaking. I am the mother.

OPERATOR: Oh, all right. Then you are Mrs. Lao?

PATIENT: No, my last name is Ying. My daughter's last name is Lao. Why are you calling?

OPERATOR: Well, I'm calling because we have a referral here for Shee to see the dermatologist. Can we go ahead and schedule that appointment?

PATIENT: Oh, well, not anymore. I don't think she needs it. Her bones aren't hurting her anymore.

OPERATOR: All right, then, we won't schedule it.

INTERPRETER: *(after interpreting)* Excuse me, as the interpreter I need to let you know that there may be some miscommunication that you might want to clear up. *(Interpreter tells the patient, in the patient's language, what she told the operator.)*

OPERATOR: Oh, really, what's that? *(Interpreter interprets.)*

INTERPRETER: *(In English, to operator.)* Well, I noticed that you offered Mom an appointment for a dermatology consultation, but Mom said it wasn't necessary because the child's bones aren't hurting anymore. It seems like there is some confusion here. You said dermatology, but she said bones. *(Interpreter tells the patient, in the patient's language, what she told the operator.)*

OPERATOR: Oh, right. Well, go ahead.

INTERPRETER: Did you want to clarify? *(Interpreter tells the patient, in the patient's language, what she told the operator.)*

OPERATOR: Yes, can you do that please? *(Interpreter tells the patient, in the patient's language, what she told the operator.)*

INTERPRET: Why don't I let you do that and I'll interpret for you. *(Interpreter tells the patient, in the patient's language, what she told the operator.)*

OPERATOR: All right, Mrs. Lao, I mean Mrs. Ying, did you know that Dr. Petersen, the pediatrician, had sent out a referral to us for Shee to see a dermatologist for the skin, not for the bones?

PATIENT: I don't know anything about that. She had pain in her bones.

OPERATOR: So she didn't have any kind of a skin problem?

PATIENT: No, she had pain in her bones, but the pain went away. She doesn't need the appointment anymore. She never had problems with her skin.

OPERATOR: Would you like me to call her doctor's office and ask what this is about?

PATIENT: Yes, please. Thank you.

OPERATOR: Well, all right. And I'll just write a note here that she no longer has pain in her joints.

INTERPRETER: As the interpreter, I'd like to make a correction. The mother said she had pain in her *bones*, rather than joints, but the pain went away. She doesn't need the appointment anymore. She never had problems with her skin.

OPERATOR: All right, I'll put in my note here that she had pain in her bones, but the pain went away and she doesn't want the appointment. And she never had problems with her skin.

PATIENT: Thank you. So will someone call me?

OPERATOR: Yes, as soon as I figure out what this is about I'll give you a call to let you know and see if we still need to schedule an appointment.

PATIENT: OK, thank you.

OPERATOR: Thank you.

What's important to know about this chapter?

Overview

Remote interpreting refers to telephone or video interpreting. This book does not address how to perform such interpreting. However, the content of the two dialogues just presented is addressed and also some of the particular challenges that healthcare interpreters face when they perform over-the-phone interpreting (OPI) or video remote interpreting (VRI).

It would be impossible to overestimate the impact of remote interpreting technology and practices on the delivery of interpreting and of healthcare itself. There are still no national qualifications or training requirements for performing remote interpreting, despite its substantial challenges. Remote interpreting in the United States and elsewhere has also begun to take a significant toll on interpreter salaries, schedules, working conditions, fatigue and well-being—and on patient satisfaction. Much research needs to be done to determine how these swift changes have affected patient understanding, treatment plans and health outcomes.

Remote interpreting has a great potential for good and for harm. None of it can be addressed here, but these are urgent matters. Such swift and massive changes in the field should be carefully considered by all interpreters in healthcare and their professional associations.

Dialogue I: Pediatric inpatient pharmacology

Red Flags

When you see a red flag on a beach, it indicates a hazard such as a riptide or undertow. A red flag means *caution!*

When you are interpreting and a "red flag" pops up in your mind, pay attention. Perhaps there is a problem.

Speaking with a minor without a parent or guardian

After a brief introduction from the pharmacist, it becomes clear that potential problems are emerging for this interpreting assignment—and for the patient. What might they be? Which laws, regulations and best medical practices address communication with minors that involves medical information?

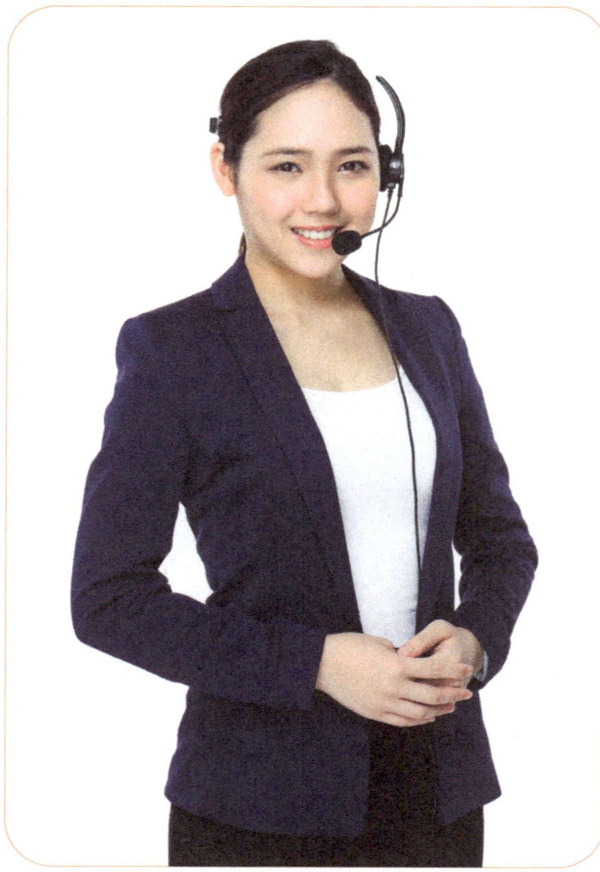

Is it legal and ethical for a health practitioner on a pediatric ward to ask a child about important medical information without a parent present? Usually not. What are the possible medical consequences of a flu shot for a person who is allergic to eggs or who has compromised immunity? What might the legal consequences be for a pharmacist, a doctor or an institution if a medical error were made because a child, rather than an adult and legal guardian, was consulted and gave wrong information?

Under some circumstances, practitioners will want to speak privately to a minor (especially a teen) about topics such as use of controlled or illegal substances, sexual activity, abuse, mental health or self-harm. If so, providers will usually advise the parent first. In the United States, this type of encounter is permissible in some states but not all. It can be helpful to know the laws governing health information and minors in the state you are interpreting in. You might also ask if interpreters can be held liable for a provider or staff member's decision to speak with a minor without a parent or guardian present.

When remote interpreting isn't enough

What can an interpreter do when she senses that remote (telephone or video) is inadequate for clear communication? Besides saying so to the provider, the interpreter's concerns should be documented. If a miscommunication should result in a negative consequence or health outcome (for example, an undocumented allergic reaction, denial of a health benefit or a misunderstanding that sabotages a treatment plan) it's important that the interpreter has documented the concern.

Extra-linguistic information

What might the interpreter miss over the phone? In this dialogue, the interpreter cannot see the patient but has access to other information from speech cues and speech patterns. What can an interpreter infer over the phone about the patient from his inflection, voice, pitch, pauses and other nonvisual information? When you speak with someone over the phone, can you assess that person's age, gender, cognition, socioeconomic status, race or ethnicity? For further information, see the suggested readings for the exercises in this chapter.

Interpreters speaking with children

As the interpreter, how should you speak to the patient? If your other working language has formal and informal pronouns or speech, which do you use, and at what age or circumstance does it change? If you would use the formal form of speech with an adult, which form would you use with a 12-year-old girl? What if she were pregnant or a mother? Consider that sometimes the formal mode of addressing a teen or young adult might seem respectful and empowering and at other times simply confusing. If your language has different pronouns, register, grammar or other markers to denote social standing, and you typically use the formal style when interpreting, it can still be inappropriate for younger children and confusing for adolescents or adults with developmental disabilities. They might not be used to being spoken to this way, even if an interpreter finds it appropriate. As the interpreter, you may have to make a decision case by case. That decision could be a bigger challenge by telephone or video.

When you speak to a young person (especially a child under eight) or a person with a developmental disability, the typical interpreter usage of the first person (direct speech) may also be disconcerting. Be sure to assess the situation as you go and monitor for understanding and comfort or confusion.

Switching languages midstream

In this dialogue, the interpreter repeated the question as spoken by the provider in English for this pediatric patient. Depending on many factors, a child may be more comfortable in the language of the new country because it is used in school, on television, with siblings and friends, rather than the language spoken at home by parents. In this case the interpreter senses some difficulty with understanding, so she tried out the question in English. Should she have made this decision and done this on her own? How else might she have handled her concern?

Interpreter role

What do you think of how the interpreter handled this situation? Assess her performance in terms of NCIHC standard 31 on advocacy.

Intuition

In much of the United States, depending on one's culture and personal upbringing, intuition isn't valued or seen as "scientific." In some cultures, intuition is regarded as being of great value. For an interpreter, it is important to pay attention to your intuition and all the nonverbal cues you sense. Though you may not always be right in your perceptions (or your actions), it's important to pay attention to situations that make you think there is a problem. Your intuition is a valuable gift at your disposal. One question this chapter explores is how to act on it.

Dialogue II: Pediatric referral service and scheduling

Performance protocols

In this dialogue, the interpreter calls attention to the need for clarification in the face of a suspected misunderstanding. Why doesn't the interpreter simply clarify the miscommunication with the mother herself?

After there has been a formal request from the operator for the interpreter to clarify, why does the interpreter respond by asking the operator to take over and ask for clarification? Assess the interpreter's performance.

Professional boundaries and advocacy

What is inappropriate or incomplete about the operator's plans for her notations? Why might her plan for documentation be problematic? As an interpreter, your role is often limited. For some, it may seem in this case that the interpreter has overstepped her bounds.

What concerns the interpreter, and what problem is she calling attention to? Should she ask for clarification at all? Should she leave it to the patient's mother or the operator to rectify the information?

Caution

Sometimes it may appear that there is a straightforward miscommunication. (For bones or joint problems, a person usually sees an orthopedist). But sometimes a situation isn't what it seems. A patient may have a disease such as gout, or an autoimmune condition such as lupus, dermatomyositis or scleroderma that causes symptoms in many parts of the body such as in the joints, kidneys or the skin. Maybe it is indeed a dermatologist who needs to see the patient and add clarity to a diagnosis.

How might an interpreter verify that there is no miscommunication, yet not cross her professional boundaries? Critique her performance from this perspective.

Ethics and standards: Reflect and practice

Goal: Review of standards (part 1)

In the following exercise, consider all 32 standards of the NCIHC *National Standards of Practice for Interpreters in Health Care.* Make a decision for each excerpt from the dialogue about which standards might apply to the situation. Then use the information you find in the standards themselves to help you answer the questions that follow each excerpt.

Note: In your answers, answer the question and then list the *number* of the NCIHC standard, e.g., #6, #14 or #21, that you find is relevant for that situation.

EXCERPT 1

PHARMACIST: Yes, we're on the eighth floor. We're using a dual-set-interpreter telephone so we won't have to pass the telephone back and forth. I'll hand him his line now. *(gives patient his telephone)* Now, could you ask the patient, let's see, if he's had a flu shot this year?

INTERPRETER: Bilal, did you get a flu shot this year?

How should you speak to the patient with a form mode of address (e.g., su/usted) or informal speech (e.g., tu/tú)? Why? Which standard(s) of practice might apply here?

When you interpret for a young person or a person with a developmental disability, can it sometimes be confusing if you use first person when you speak to that patient? Why? Which standard(s) of practice might apply here?

EXCERPT 2

INTERPRETER: Bilal, did you get a flu shot this year?

PATIENT: ¿Mm?

INTERPRETER: Bilal, did you get a flu shot this year? *(tries in English.)* Did you get a flu shot this year, Bilal?

Why might the interpreter be repeating the question in English for this pediatric patient? Which standard(s) of practice might apply here?

EXCERPT 3

INTERPRETER: Do you know what I mean when I say shot or injection? Do you know what vaccination is? Did they stick you with a needle or give you a shot recently?

PATIENT: Yes.

INTERPRETER: Do you know what it was for?

PATIENT: No.

INTERPRETER: *(switches to English, speaking to the pharmacist)* As the interpreter, Bridget, I'm not really sure he's understanding. He can just tell me he's been injected, or stuck with needles recently, but he's been to the doctor a lot and he is now in the hospital. It could be anything, including blood draws or IVs or blood sugar sticks in the finger.

Do you agree with how the interpreter handled this concern? Why or why not? Which standard(s) of practice might apply here?

EXCERPT 4

INTERPRETER: *(switches to English, speaking to the pharmacist)* You know, Bridget, speaking as the interpreter, he sounds a little out of it or confused. He's having trouble understanding or answering really basic questions. I can't see his face, but is there any kind of a problem? He really doesn't seem to be responding normally.

Do you agree with how the interpreter handled this concern? Why or why not? Which standard(s) of practice might apply here?

EXCERPT 5

INTERPRETER: As the interpreter, I need to clarify a little bit. He says he's not allergic to eggs and he eats them at home, but I need to let you know I'm really uncomfortable with this. I sense there is something going on and it's definitely more than just shyness. There's something else going on here. He's a minor. I would be really hesitant to count on any of this information without talking to a parent.

What are the possible medical consequences of a flu shot for a person who is allergic to eggs? What might be some legal consequences for the institution if the interpreter says nothing here and the patient is in fact allergic to eggs? What would you say or do (if anything) as the interpreter in this situation? Which standard(s) of practice might apply here?

EXCERPT 6

PHARMACIST: Well, we really need to give him a flu shot, I think it'll be OK.

> **INTERPRETER:** Well, it's your decision, I just have to tell you what I'm picking up, and I really believe there is something going on here. Something's not quite right with his responses, and he's a minor.

Why do you think the interpreter says this? Do you agree that she should? Why or why not? Which standard(s) of practice might apply here?

EXCERPT 7

> **INTERPRETER:** *(after interpreting)* Excuse me, as the interpreter I need to let you know that there may be some miscommunication that you might want to clear up. *(Interpreter repeats in parent's language.)*

OPERATOR: Oh, really, what's that? *(Interpreter interprets.)*

> **INTERPRETER:** *(in English to operator.)* Well, I noticed that you offered Mom an appointment for a dermatology consultation, but Mom said it wasn't necessary because the child's bones aren't hurting anymore. It seems like there is some confusion here. You said dermatology, but she said bones. *(Interpreter tells the patient, in the patient's language, what she told the operator.)*

OPERATOR: Oh, right. Well go ahead.

> **INTERPRETER:** Did you want to clarify? *(Interpreter tells the patient, in Spanish, what she told the operator.)*

OPERATOR: Yes, can you do that please? *(Interpreter tells the patient, in Spanish, what she told the operator.)*

> **INTERPRET:** Why don't I let you do that and I'll interpret for you. *(Interpreter tells the patient, in Spanish, what she told the operator.)*

Do you agree with how the interpreter handled this concern? Why or why not? Which standard(s) of practice might apply here?

EXCERPT 8

PARENT: No, she had pain in her bones, but the pain went away. She doesn't need the appointment anymore. She never had problems with her skin.

OPERATOR: Would you like me to call her doctor's office and ask what this is about?

PARENT: Yes, please. Thank you.

OPERATOR: Well, all right. And I'll just write a note here that she no longer has pain in her joints.

INTERPRETER: As the interpreter, I'd like to make a correction... The mother said she had pain in her *bones,* rather than joints, but the pain went away. She doesn't need the appointment anymore. She never had problems with her skin.

OPERATOR: All right, I'll put in my note here that she had pain in her bones, but the pain went away and she doesn't want the appointment. And she never had problems with her skin.

Do you agree with how the interpreter handled this concern? Why or why not? Which standard(s) of practice might apply here?

Occupational therapy for interpreters

EXERCISES FOR THE TONGUE, HEART AND MIND

Suggested reading

Kelly, N. (2008). The voice on the other end of the phone. *Health Affairs*, *27*(6): 1701-1706.[44]

Consider and discuss

This informative article by Nataly Kelly discusses how professional medical interpreters provide accurate, sometimes life-saving language support from a knowledgeable, personal and practical perspective. It describes many other important aspects of medical interpreting and important developments in the field.

1. In the first paragraph, which three tasks does the author describe performing during telephone interpreting?
2. The author also refers to the last of these three tasks as "inflection." Why is it important and what does the interpreter learn from the speaker's inflection?
3. What would you say to participants in a telephone conversation (providers, patients, family) in order to give an introduction or orientation to telephone interpreting and how to work together? Start with "Hello," then identify yourself and finish the introduction.
4. High stress, speed and emotional levels among health providers and patients/family in the emergency room (ER) influence communication, the interpreting experience and the provision of care. What other ambient factors does the author describe that have a direct impact on her ability to interpret for the ER over the phone?
5. Why is the professional interpreter standard of impartiality important in the ER? Where else besides the ER is it relevant?
6. In the first ER example in this article, an interpreter arrives in-person to take over for the phone interpreter (author). The telephone interpreter may have lost work and income as a result, yet she conveys no sense of offense or disappointment at being replaced. Why might this be?
7. In the section in the article titled, "Conveying More Than Words," what are some of the challenges the author describes in terms of diversity of settings and terminology? (What's required to perform her job? Make a list.)
8. In the same section, the interpreter makes a suggestion to a visiting nurse on how to instruct young parents on use of a thermometer. In view of interpreter standards regarding impartiality, role boundaries and advocacy, how is the interpreter's intervention acceptable?
9. Briefly describe the range of socioeconomic backgrounds of some of the patients in this article. How does this influence communication and what is the challenge for the interpreter?
10. What are some of the pleasures or joys this interpreter experiences through her work?

44 Retrieved from http://content.healthaffairs.org/content/27/6/1701.full.pdf+html

11. The author reports the following exchanges, which might be uncomfortable to interpret: a patient who asks, "Why is the doctor speaking so slowly to me? Does he think I am stupid?"; a patient who says, "Please tell the nurse not to yell at me. I don't have a hearing problem—I just don't speak English" and a clinician who instructs, "Next time you come, you speak *inglés*, understand?" Why interpret these utterances at all?
12. In the section titled, "The Complexity And The Frustration," how does the author describe some of the differences between in-person and telephone interpreters?
13. Does the passage below refer to telephone interpreters or in-person interpreters?

    > "Those of us who work within the interpreting field also face a lack of awareness within the health care community at large of the importance of professional medical interpreters, what it means to provide professional interpreting services, and the enormous effect that professional interpreters have on the delivery of high quality health care services" (Kelly, p. 1705).

14. What common misperception does the author describe and why is it potentially deadly?
15. According to the author, how does the NCIHC provide support or advocate so that interpreters can do their jobs?
16. Comment on the author's final statement below. What does it say to you?

    > "Even when I hear the words, "You're going to be disconnected," I silently know that, in reality, I couldn't be more connected" (Kelly, p. 1706).

Suggested reading

Mikkelson, H. (2003). Telephone interpreting: Boon or bane? In González, L.P. (Ed.). *Speaking in Tongues: Language across Contexts and Users.* Valencia, Spain, Universitat de València. pp. 251-269.[45]

Consider and discuss

What are some of the most interesting or compelling issues discussed by Holly Mikkelson in this article? How do they compare or contrast with points raised in the article by Nataly Kelly?

1. Choose two of the important issues raised by the two authors mentioned above. Describe how they support, complement and challenge each other.
2. Perform an Internet search and cite three articles that appear to discuss some aspect of telephone or remote interpreting.
3. Review the following sampling of literature. From the title or minimal information in the citation, identify which two articles seem the most intriguing if you were to read them for a homework assignment. Explain why.

45 Retrieved from www.acebo.com/pages/telephone-interpreting-boon-or-bane

Remote interpreting: A sampling of the literature

Advisory

Inclusion of the following articles in this short sampling does not necessarily constitute endorsement by the author or publisher of research methodologies or the accuracy of claims or conclusions.

Video remote interpreting research: Medical

Azarmina, P., & Wallace, P. (2005). Remote interpretation in medical encounters: A systematic review. *Journal of Telemedicine and Telecare, 11*(3), 140-145.

Gany, F., Kapelusznik, L., Prakash, K., Gonzalez, J., Orta, L.Y., Tseng, C.H., & Changrani, J. (2007). The impact of medical interpretation method on time and errors. *Journal of General Internal Medicine*, *22* Suppl 2, 319-323.

Karliner, L.S., & Mutha, S. (2010). Achieving quality in healthcare through language access services: Lessons from a California public hospital. *American Journal of Medical Quality, 25*(1), 51-59.

Kelly, N. (2009). *Meddling with Medical Machine Translation*. Cambridge, Massachusetts: Common Sense Advisory.

Lee, L.J., Batal, H.A., Maselli, J.H., & Kutner, J.S. (2002). Effect of Spanish interpretation method on patient satisfaction in an urban walk-in clinic. *Journal of General Internal Medicine*, *17*(8), 641-646

Moser-Mercer, B. (2003). *Remote interpreting: Assessment of human factors and performance parameters*. Geneva: Joint project International Telecommunication Union (ITU)-Ecole de Traduction et d'Interpretation, Université de Genève.

Nápoles, A.M., Santoyo-Olsson, J., Karliner, L.S., O'Brien, H., Gregorich, S.E., & Pérez-Stable, E.J. (2010). Clinic ratings of interpreter mediated visits in underserved primary care settings with ad hoc, in-person professional and videoconferencing modes. *Journal of Healthcare for the Poor and Underserved*, *21*(1), 301-317.

Price, E.L., Pérez-Stable, E.J., Nickleach, D., López, M., & Karliner, L.S. (2012). Interpreter perspectives of in-person, telephonic and videoconferencing medical interpretation in clinical encounters. *Patient Education and Counseling*, *87*(2), 226-232.

Saint-Louis, L., Friedman, E., Chiasson, E., Quessa, A., & Novaes, F. (2003). *Testing New Technologies in Medical Interpreting*. Somerville, Massachusetts: Cambridge Health Alliance.

Wofford, J.L., Campos, C.L., Johnson, D.A., & Brown, M.T. (2012). Providing a Spanish interpreter using low-cost videoconferencing in a community health centre: A pilot study using tablet computers. *Journal of Information in Health Informatics* (formerly *Informatics in Primary Care), 20*(2), 141-146.

Video remote interpreting research: Nonmedical interpreting

Braun, S. (2013). Keep your distance? Remote interpreting in legal proceedings: A critical assessment of a growing practice. *Interpreting, 15*(2), 200-228.

Braun, S. (2014). Comparing traditional and remote interpreting in police settings: Quality and impact factors. In Viezzi, M., & Falbo, C. (Eds.), *Traduzione e interpretazione per la società e le istituzioni.* Trieste: Edizioni Università di Trieste, 161-176.

Braun, S. (2015). Remote interpreting. In Mikkelson, H., & Jourdenais, R. (Eds.), *Routledge Handbook of Interpreting*. New York: Routledge, 352-367.

Braun, S. (2016). The European AVIDICUS projects: Collaborating to assess the viability of video-mediated interpreting in legal proceedings. *European Journal of Applied Linguistics*, 1-7.

Braun, S., & Taylor, J.L. (2011). Video-mediated interpreting: An overview of current practice and research. In Braun, S., & Taylor, J.L. (Eds.), *Videoconference and remote interpreting in criminal proceedings*. Guildford: University of Surrey, 27-57.

Braun, S., & Taylor, J. (Eds.). (2012). *Videoconference and remote interpreting in criminal proceedings.* Antwerp: Intersentia.

Licoppe, C., & Verdier, M. (2015). L'interprétariat par visioconférence au sein des chambres de l'instruction en France: Une étude conversationnelle de l'activité d'interprétariat dans un dispositif interactionnel médiatisé. *Langage et société, 153*(3), 109-131.

Napier, J. (2013). "You get that vibe": A pragmatic analysis of clarification and communicative accommodation in legal video remote interpreting. In Meurant, L., Sinte, A., Van Herreweghe, M., & Vermeerbergen. M. (Eds). *Sign Language Research, Uses and Practices: Crossing Views on Theoretical and Applied Sign Language Linguistics.* Sign Languages and Deaf Communities, vol. 1, Berlin: Walter de Gruyter, 85-110.

Napier, J., Braun, S., & Skinner, R. (Eds.) (2017, in press). Here or there: Research on remote interpreting. Washington, DC: Gallaudet Press.

NCIEC. (2010). *Steps Toward Identifying Best Practices in Video Remote Interpreting: 2010 Report.* Boston, Massachusetts: National Consortium of Interpreter Education Centers.

Genetics Counseling 11

Advisory

This chapter involves some material related to prenatal diagnosis and procedures, Down syndrome, race and infant death.

This is a genetics consultation and prenatal diagnosis appointment for a 36-year-old, pregnant, Afro-Peruvian woman. The interpreter introduces herself and the encounter begins.

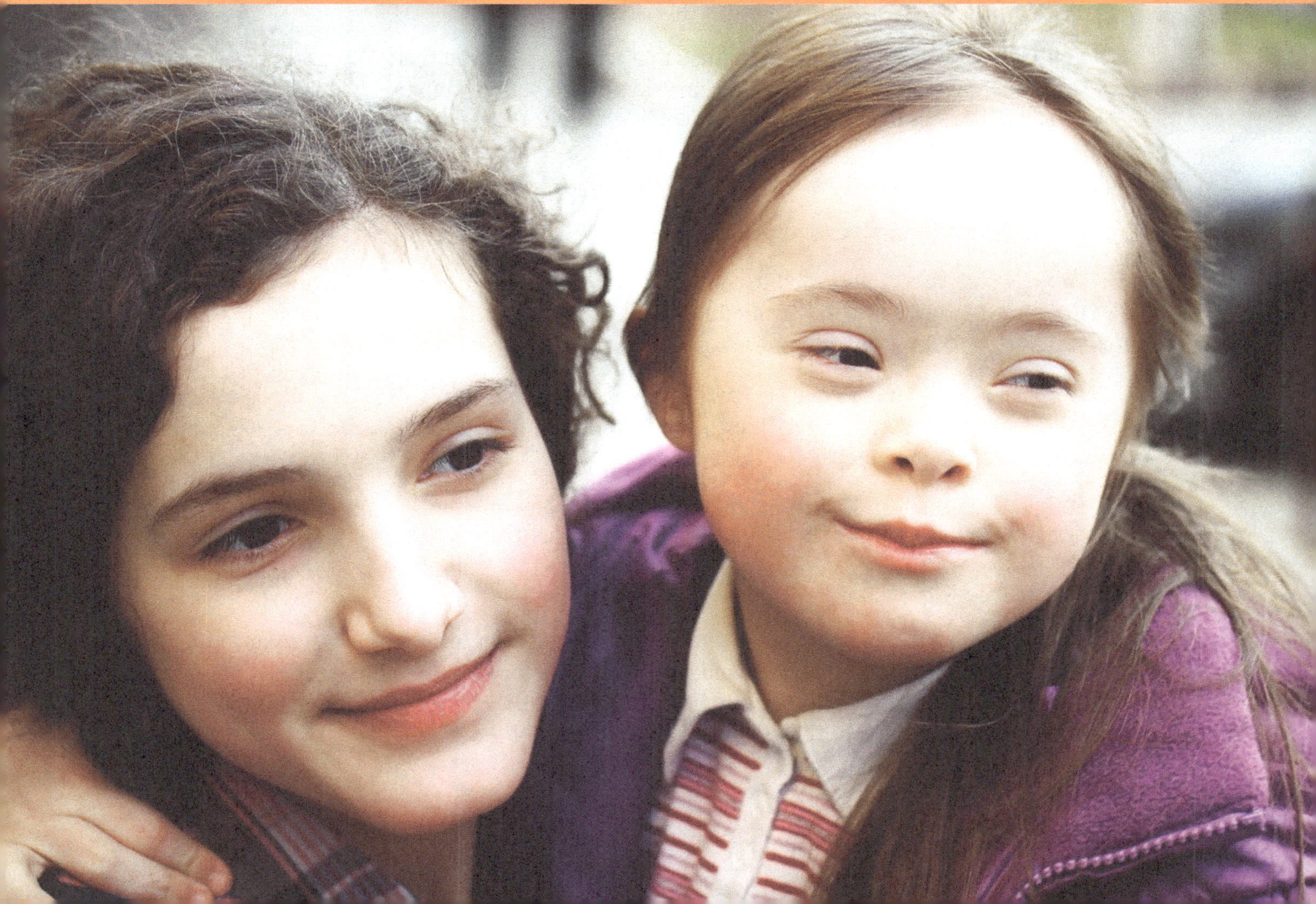

Prenatal diagnosis and genetics counseling role play (English-Spanish)

PART 1

GENETIC COUNSELOR: Good afternoon, Lorenza. I'm Kelly, a genetic counselor. Did your doctor at the clinic explain to you why they asked you to come here today?

PATIENT: Sí, Señorita. Me dijeron que podría haber un problema con mi bebé, según el resultado de laboratorio.

GENETIC COUNSELOR: That's exactly right. Now, what I'd like to do is explain a little bit more about the blood test that you had done with your doctor. What that test does is look at a level of protein in the blood, and according to the calculation that the laboratory did, the level of protein in your blood suggests there may be a higher risk that your baby has something called Down syndrome. Have you ever heard of Down syndrome?

PATIENT: Es como esos mongolitos que se ven en la calle, ¿no?

GENETIC COUNSELOR: Well, we usually don't use that word to describe them anymore, but yes. That's right. I want to show you this chart. This chart says that when a woman is your age, she has about 1 in 187 chances of having a baby with Down syndrome. But in your case, at this point in your pregnancy, your blood test suggests that there is about a 1 in 21 chance that your baby could have Down syndrome. That's different than what's typical for other women your age.

PATIENT: Ya, pero no es seguro, ¿verdad?

GENETIC COUNSELOR: Right. This blood test doesn't give us a definite answer, it just *suggests* that this may be the case. Let me just verify something here. Your doctor and the lab calculated that you are approximately 11 weeks along in your pregnancy. Is that what you think?

PATIENT: Pues, yo creo que sí. Tuve la última regla entre el 6 y el 11 de julio, así que tengo como tres meses. Pero luego el mes después sangré un poquito y tuve cólicos, así que puede ser que esté equivocada.

GENETIC COUNSELOR: OK. Let me just calculate that on my wheel...You are...Let me see...According to your last full period, you are eleven weeks and two days along in your pregnancy.

PATIENT: Sí.

GENETIC COUNSELOR: Now, the first thing we will do today is talk a little more about your pregnancy and also about the family health history and the medical history of the baby's father. After that, the technician will do an ultrasound. Many times a woman finds that she was wrong about the date of her pregnancy, and that clears up the whole question of the blood result.

PATIENT: ¿Puede explicar un poco más de eso acerca del análisis de sangre?

GENETIC COUNSELOR: Yes. The blood test measures the level of a protein and two hormones in your blood. Depending how far along you are in your pregnancy, the level of the protein can tell us if there might be a problem. At a different point in your pregnancy, let's say if you are not as far along, or further along than you think, the levels shown in the blood test may mean nothing.

PATIENT: Ah, ya, ya.

GENETIC COUNSELOR: Now, if it doesn't answer that question, then we can offer you some other tests. One of these is called chorionic villus sampling (CVS). This test can be done between 10 and 12 weeks of pregnancy, which is where your lab test thought you were at the time of the analysis.

PATIENT: Entonces, ¿esto no va a ser para un amniocentesis?

GENETIC COUNSELOR: Well, if you want to do the amnio, usually you'd have to wait until you're at least 16 weeks along, between 16 and 18 weeks is best. What we can offer you is the CVS. I understand you didn't want to wait that long, until 16 weeks like you'd have to for an amnio.

PATIENT: ¿Y por qué no pueden hacerme otra prueba de sangre y así saber si es que creen que mi bebé tenga eso?

GENETIC COUNSELOR: As I said, the blood test just tells us if there's a greater chance statistically that something might be wrong. It isn't anything conclusive, nothing definite. If you want to be sure, then we need to do one of these other tests, the CVS or the amnio. What the CVS does is go in, either through the abdomen with a fine needle, or through the cervix with a thin tube, and take cells from the placenta. If it were an amnio, we would take some of the baby's skin cells that slough off and are floating around in the amniotic fluid.

PATIENT: ¿Quiere decir que van a picar al bebé?

GENETIC COUNSELOR: No, we don't touch the baby. The doctor first looks at the baby with ultrasound to see exactly where it is and where the placenta is lying so she knows which way to go in, either through the abdomen or through the vagina and cervix. Then she uses ultrasound the entire time to guide her. The needle or catheter never touches the baby.

PATIENT: Ah, ya. Pensé que iban a picar al bebé.

GENETIC COUNSELOR: No, no. The needle never touches the baby. They take those cells from the amniotic fluid and then these cells from the baby are cultured in the lab and grown out.

PATIENT: Entonces sí, ¿me podrán dar una respuesta definitiva?

GENETIC COUNSELOR: Yes. In the lab, they'll look at the chromosomes in the cells. They will be sorted and lined up like this *(shows a chart in a book to the patient)*. There are 23 pairs of chromosomes. The baby inherits one of each of these from the mother from the ovum, and one from the father from the sperm cell. Each of these pairs has a number. The last pair is either an XX for a boy, or an XY for a girl.

PATIENT: También me podrán decir sobre la existencia de ciertas enfermedades, ¿no?

GENETIC COUNSELOR: Yes. For example, all the chromosomes will be looked at. If your baby had a problem with this pair for example *(points to the chart)*, and we see an alteration, if something is missing, for example, we would know there is a problem. Or if, for example, with this pair *(points to the chart)*, pair 18, if we see an extra chromosome here, then we know there is a problem.

PATIENT: Ya.

GENETIC COUNSELOR: Now, depending on our consultation today and your family health history, we would test for anything else we might think there's a higher risk for. We will then be able to tell you about any change, alteration or mutation in the chromosomes and about any genetic disease or condition your baby has.

PATIENT: Ya, entonces es una cuestión de la genética. Pero no entiendo entonces. ¿Por qué no podrían decirme si el bebé tiene alguna condición, si van a hacer una prueba genética?

GENETIC COUNSELOR: Well, we can check for many of the conditions, especially if there is any indication from the blood test that you run a higher risk for that particular condition in your pregnancy, or if there is something in your family health history that indicates a higher risk for something. Then we can check for that particular thing, if a test for it exists. But we each have over 100,000 genetic instructions, in every cell in our bodies, and we can't check for all of them.

PART 2

PATIENT: Ah, ya estoy comprendiendo.

GENETIC COUNSELOR: Now, I have to advise you, there is some risk associated with the exams. The risk of a miscarriage due to the CVS is about 0.5 percent to 1 percent, or 1 or 2 women for every 200 that have a CVS. With amniocentesis, it's less than one half of 1 percent. That's less than 1 in 200 women. But the reason they've called you to offer these tests is because according to your blood test, the risk that your baby might have Down syndrome is slightly higher than for a woman of your same age in the general population and higher than the risk associated with an amnio.

PATIENT: Pero usted también dijo que si con el sonograma pueden confirmar que la fecha del embarazo es diferente, entonces no tendría que someterme a ningún examen, ¿verdad?

GENETIC COUNSELOR: Correct, there would be less of a reason to do it. But either way, it is absolutely your choice and I'm obligated to explain the risks to you. Now, if the ultrasound shows that we were mistaken about the date of the pregnancy, then that would change the percentage of risk and the recommendation for the exam. Or in other words, you might turn out to have the same risk as any other woman in your age group. Is that all clear?

PATIENT: Ya.

GENETIC COUNSELOR: So let's talk about your family history. Let's see if there's anything else we need to think about. You're from what country originally, Lorenza—Perú is it?

PATIENT: Sí. Soy del Perú.

GENETIC COUNSELOR: And the baby's father?

PATIENT: Él también es peruano.

GENETIC COUNSELOR: All right, and it says here you're 36 years old, right?

PATIENT: Correcto.

GENETIC COUNSELOR: Lorenza, your last name is Barillette. That's a French name, isn't it?

PATIENT: Sí.

GENETIC COUNSELOR: And the baby's father?

PATIENT: Barillette también, Gustavo.

GENETIC COUNSELOR: Is there any way you and the baby's father, uh, Gustavo, could be related?

PATIENT: No, no somos parientes.

GENETIC COUNSELOR: You're sure you aren't distant cousins, or don't have a great-grandparent in common?

PATIENT: No, no, doctora. No somos parientes.

GENETIC COUNSELOR: It's just that it's a French name, so uncommon, and you are from the same country and have the same last name.

PATIENT: Cómo no, doctora, es curioso. Nosotros también nos hemos preguntado lo mismo, pero no.

GENETIC COUNSELOR: OK. Well, we ask all our patients if they are related. So, you are Peruvian and I'm guessing you have Spanish ancestry and French ancestry, and I imagine there could be some native Peruvian or Indian blood as well. That's about it, right? *(The patient has dark skin and her hair and features suggest African descent.)*

PATIENT: También tengo sangre china. Mi mamá se apellida Quan.

GENETIC COUNSELOR: Well, you've got a little of the entire world in you! All right, Lorenza. Now, do you have brothers or sisters?

PATIENT: Tengo cuatro.

GENETIC COUNSELOR: Can you tell me their ages and if they are boys or girls?

PATIENT: Si. Tengo tres hermanos y una hermana. El primero tiene 41 años, los siguientes son mellizos y tienen 39 años. Después sigo yo y después una hermana.

GENETIC COUNSELOR: And how old is your sister?

PATIENT: Bueno, ya falleció.

GENETIC COUNSELOR: Oh, I'm sorry. And how old was she when she died?

PATIENT: Oh, ella murió cuando tenía 13 años.

GENETIC COUNSELOR: And how did she die?

PATIENT: Se murió de repente. Dicen que fue un susto, pero yo creo que nació con problemas del corazón.

GENETIC COUNSELOR: I'm very sorry. Now what makes you think she had a heart problem? Were you ever told that by a doctor?

PATIENT: No me acuerdo exactamente, pero creo que mi mami me dijo algo así. También mi hermana siempre fue enfermiza. Se agitaba fácilmente y se cansaba demasiado pronto.

GENETIC COUNSELOR: Lorenza, did your mother have any other pregnancies? Did she have any abortions or miscarriages, or did she have any babies that were stillborn or babies that died shortly after birth?

PATIENT: Sí. Perdió un bebé entre mi hermana y yo. Lo abortó.

GENETIC COUNSELOR: Do you know how far along she was or why it happened?

PATIENT: No, nunca habló de los detalles. Solamente sé que perdió un bebé.

GENETIC COUNSELOR: All right. Do all of your brothers have children?

PATIENT: Sí.

GENETIC COUNSELOR: Can you tell me how many each one has, and if they're boys or girls?

PATIENT: El primero, Leonel, tiene dos niñas y un niño. Los otros dos tienen un niño y una niña, ambos.

GENETIC COUNSELOR: And is everyone in good health?

PATIENT: Sí.

GENETIC COUNSELOR: Lorenza, if you think about all your relatives—brothers, sisters, aunts, uncles, mother, father, grandparents, nieces and nephews—is there anyone who has a birth defect, a deformity, a learning disability, any developmental delays or any major diseases or problems with their heart, liver, lungs, any kind of a health condition or anything like that?

PATIENT: No, todos están muy bien de salud, gracias al Señor.

GENETIC COUNSELOR: Very good. And how about your parents, Lorenza, are they still alive?

PATIENT: Si. Están en el Perú.

GENETIC COUNSELOR: And how old are they?

PATIENT: A ver, creo que mi mami tiene unos 65 años y papi unos 68.

GENETIC COUNSELOR: And how is their health?

PATIENT: Mi mamá sufre de alta presión, pero está controlada. Y mi papi tiene artritis, pero creo que es cuestión de la vejez, ya son ancianitos.

GENETIC COUNSELOR: All right. Now Lorenza, this is your third pregnancy?

PATIENT: Sí, doctora. Tengo una mujercita de 9 años y un varón de 11 años.

GENETIC COUNSELOR: And are they in good health?

PATIENT: Sí, gracias a Dios están muy bien de salud.

GENETIC COUNSELOR: Very good. Now, Lorenza, I want to ask you about Gustavo...*(The genetic counselor proceeds with the family health history of the father of the baby.)*

PART 3

GENETIC COUNSELOR: Well, Lorenza, I don't see anything in your family health history that makes me think there is anything special we might want to look out for. It looks like a very healthy family. So do you think you want to go ahead and have the CVS?

PATIENT: Pues, yo creo que sí doctora. Pero, ¿primero van a hacer el sonograma?

GENETIC COUNSELOR: Yes, first they'll do the ultrasound and take a look at how the baby's doing. They'll take some measurements and see if they want to change the due date and age of the baby. But if you think you want to go ahead with it in case the date doesn't change, you could sign the consent form and then we wouldn't have to stop for that.

PATIENT: Ya, pero no sé, es que me da miedo. ¿Si todo está bien con el bebé y después sufro un aborto?

GENETIC COUNSELOR: Well, there's always that risk. It's a small risk. You know, some women know that if something were seriously wrong with the baby, they would like to know ahead of time. Then they can consider their alternatives, either to go ahead with the pregnancy and be prepared for whatever type of problem the baby might have, or they would have the option to terminate the pregnancy, in which case we would help with the arrangements. Other women know that they would never terminate a pregnancy under any circumstances and they don't want to take the risk.

PATIENT: Ah, ya.

GENETIC COUNSELOR: But I can assure you that we've done thousands of these procedures here. The doctors have lots of experience, and I've almost never seen a problem. We tell you a lot of scary statistics but it's because we're obligated to do that, by law.

PATIENT: ¿Y duele mucho?

GENETIC COUNSELOR: Well, most women say it is a little uncomfortable, but not especially painful. Most women have also told me that the anticipation is far worse than the actual procedure. It's also over pretty quickly. It only takes a minute or two.

PATIENT: ¿Y no le va a hacer daño al bebe, si quitamos tanto líquido amniótico?

GENETIC COUNSELOR: It's really not much, just a couple of tablespoons, and your body will replace it in about 24 hours. But you're not at a stage when you can have an amniocentesis. You could go ahead with a CVS, and that's just a few cells from the placenta.

PATIENT: Ya. Bueno, está bien entonces. ¿Y tengo que estar en reposo?

GENETIC COUNSELOR: No, you don't really have to be on bed rest. We just ask you to take it easy for the next 24 hours. You shouldn't work or do anything that requires a lot of physical exertion. You don't have small children, so that's good, but no lifting anything heavy, nothing over 10 pounds for the next 24 hours.

PATIENT: ¿Y si el bebé empieza a venir, no hay nada que se pueda hacer?

GENETIC COUNSELOR: No, it doesn't necessarily mean there's nothing that can be done, but you need to call your doctor or go to an emergency room right away. Now, there are just a couple of other things I need to tell you.

PATIENT: Oh, perdón, doctora.

GENETIC COUNSELOR: Oh, that's OK. I just want to let you know what the things are that you need to watch out for. Now, it's normal to have some slight cramping. But if you have anything more severe, or any vaginal bleeding or fluid of any kind, you should call your doctor, or if it's after hours go to an emergency room. Also, if you have a fever at any time during the next two weeks, you need to come in and see a doctor even if you think it's a flu or something else. I'm going to give you something in writing with all this information, but did you understand all that?

PATIENT: Sí, doctora.

GENETIC COUNSELOR: I'm sure everything is going to be just fine. If you'll sign this and have a seat in the waiting room, the sonographer will call you in a few minutes.

PATIENT: Gracias doctora, muchas gracias.

GENETIC COUNSELOR: My pleasure, Lorenza, it was very nice to meet you.

Prenatal diagnosis and genetics counseling role play (English only)

PART 1

GENETIC COUNSELOR: Good afternoon, Lorenza. I'm Kelly, a genetics counselor. Did your doctor at the clinic explain to you why they asked you to come here today?

PATIENT: Yes, Miss. They told me there could be a problem with my baby, according to the laboratory results.

GENETIC COUNSELOR: That's exactly right. Now, what I'd like to do is explain a little bit more about the blood test that you had done with your doctor. What that test does is look at a level of protein in the blood, and according to the calculation that the laboratory did, the level of protein in your blood suggests there may be a higher risk that your baby has something called Down syndrome. Have you ever heard of Down syndrome?

PATIENT: It's like those little mongoloid children you see in the playground sometimes, right?

GENETIC COUNSELOR: Well, we usually don't use that word to describe them anymore, but yes. That's right. I want to show you this chart. This chart says that when a woman is your age, she has about 1 in 187 chances of having a baby with Down syndrome. But in your case, at this point in your pregnancy, your blood test suggests that there is about a 1 in 21 chance that your baby could have Down syndrome. That's different than what's typical for other women your age.

PATIENT: I understand, but it's not for sure, right?

GENETIC COUNSELOR: Right. This blood test doesn't give us a definite answer, it just *suggests* that this may be the case. Let me just verify something here. Your doctor and the lab calculated that you are approximately 11 weeks along in your pregnancy. Is that what you think?

PATIENT: Well, I think so. I had my last period from July 6 to 11, so I'm about three months along. But later, the month after, I did bleed just a little and had cramps, so it could be that I'm mistaken.

GENETIC COUNSELOR: OK. Let me just calculate that on my wheel... You are...Let me see...According to your last full period, you are eleven weeks and two days along in your pregnancy.

PATIENT: Yes.

GENETIC COUNSELOR: Now, the first thing we will do today is talk a little more about your pregnancy, and also about the family health history, and the medical history of the baby's father. After that, the technician will do an ultrasound. Many times a woman finds that she was wrong about the date of her pregnancy, and that clears up the whole question of the blood result.

PATIENT: Can you explain a little more about that part about the blood test results?

GENETIC COUNSELOR: Yes. The blood test measures the level of a protein and two hormones in your blood. Depending how far along you are in your pregnancy, the level of the protein can tell us if there might be a problem. At a different point in your pregnancy, let's say if you are not as far along, or further along than you think, the levels shown in the blood test may mean nothing.

PATIENT: Ah, right, right, now I get it.

GENETIC COUNSELOR: Now, if it doesn't answer that question, then we can offer you some other tests. One of these is called chorionic villus sampling (CVS). This test can be done between 10 and 12 weeks of pregnancy, which is where your lab test thought you were at the time of the analysis.

PATIENT: So then this isn't for an amniocentesis

GENETIC COUNSELOR: Well, if you want to do the amnio, usually you'd have to wait until you're at least 16 weeks along, between 16 and 18 weeks is best. What we can offer you is the CVS. I understand you didn't want to wait that long, until 16 weeks like you'd have to for an amnio.

PATIENT: And why can't you do another blood test to see if you think my baby has that?

GENETIC COUNSELOR: As I said, the blood test just tells us if there's a greater chance statistically that something might be wrong. It isn't anything conclusive, nothing definite. If you want to be sure, then we need to do one of these other tests, the CVS or the amnio. What the CVS does is go in, either through the abdomen with a fine needle, or through the cervix with a thin tube, and take cells from the placenta. If it were an amnio, we would take some of the baby's skin cells that slough off and are floating around in the amniotic fluid.

PATIENT: You mean you'll stick the baby with a needle?

GENETIC COUNSELOR: No, we don't touch the baby. The doctor first looks at the baby with ultrasound to see exactly where it is and where the placenta is lying so she knows which way to go in, either through the abdomen or through the vagina and cervix. Then she uses ultrasound the entire time to guide her. The needle or catheter never touches the baby.

PATIENT: Ah, I get it. I thought you were going to stick the baby.

GENETIC COUNSELOR: No, no. The needle never touches the baby. They take those cells from the amniotic fluid, and then these cells from the baby are cultured in the lab and grown out.

PATIENT: So then you could give me a definite answer?

GENETIC COUNSELOR: Yes. In the lab, they'll look at the chromosomes in the cells. They will be sorted and lined up like this. *(shows a chart in a book to the patient).* There are 23 pairs of chromosomes. The baby inherits one of each of these from the mother from the ovum, and one from the father from the sperm cell. Each of these pairs has a number. The last pair is either an XX for a boy, or an XY for a girl.

PATIENT: And you could also tell me if you think the baby has other diseases, right?

GENETIC COUNSELOR: Yes. For example, all the chromosomes will be looked at. If your baby had a problem with this pair for example *(points to the chart)*, and we see an alteration, if something is missing for example, we would know there is a problem. Or if, for example, with this pair *(points to the chart)*, pair 18, if we see an extra chromosome here, then we know there is a problem.

PATIENT: Right.

GENETIC COUNSELOR: Now, depending on our consultation today and your family health history, we would test for anything else we might think there's a higher risk for. We will then be able to tell you about any change, alteration or mutation in the chromosomes and about any genetic disease or condition your baby has.

PATIENT: Right, so then it's about genetics. But then I don't understand. Why won't you be able to tell me if the baby has a condition, if you're going to do that genetic test?

GENETIC COUNSELOR: Well, we can check for many of the conditions, especially if there is any indication from the blood test that you run a higher risk for that particular condition in your pregnancy, or if there is something in your family health history that indicates a higher risk for something. Then we can check for that particular thing, if a test for it exists. But we each have over 100,000 genetic instructions, in every cell in our bodies, and we can't check for all of them.

PART 2

PATIENT: Oh, now I'm getting it.

GENETIC COUNSELOR: Now, I have to advise you, there is some risk associated with the exams. The risk of a miscarriage due to the CVS is about 0.5 percent to 1 percent, or 1 or 2 women for every 200 that have a CVS. With amniocentesis, it's less than one half of 1 percent. That's less than 1 in 200 women. But the reason they've called you to offer these tests is because according to your blood test, the risk that your baby might have Down syndrome is slightly higher than for a woman of your same age in the general population, and higher than the risk associated with an amnio.

PATIENT: But you also said that with the sonogram you can confirm if the due date is different, if whether the date I think I got pregnant is right, so then I wouldn't have to have any kind of a test, right?

GENETIC COUNSELOR: Correct, there would be less of a reason to do it. But either way, it is absolutely your choice, and I'm obligated to explain the risks to you. Now, if the ultrasound shows that we were mistaken about the date of the pregnancy, then that would change the percentage of risk and the recommendation for the exam. Or in other words, you might turn out to have the same risk as any other woman in your age group. Is that all clear?

PATIENT: Yes.

GENETIC COUNSELOR: So let's talk about your family history. Let's see if there's anything else we need to think about. You're from what country originally, Lorenza—Perú is it?

PATIENT: Yes, I'm from Perú.

GENETIC COUNSELOR: And the baby's father?

PATIENT: He's also Peruvian.

GENETIC COUNSELOR: All right, and it says here you're 36 years old, right?

PATIENT: Correct.

GENETIC COUNSELOR: Lorenza, your last name is Barillette. That's a French name, isn't it?

PATIENT: Yes.

GENETIC COUNSELOR: And the baby's father?

PATIENT: Barillette as well, Gustavo.

GENETIC COUNSELOR: Is there any way you and the baby's father, uh, Gustavo, could be related?

PATIENT: No, we're not related to each other.

GENETIC COUNSELOR: You're sure you aren't distant cousins, or don't have a great-grandparent in common?

PATIENT: No, no, doctor. We aren't related.

GENETIC COUNSELOR: It's just that it's a French name, so uncommon, and you are from the same country and have the same last name.

PATIENT: You're right, doctor, it's pretty uncommon. We've also wondered if we're related, but we're not.

GENETIC COUNSELOR: OK. Well, we ask all our patients if they are related. So you're Peruvian and I'm guessing you have Spanish ancestry and French ancestry, and I imagine there could be some native Peruvian or Indian blood as well. That's about it, right? *(The patient has dark skin and her hair and features suggest African descent.)*

PATIENT: I also have some Chinese blood. My mother's last name is Quan.

GENETIC COUNSELOR: Well, you've got a little of the entire world in you! All right, Lorenza. Now, do you have brothers or sisters?

PATIENT: I have four.

GENETIC COUNSELOR: Can you tell me their ages and if they are boys or girls?

PATIENT: Yes. I have three brothers and a sister. The first brother is 41 years old, the next ones are twins. They're 39. Then comes me, and then my sister.

GENETIC COUNSELOR: And how old is your sister?

PATIENT: Well, she died.

GENETIC COUNSELOR: Oh, I'm sorry. And how old was she when she died?

PATIENT: She died when she was 13 years old.

GENETIC COUNSELOR: And how did she die?

PATIENT: She died suddenly. They say she had a shock, but I think she was born with heart problems.

GENETIC COUNSELOR: I'm very sorry. Now what makes you think she had a heart problem? Were you ever told that by a doctor?

PATIENT: I don't remember exactly, but I think my mom told me something like that. My sister was also always sickly. She got out of breath easily and she got tired really quickly.

GENETIC COUNSELOR: Lorenza, did your mother have any other pregnancies? Did she have any abortions or miscarriages, or did she have any babies that were stillborn or babies that died shortly after birth?

PATIENT: Yes. She lost a baby between my sister and me. She suffered a miscarriage.

GENETIC COUNSELOR: Do you know how far along she was or why it happened?

PATIENT: No, she never told me the details. Just that she lost a baby.

GENETIC COUNSELOR: All right. Do all of your brothers have children?

PATIENT: Yes.

GENETIC COUNSELOR: Can you tell me how many each one has, and if they're boys or girls?

PATIENT: The first one, Leonel, has two girls and a boy. The other two have a boy and a girl each.

GENETIC COUNSELOR: And is everyone in good health?

PATIENT: Yes.

GENETIC COUNSELOR: Lorenza, if you think about all of your relatives—brothers, sisters, aunts, uncles, mother, father, grandparents, nieces and nephews—is there anyone that has a birth defect, a deformity, a learning disability, any mental developmental delays or any major diseases or problems with their heart, liver, lungs, any kind of a health condition or anything like that?

PATIENT: No, everyone is in good health, thank the Lord.

GENETIC COUNSELOR: Very good. And how about your parents, Lorenza, are they still alive?

PATIENT: Yes, they're in Perú.

GENETIC COUNSELOR: And how old are they?

PATIENT: Let's see, I think that my mom is 65 and my dad is 68.

GENETIC COUNSELOR: And how is their health?

PATIENT: My mom suffers from high blood pressure, but it's under control. My dad has arthritis, but it's because of his age, they're both really old now.

GENETIC COUNSELOR: All right. Now Lorenza, this is your third pregnancy?

PATIENT: Yes, doctor. I have a girl, she's 9 years old, and I have a little man, he's 11.

GENETIC COUNSELOR: And are they in good health?

PATIENT: Yes, thanks to God they're in very good health.

GENETIC COUNSELOR: Very good. Now, Lorenza, I want to ask you about Gustavo...*(The genetic counselor proceeds with the family health history of the father of the baby.)*

PART 3

GENETIC COUNSELOR: Well, Lorenza, I don't see anything in your family health history that makes me think there is anything special we might want to look out for. It looks like a very healthy family. So do you think you want to go ahead and have the CVS?

PATIENT: Well, I think so, doctor. But will they do the sonogram first?

GENETIC COUNSELOR: Yes, first they'll do the ultrasound and take a look at how the baby's doing. They'll take some measurements and see if they want to change the due date and age of the baby. But if you think you want to go ahead with it in case the date doesn't change, you could sign the consent form and then we wouldn't have to stop for that.

PATIENT: All right, but I don't know, I'm scared. What if everything is fine with the baby, and then I have a miscarriage?

GENETIC COUNSELOR: Well, there's always that risk. It's a small risk. You know, some women know that if something were seriously wrong with the baby, they would like to know ahead of time. Then they can consider their alternatives, either to go ahead with the pregnancy and be prepared for whatever type of problem the baby might have, or they would have the option to terminate the pregnancy, in which case we would help with the arrangements. Other women know that they would never terminate a pregnancy under any circumstances and they don't want to take the risk.

PATIENT: Ah, right.

GENETIC COUNSELOR: But I can assure you that we've done thousands of these procedures here. The doctors have lots of experience, and I've almost never seen a problem. We tell you a lot of scary statistics but it's because we're obligated to do that, by law.

PATIENT: Does it hurt a lot?

GENETIC COUNSELOR: Well, most women say it is a little uncomfortable, but not especially painful. Most women have also told me that the anticipation is far worse than the actual procedure. It's also over pretty quickly. It only takes a minute or two.

PATIENT: And it won't hurt the baby, if we take away so much amniotic fluid?

GENETIC COUNSELOR: It's really not much, just a couple of tablespoons, and your body will replace it in about 24 hours. But you're not at a stage when you can have an amniocentesis. You could go ahead with a CVS, and that's just a few cells from the placenta.

PATIENT: Right, well, it's all right then. And do I have to be on bed rest after?

GENETIC COUNSELOR: No, you don't really have to be on bed rest. We just ask you to take it easy for the next 24 hours. You shouldn't work or do anything that requires a lot of physical exertion. You don't have small children, so that's good, but no lifting anything heavy, nothing over 10 pounds for the next 24 hours.

PATIENT: And if I start to go into labor, then there's nothing that can be done?

GENETIC COUNSELOR: No, it doesn't necessarily mean there's nothing that can be done, but you need to call your doctor or go to an emergency room right away. Now, there are just a couple of other things I need to tell you.

PATIENT: Oh, pardon me, doctor.

GENETIC COUNSELOR: Oh, that's OK. I just want to let you know what the things are that you need to watch out for. Now, it's normal to have some slight cramping. But if you have anything more severe, or any vaginal bleeding or fluid of any kind, you should call your doctor, or if it's after hours go to an emergency room. Also, if you have a fever at any time during the next two weeks, you need to come in and see a doctor even if you think it's a flu or something else. I'm going to give you something in writing with all this information, but did you understand all that?

PATIENT: Yes, doctor.

GENETIC COUNSELOR: I'm sure everything is going to be just fine. If you'll sign this and have a seat in the waiting room, the sonographer will call you in a few minutes.

PATIENT: Thank you, doctor, thank you very much.

GENETIC COUNSELOR: My pleasure, Lorenza, it was very nice to meet you.

What's important to know about this chapter?

Socially acceptable terms

In this dialogue, the genetic counselor is discussing Down syndrome with the patient, who refers to it as "mongolism." This term was once common in the United States. Is there a cultural, social or political point of view being discussed here? What is the position? How does language evolve as a reflection of social values, or do social values change as a result of the evolution of language?

While the provider in this dialogue indicates that using "mongolism" for Down syndrome is socially unacceptable, many people object to changes where a term once widely used is seen as inappropriate. Why do they object?

Consider the word "gyp" as in "to get gypped" (robbed or cheated). For some, this word is profoundly offensive. What is the root word? Is it based on a stereotype, a truth or does it perpetuate one? Throughout the years, social acceptance for certain terms referring to race or ethnicity has changed in parts of the United States. For example, in the United States, people no longer tend to speak about someone as being Oriental but rather Asian. The terms Negro and Afro-American have largely been replaced by the terms Black and African American. Even whether to capitalize the word "Black" (when it refers to individuals) is a matter that is discussed, often with strong opinions.

"Middle" Easterners got this name because of English colonialism, because the Middle East was seen as halfway to the "Far East" (from England). And does it make linguistic, social or historical sense to refer to non-Spanish-speaking Native American/ First Nation/Indigenous, Triqui-speaking Mexicans as

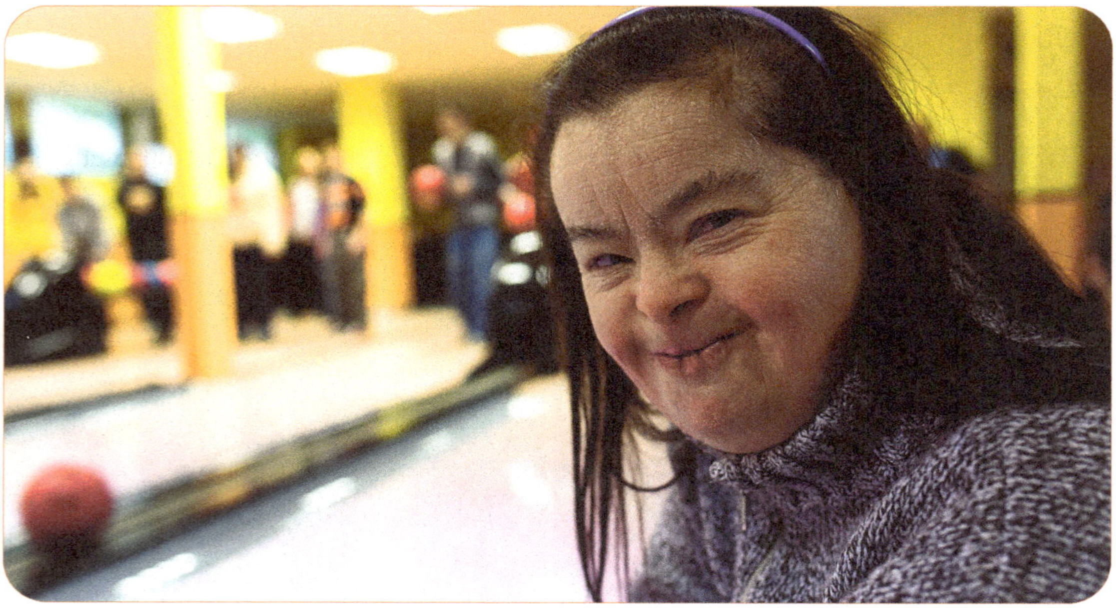

"Latinos" or "Hispanics" simply because they come from countries where Spanish is spoken? Why is a non-Indo-European language spoken in Mesoamerica commonly referred to as a "dialect" rather than a language? (There is no scientifically valid way to distinguish a dialect from a language. A language is defined as such by a particular society or social, political group and/or a group of researchers at a given point in time. The same is true for dialects. Over time, what is referred to as a dialect can change to being called language, or an Indigenous language—and vice versa.)

How do the terms we use for people and languages impact our relationships and society? In some cases, perhaps most, people who use terms that can be hurtful to others (such as "I got gypped") are not aware of the cultural slur in the word. In other cases, people use many denigrating terms intentionally. In still other cases, they might not see that to refer to Spanish as a language and Mixteco as a dialect, when linguistically they are both languages, can reflect what some consider to be ingrained racism that devalues Indigenous cultures.

As language specialists, interpreters should be aware of the impact of the language they use and make conscious decisions about such terms. They might also have to prepare to avoid showing, in their facial expressions or body language, their own anger or distress when they have to listen to—and interpret—denigrating terms and expressions.

Clarification or intervention and informed consent

An interpreter might ask for clarification about an utterance by the provider regarding the ability to check for "any genetic disease or condition," although the genetic counselor's statement in this dialogue on the surface is perfectly clear and interpretable. Look at what an interpreter might have said here.

GENETIC COUNSELOR: Now, depending on our consultation today and your family health history, we would test for anything else we might think there's a higher risk for. We will then be able to tell you about any change, alteration or mutation in the chromosomes and about any genetic disease or condition your baby has.

> **INTERPRETER:** As the interpreter, just to clarify, did you say you'd be able to tell if there was *any* genetic condition or abnormality? Como intérprete, para clarificar, ¿dijo usted que se podrá detectar la presencia de *cualquier* condición genética o anormalidad?

GENETIC COUNSELOR: Well, all the major, more common genetic conditions we see. It can't check for everything.

Consider some reasons that an interpreter might want to intervene in a case like this to request a clarification about genetics when it seems a genetic counselor's statement was clear.

First, humans are believed to have tens of thousands of genes or units of hereditary information. If typical prenatal testing looks at numbers of chromosomes, sections of chromosomes or specific genes (for duplication, absence, mutation, translocation) and doesn't find evidence of them, it does not mean there are no problems, but in this case, that none of the most *common* or *obvious* problems are apparent.

For some conditions, genetic testing does not even exist (the specific gene causing a condition has not been identified). More research is being conducted, including the impact of the environment and how genes that are present may be expressed or not. Since this interpreter has had some experience and knows that not all genetic diseases or conditions will be tested for, and therefore will not be apparent, then how does she wrestle with the obligation to "Do no harm" if the genetic counselor believes the mother understands the limitations of testing while the mother believes that *all* possible problematic conditions are being tested for?

Say that a fetus has a genetic condition that the test would not uncover, but the mother is told after the test that "everything is fine" without further discussion about the limitations of the test. What is the interpreter's role in a situation of this kind?

The genetic counselor changes and qualifies her original statement about what the test can show. This changes the equation. There are risks with any invasive procedure and with amniocentesis, there is a small risk of miscarriage. All patients must weigh the risks and the benefits and having accurate information about them is essential for making decisions. If information is incomplete or misrepresented, then a person is denied true participation in decision-making. What is "informed consent" and how is it impacted if the interpreter does or does not clarify the counselor's statement?

Race, racism and bigotry

The United States has problems of racism, like every other country in the world. Sometimes interracial incidents, public response and media coverage result in bringing conditions to the surface where they are less easily ignored. Responses to racism range from a willingness or desire to face it and reduce it to avoidance or denial.

In this dialogue there is some discomfort about racial issues, a lack of information or both. The genetic counselor sees that the patient most likely has African ancestry yet doesn't ask about it. The patient doesn't mention it.

It's also not uncommon for people in the United States to know something about the history of slavery in their own country but little about slavery in Latin America. Some are surprised to learn, for example, that there are whole regions of people of African descent in México (*los pueblos negros*) or English-speaking descendants of runaway slaves from English colonies on the east coast of Central America, or that by 1804 the population of Buenos Aires and Montevideo was 30 percent African or African-American.[46]

46 A vivid and informative portrayal of the immensity of the African presence in the Americas and its importance in the development of the continents is Greg Grandin's *The Empire of Necessity: Slavery, Freedom, and Deception in the New World* (Metropolitan, 2014).

Share with the group what you know about the history of African slavery in the Americas. What possible combinations of ancestry might a Peruvian have? If a descendant of an African slave has a European last name, is that name an indication of a slave master's ancestry, a slave's ancestry or both? What suggests that the patient in this dialogue has any Spanish ancestry? What are your thoughts about discussions of race among different people in this dialogue? Are the African contributions to and impact on Latin American society readily recognized? Are they similar to or different from the African contributions and impact in the United States?

Consanguinity: Of the same blood

In this appointment to screen for possible genetically inherited diseases, questions about consanguinity, racial and family history are central to the discussion. Different cultures have different norms regarding consanguinity and whether marriage between cousins or other family members is acceptable or legal. What are the societal rules and norms of the speakers of your other working languages? Is there acceptance or shame associated with consanguinity? Is the topic taboo or commonplace?

Plurals and inclusion

In a number of languages, there are different words for male siblings (brothers) and female siblings (sisters), yet the male term in plural can mean brothers or siblings of any gender. Sometimes if a question is asked about "brothers" (meaning siblings of both genders), a patient will only mention the male siblings. In your other working language, how could you ask the question about the number of siblings of any gender so that you'll get the information that the genetic counselor is seeking?

Twins

What are the different words for "twins" in your other language and how do they differ from country to countries (e.g., Spanish in México and Spanish in Paraguay)? Some languages differentiate between fraternal or identical twins with different words. Add all these terms to your terminology list to study.

Pregnancy termination

Pregnancies can end in many ways. Sometimes it's hard to tell because of the different medical, colloquial or common terms for pregnancy termination. Of course, a pregnancy can end with live birth, stillbirth (fetal death after 20 to 28 weeks or more of pregnancy, depending on local legal definitions) death, single or multiple births.

For termination of a pregnancy preterm, be sure to know all the terms and how to distinguish them without misinterpretations: "abortion" in English commonly refers to a medically induced or performed termination of a pregnancy, while "miscarriage" refers to the unintentional or natural loss of a pregnancy. However, "spontaneous abortion" is a term sometimes used for "miscarriage." The word abortion, even in English, technically refers to both events, whether intentional or unintentional. Healthcare providers and patients must however both be clear which meaning is intended during the interpreted encounter.

In many other languages, there is also one word for both these events, but in U.S. healthcare the end of pregnancy must be clearly qualified as intentional or unintentional when that information is needed. Be familiar with the differences and nuances.

Professional titles

The genetic counselor may be a PhD, but she is not a medical doctor. Patients often address health professionals as "doctor." In some places, "doctor" is commonly used as a simple term of respect regardless of education, but often in reference to social class. Should an interpreter correct this usage or possible misconception? Why or why not? How might it be important in the future if the patient is asked to name or identify the provider he or she saw?

Medical instructions in writing

The genetic counselor tells the patient, "I'm going to give you something in writing with all this information, but did you understand all that?" How important are these instruction? Could they make the difference in stopping a potential miscarriage? In many U.S. healthcare settings, such documents are provided only in English, or in English and one or two other languages. How meaningful will they be in English if the patient doesn't read English?

If medical instructions are given to all patients as a written reference to check in case they can't remember all the information that was orally explained to them, should everyone receive both oral and written instructions in a language they can understand? Do you know the policies or laws that address the meaningful provision of vital medical instructions to patients? If not, how can you learn them?

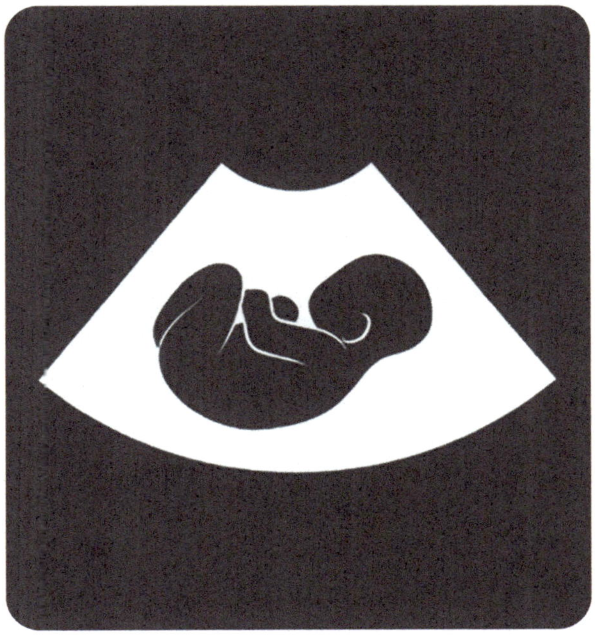

Ethics and standards: Reflect and practice

Goal: Review of standards (part 2)

In the following exercise, just as in the previous chapter, consider all 32 standards of the NCIHC *National Standards of Practice for Interpreters in Health Care.* Make a decision for each excerpt from the dialogue listed below about which standards apply. Use the information in the standards to answer the questions that follow each excerpt.

Note: In your answers, answer the question and then list the *number* of the standard, e.g., #6, #14 or #21.

EXCERPT 1

PATIENT: Es como esos mongolitos que se ven en la calle, ¿no?

GENETIC COUNSELOR: Well, we usually don't use that word to describe them anymore, but yes.

Cultural, social and political values and points of view are all present in this short excerpt. What is the responsibility of the interpreter, if any? Which standard(s) of practice might apply here?

EXCERPT 2 (discussed above)

GENETIC COUNSELOR: Now, depending on our consultation today and your family health history, we would test for anything else we might think there's a higher risk for. We will then be able to tell you about any change, alteration or mutation in the chromosomes and about any genetic disease or condition your baby has.

> **INTERPRETER:** As the interpreter, just to clarify, did you say you'd be able to tell if there was *any* genetic condition or abnormality? Como intérprete, para clarificar, ¿dijo usted que se podrá detectar la presencia de *cualquier* condición genética o anormalidad?

GENETIC COUNSELOR: Well, all the major, more common genetic conditions we see. It can't check for everything.

Why does the interpreter consider this point important to clarify? How does the genetic counselor's response change the meaning of her original statement, and how important a change is it? What is "informed consent" and how is it impacted if the interpreter does or does not clarify the counselor's statement? Finally, which standard(s) of practice might apply here?

EXCERPT 3

GENETIC COUNSELOR: OK. Well, we ask all our patients if they are related. So, you are Peruvian and I guess you have Spanish ancestry and French ancestry, and I guess there would be some native Peruvian or Indian blood as well. I guess that's about it, right? *(The patient has dark skin and her hair and features suggest African descent.)*

PATIENT: Yes.

INTERPRETER: *(to patient)* And you are also of African descent, right?

PATIENT: Oh, yes.

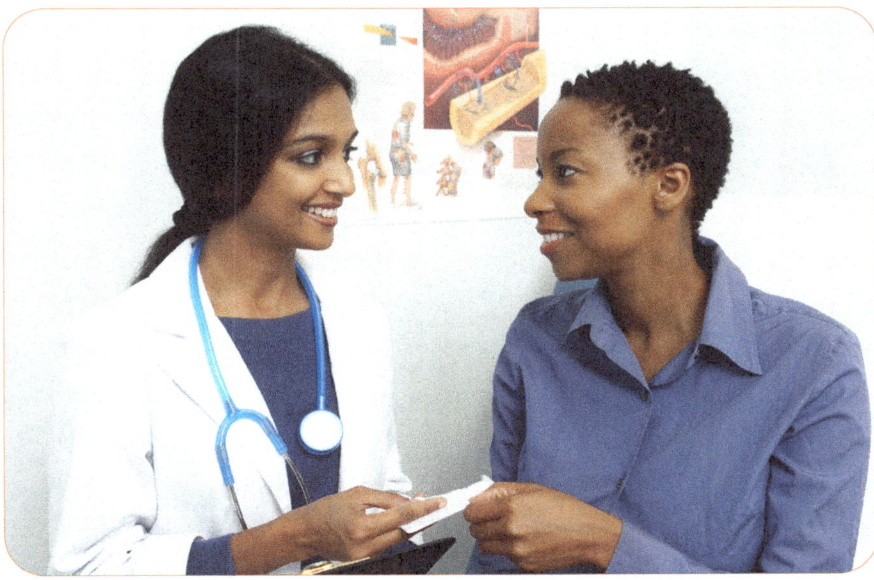

INTERPRETER: *(to genetic counselor)* She is also of African descent.

What was left unsaid here by the genetic counselor? Why, in your opinion? Which standard(s) of practice apply here?

How is this interpreter deviating from professional protocols? How could she do manage the situation differently? Which standard(s) of practice might apply to her intervention?

Occupational therapy for interpreters

EXERCISES FOR THE TONGUE, HEART AND MIND

Suggested reading

Ku, L., and Flores, G. (2005). Pay now or pay later: Providing interpreter services in health care. *Health Affairs*, *24*(2), pp. 435-444.[47]

Consider and discuss

1. How are the statements below, describing negative impacts on health as a result of language barriers, connected to costs? What is meant by the idea of "pay now or later"? How can this information be used to advocate for appropriate language access services from an economic perspective?

   "Research amply documents that language barriers impede access to health care, compromise quality of care, and increase the risk of adverse health outcomes among patients with limited English proficiency" (Ku & Flores, p. 435).

   "Language barriers can lead to inefficient care because clinicians are unable to elicit LEP patients' symptoms and, thus, use more diagnostic resources or invasive procedures" (Ku & Flores, p. 436).

2. The authors of this article refer to Title VI of the Civil Rights Act and a key term in that law, "national origin." What is meant by "national origin," and where is it defined? (Try an Internet search for the answer.)

3. How can the information below from this article be used to advocate for appropriate language access services from a legal or moral perspective?

   "Title VI of the Civil Rights Act obligates medical caregivers to provide interpretation and translation services so that LEP patients can have access to health care services equal to that of English speakers; this constitutes a protection against discrimination based on national origin. But the regrettable truth is that thousands of patients face language barriers every day, either because they cannot communicate with their medical caregivers or because communication is distorted by poorly trained, inexperienced, or inappropriate (for example, child) interpreters" (Ku & Flores, p. 435).

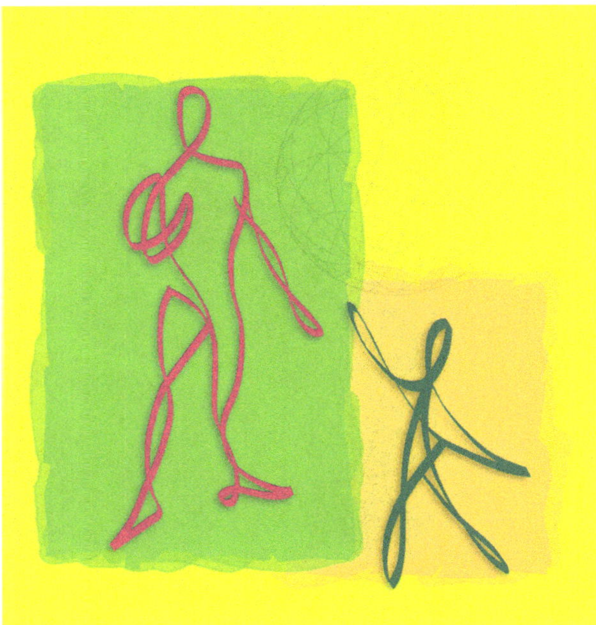

47 Retrieved from http://content.healthaffairs.org/content/24/2/435.full

4. Ku and Flores, in this article, identify multiple research studies that demonstrate health impacts. In which real-life context or situation and with whom can this information be used to advocate for appropriate language access services from a health perspective?

   > "Patients with limited English proficiency experience barriers to health care access; they also risk misdiagnosis, medical errors, and poor quality of care" (Ku & Flores, p. 436).

   > "LEP patients are more likely than others to report being in fair or poor health, defer needed medical care, leave the hospital against medical advice, miss follow-up appointments, or experience drug complications; they are also less likely to have a regular health care provider" (Ku & Flores, p. 436).

5. The authors cite many reasons for gaps in the provision of services despite legal requirements to provide language assistance. Is providing such services legally optional? Who is responsible for providing language access services?
6. In your opinion, is providing language access services a cost of doing business, or should it be the responsibility of the patient?
7. How interpreters matter: Review the two passages below and all the passages quoted above. Make a list of all the negative health impacts that can result from inadequate provision of language assistance in healthcare.

   > "Numerous studies document the profound adverse impact of language barriers across many dimensions of access to and quality of care. LEP patients are more likely than others to report being in fair or poor health, defer needed medical care, leave the hospital against medical advice, miss follow-up appointments, or experience drug complications; they are also less likely to have a regular health care provider" (Ku & Flores, p. 436).

   > "A survey of Latino parents revealed that language issues were cited as the single

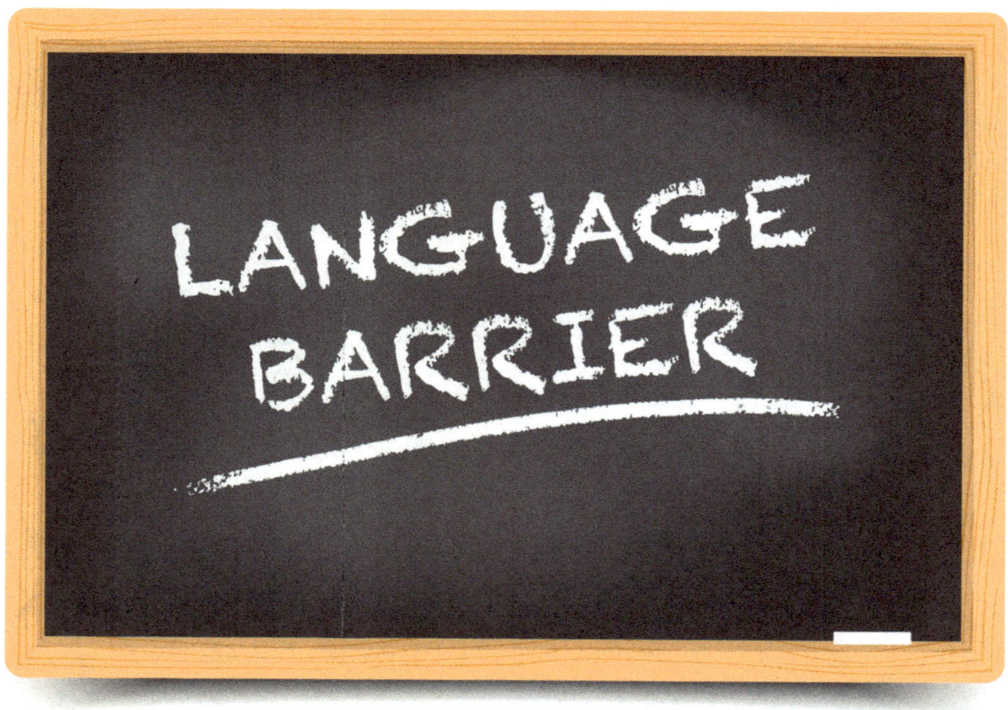

greatest barrier to healthcare access for their children...Six percent of parents reported not bringing their child in for needed medical care because of language barriers. Also, a growing body of research shows that lack of adequate interpreter services compromises the quality of care for patients with Limited English Proficiency" (Ku & Flores, p. 436).

8. Are the *results* of inadequate provision of language access services discriminatory? How?
9. Are the results of not providing interpreters to patients who need them intended or unintended?
10. Does intent or lack of intent justify or excuse the impacts on LEP patients?
11. In this short article, the authors provide more precise information from the U.S. Office of Management and Budget (OMB) about the estimated cost of provision of interpreters nationally: $268 million for inpatient hospital, outpatient physician, emergency department and dental visits. With some variation, interpretation for LEP patients would cost an estimated $4.04, or 0.5 percent (half of 1 percent) of the cost of a visit (Ku & Flores, p. 439).

    Ku and Flores also explore different strategies for covering these costs in the United States and how government Medicare or Medicaid payment policies may support or undermine the civil rights of LEP patients.

    In 2002, the OMB estimated that interpreters received $20–$26 per hour and that telephone interpretation costs $132 per hour, (Ku & Flores, p. 439). Technological change and globalization have had an impact on costs since then, but they have also opened up a wide array of quality control concerns.

    Among your study mates and colleagues, discuss what questions you have or opinions you have formed about the costs and benefits of providing interpreters for LEP patients.

12. In case you have not been able to read the whole article, here is the authors' summary, explaining the title, "Pay now or pay later."

    "The United States has already established the legal and ethical obligation of health care providers to offer language services to patients with limited English proficiency. The system should catch up and begin paying for these services. We can either pay a small amount up front to ensure that all patients receive equitable, high-quality care, or pay a lot more later for unnecessary tests and procedures, preventable hospitalizations, medical errors and injuries, and expensive lawsuits (Ku & Flores, p. 442).

Suggested reading

Green, D. (2009). The economics of language services: Or how to save healthcare in Texas. Presentation at the Texas Association of Healthcare Interpreters and Translators 3rd Annual Symposium on Language Access and Healthcare, April 2009.[48]

Consider and discuss

This is a powerful slide presentation from a conference. The first few slides target language demographics in Texas, but you may find those statistics either relevant or similar to the state where you live. Pay particular attention to slides 8-38. View them with colleagues.

1. Discuss how the information in this slide show corroborates or contradicts the thesis of Ku and Flores in the previous article. Include information that you feel makes the strongest or most impressive case for your point of view.
2. Write a list of at least five stakeholders who might benefit or be impacted by viewing this slide show.
3. Which slide(s) do you find the most compelling? Describe why and how you might use this information as an interpreter.

48 Retrieved from www.slideshare.net/DouglasGreen/the-economics-of-language-services-in-healthcarefinal

Medical terminology: Prenatal genetic testing

Below you will find anatomical drawings relevant to the content of this chapter. Follow the instructions found at the end of Chapter 1 to study the terminology in this section.

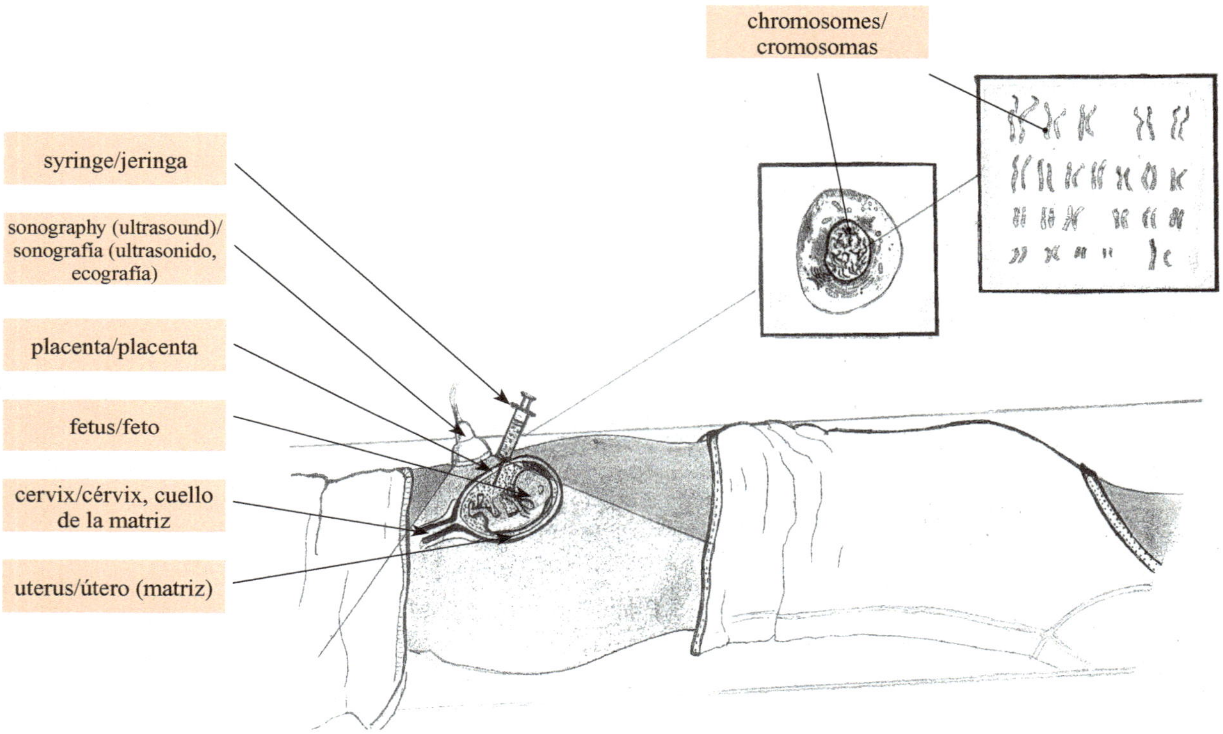

Figure 11-A: Prenatal genetics (English and Spanish)

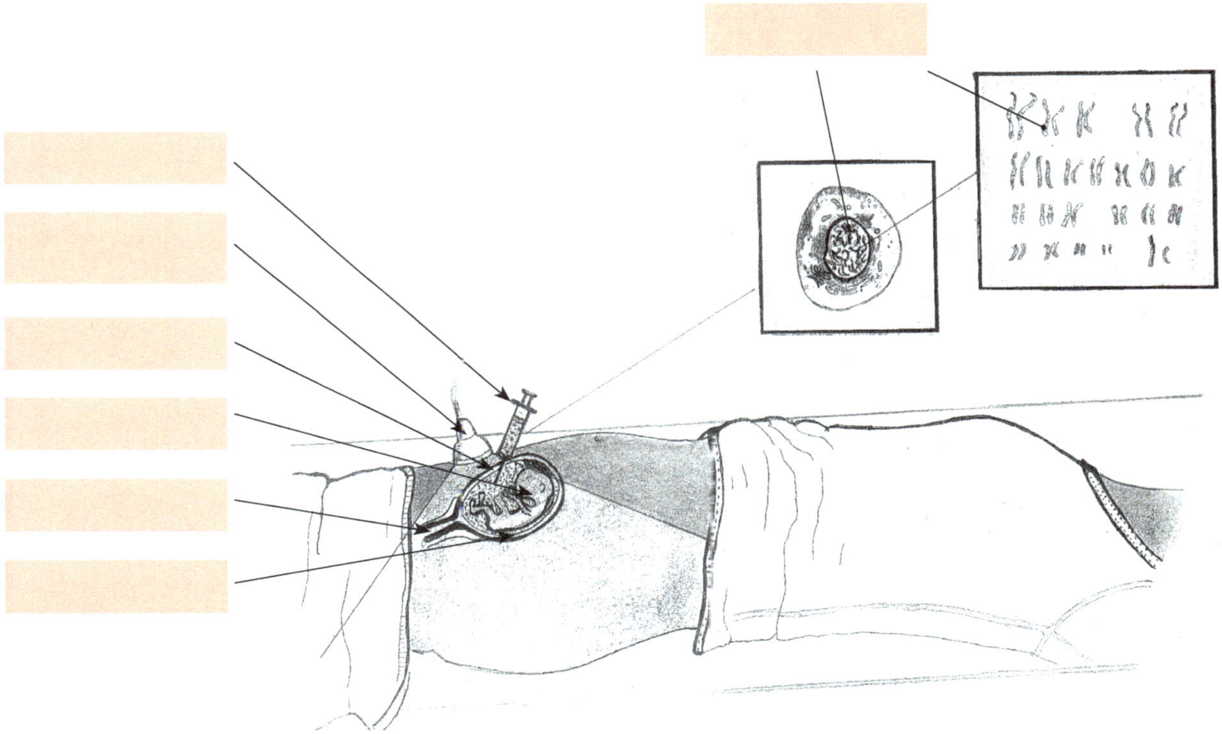

Figure 11-B: Prenatal genetics (blank labels)

Medical terminology list

Prenatal genetics

VOCABULARY FOR GRAPHIC–IN ENGLISH	VOCABULARY FOR GRAPHIC–IN SPANISH	ANY OTHER LANGUAGE
absence (of a gene)	ausencia	
AFP (alpha-fetoprotein)	AFP (alfafetoproteína)	
amniocentesis	amniocentesis	
amniotic fluid	líquido amniótico	
cell	célula	
cervix	cervix, cuello de la matriz	
cfDNA (cell-free DNA)	ADN fetal en sangre materna	
Chorionic villus sampling	muestras de vellosidad coriónica	
chromosomes	cromosomas	
condition	trastorno, condición	
deletion	deleción	
deoxyribonucleic acid	Ácido Desoxirribo Nucleico	
DNA	ADN	
duplication	duplicación	
fetus	feto	
gene, genes	gen, genes	
genetics	La genetica	
informed consent	Consentimiento informado	
mutation	mutación	
nuchal translucency	translucencia nucal	
placenta	placenta	
prenatal	prenatal	
scanner	escáner	
sonography (ultrasound)	sonografía (ultrasonido, ecografía)	
syndrome	síndrome	
Syringe	geringa	
translocation	translocación cromosómico	
ultrasound (sonography)	ultrasonido (sonografía, ecografiía)	
uterus	útero (matriz)	

Appendix 1

Resources for medical interpreters

Note: These resources were developed by Cross-Cultural Communications for medical interpreters in the United States and are used here by permission.

WEBSITES

All U.S. medical interpreters should be familiar with the following influential and important websites:

- National Council on Interpreting in Health Care: www.ncihc.org
- International Medical Interpreters Association: www.imiaweb.org
- California Healthcare Interpreting Association: www.chiaonline.org
- Texas Association of Healthcare Interpreters and Translators: www.tahit.us
- Diversity Rx, a website devoted to improving access to quality healthcare for diverse populations: www.diversityrx.org

In addition, here is a listing of many important U.S. healthcare interpreting associations hosted by NCIHC: www.ncihc.org/interpreter-associations

NATIONAL CERTIFICATION

All U.S. medical interpreters should be informed about the two national programs for certifying interpreters in healthcare. The websites for the two programs offer valuable information and are the best source for accurate, up-to-date information about these certification entities.

The two websites are listed here:

- Certification Commission for Healthcare Interpreters: www.cchicertification.org
- The National Board of Certification for Medical Interpreters (NBCMI): www.certifiedmedicalinterpreters.org

INTERPRETING STANDARDS

International standards

ISO 13611:2014. *Interpreting—Guidelines for community interpreting* (including medical). The International Organization for Standardization published its first international standard for any specialization of interpreting in 2014, after five years of development by 22 national member delegations. This document represents the first international standard for community interpreting. The document is a guideline standard, meaning that it contains no requirements but offers valuable information about international consensus on the profession and the industry. Purchase and download at www.iso.org/

ASTM International, F2089-15 *Standard Practice for Language Interpreting*. West Conshohocken, Pennsylvania: ASTM International. These industry standards were developed in 2001; the current revised standard was published in 2015. These standards are not mandatory but critically important: the requirements offer a national charter for the development of voluntary standards for all specializations of interpreting, including medical.

In addition, this requirements-based ASTM standard identifies components of quality language interpreting. ASTM International's standards are used in more than 100 countries. To order or download a copy, contact—

ASTM International
100 Barr Harbor Drive
PO Box C700
West Conshohocken, PA 19428-2959.
E-mail inquiries: service@astm.org
Website: www.astm.org

(ASTM International was formerly known as the American Society for Testing and Materials.)

Interpreting standards of practice

National Council of Interpreting in Health Care (NCIHC), *National Standards of Practice for Interpreters in Health Care* (NCIHC, 2005). To download a copy at no charge, go to www.ncihc.org

Massachusetts Medical Interpreters Association (now the International Medical Interpreters Association, and Educational Development Center, Inc. (MMIA & EDC, 1995). *Medical Interpreting Standards* of Practice. Available at www.imiaweb.org

The California Healthcare Interpreting Association (CHIA), *Standards of practice for healthcare interpreters* (CHIA, 2002). CHIA produced the other set of highly influential standards of practice for interpreters in healthcare in the U.S. Available at www.chiaonline.org

Bancroft, M.A. (2005). *The Interpreter's World Tour: An Environmental Scan of Standards of Practice for Interpreters,* California Endowment. Prepared for the National Council on Interpreting in Health Care. The review offers a detailed analysis of codes of ethics and standards of practice for medical, legal, community, conference, sign language and general interpreters around the world. Available at www.ncihc.org

Interpreting skill level descriptors

Interagency Language Roundtable (ILR) Skill Level Descriptions for Interpreter Performance

Federal standards for interpreter performance were developed in 2007. They are available at www.govtilr.org/skills/interpretationSLDsapproved.htm. The following information about these standards is taken from the website:

"These Skill Level Descriptions are primarily intended to serve as guidelines for use in government settings. They are separate and distinct from the ILR Language Skill Level Descriptions for Speaking, Listening, Reading, and Writing...

Interpreting is a complex task that combines several abilities beyond language competence in order to enable delivery of an effective professional interpretation in a given setting. Consequently, extreme care must be exercised in hiring interpreters and interpreting duties should be assigned to individuals within their performance level.

To facilitate this correspondence, the Skill Level Descriptions characterize interpreting performance in three bands: Professional Performance (Levels 3 to 5), Limited Performance (Levels 2 and 2+), and Minimal Performance (Levels 1 and 1+). Only individuals performing at the Professional Performance levels are properly termed "interpreters"...

From the standpoint of the user, a successful interpretation is one that faithfully and accurately conveys the meaning of the source language orally, reflecting the style, register, and cultural context of the source message, without omissions, additions or embellishments on the part of the interpreter."

ONLINE DICTIONARIES AND GLOSSARIES

The following are only a sampling of the many valuable multilingual glossary resources available online. Some are of higher quality than others. Be careful.

Multilingual sites

- www.wordreference.com: A user-friendly online multilingual dictionary. Select the two languages, type in the word for which a translation is desired in one language, and the translation of that word (and other information) appears. Study the forums that discuss particular usage for details useful for interpreters and translators.
- www.lexicool.com: An online dictionary search engine that currently has links to over 8,000 bilingual and multilingual dictionaries and glossaries in 70 languages.
- www.freedict.com offers links to bidirectional dictionaries in 16 languages.

Medical dictionaries and glossaries online

Spanish medical dictionaries

- *Manual Merck de información médica para el hogar:* The entire manual is available for free consultation online at www.msd.es/publicaciones/mmerck_hogar/
- For Spanish medical glossaries, go to www.onelook.com/?d=all_med&v=&sort=&langdf=spanish Spanish medical glossaries
- You can find an online searchable dictionary of 4,748 Spanish medical terms and abbreviations (as of June 2016) at www.msc.es/estadEstudios/estadisticas/docs/diccionarioSiglasMedicas.pdf
- Medline Plus, a service offered by the U.S. Department of Health and Human Services National Institutes of Health and the U.S. National Library of Medicine, provides high-quality information on healthcare and health terms in Spanish at www.nlm.nih.gov/medlineplus/spanish/anatomy.html

Medical dictionaries in other languages

- English: Medline Plus offers a medical dictionary at www.medlineplus.gov/mplusdictionary.html
- In addition, www.online-medical-dictionary.org, is a free online medical dictionary search engine to research and learn about medical terminology, pharmaceutical drugs, healthcare equipment, health conditions, medical devices, medical abbreviations and more, with information from more than 40,000 dictionaries, encyclopedias, research articles and books.
- Chinese: www.esaurus.org/ offers bilingual medical dictionaries and glossaries from the People's Republic of China, Taiwan and Hong Kong.
- For medical and technical online multilingual dictionaries in 34 languages, access www.multi-lingualbooks.com/onlinedicts-medtech.html
- Multiple languages: for a listing of multilingual online medical dictionaries hosted by the University of Vigo in Spain, go to http://sli.webs.uvigo.es/virtual/dicten.htm#medicine or another listing created by nurses at www.nurses.info/multilinguil_medical_dictionaries.htm
- For *print* medical glossaries for purchase in 24 languages, including refugee languages, to go www.xculture.org

Social and human services glossaries

- http://languagedoc.sfhsa.org: Links to glossaries of commonly used terms in human and social services that can be useful to interpreters in healthcare. Available in Chinese, Russian, Spanish and Vietnamese and put out by the San Francisco Department of Human Services.
- www.fns.usda.gov/documents-available-other-languages: U.S. Supplemental Nutrition Assistance Program informational materials in 48 languages.
- www.ssa.gov/espanol/agencia/glosario/: A Spanish-English glossary of Social Security terms from by the U.S. Social Security Administration.

Public health

- www.mass.gov/eohhs/gov/departments/dph/programs/admin/health-equity/translation-services-and-materials.html: This glossary, available in Spanish, French and Portuguese, is on a website with many other tools for translation. It was developed by the Massachusetts Department of Health and Human Services.

Colloquial and vulgar language

Interpreters often say they cannot interpret the "bad words" because they don't know them. Yet obscenities, vulgarities and coarse language do arise often in healthcare settings. Many bilingual print and online glossaries for the "bad words" exist in a variety of language pairs.

For Spanish interpreters, the following is just one example of what might be a helpful resource, particularly because it addresses so many Spanish-speaking countries: the *Glosario de Términos Vulgares e Insultos. Malas Palabras*, available at http://avizora.com/glosarios/glosarios_i/textos_i/insultos_eufemismos_i_0001.htm

Language access laws

Title VI of the Civil Rights Act of 1964

This is the text of the law:

> "No person in the United States shall, on ground of race, color, or national origin, be excluded from participation in, or be denied the benefits of, or be subjected to discrimination under any program or activity receiving federal financial assistance."

For the summary guidance on how recipients of federal funding through HHS are to respect Title VI, which was issued on August 4, 2003, go to www.gpo.gov/fdsys/pkg/FR-2003-08-08/html/03-20179.htm

State and local language access laws

All states

For an overview of state language access laws that affect healthcare, see Perkins and Youdelman (2008), *Summary of State Law Requirements Addressing Language Needs in Healthcare.*

National CLAS standards

Federal standards for Culturally and Linguistically Appropriate Services (National CLAS Standards) were developed by the Office of Minority Health of the U.S. Department of Health and Human Services. National CLAS Standards were created for organizations that offer health services.

The 15 standards target health services and are a critical resource for other community services. Four standards target language access; others target cultural barriers, cultural competence and institutional access.

For information about the standards, go to www.thinkculturalhealth.hhs.gov

To read the standards, go to www.thinkculturalhealth.hhs.gov/pdfs/enhancednationalclasstandards.pdf

Training for medical interpreters

An increasing number of community colleges and universities offer certificate programs in interpreting. Short training programs and workshops of almost any length are now widely available across the United States.

For a directory of U.S. healthcare interpreter training programs, go to the IMIA website, www.imiaweb.org, and click on *Education*, then on the *Education Registry*. You can search for programs by state, by type of program and whether the program is online or face-to-face.

Before you select a program and register, be sure to contact the training organization and ask questions about the program, for example:

- Who developed the program? What are the credentials of the developers?
- Who teaches the program? What are the credentials of the instructors?
- Is this program recognized by professional organizations?
- Will the program meet requirements to apply for national medical interpreter certification?
- How will this program prepare me to perform medical interpreting?

Appendix 2

Language access resources

Toolkit index

This informative document was circulated on the listserv of the National Council on Interpreting in Health Care (www.ncihc.org) in 2011 and 2012 by an unknown author. Note: Number 8 has been changed by the author of this book. The original recommendation 8 appears at the end of the document.

APPENDIX 2.1

Ten recommendations for medical professionals to consider when working with medical interpreters

1. **Being bilingual is not enough to ensure the quality of a medical interpreter**. Interpreting is a skill and not even being able to speak two languages *fluently* can guarantee that professional medical interpreting is what is taking place.
2. **Don't ask medical interpreters to provide word-for-word interpreting.** Interpreters relay the meaning of the words. A word-for-word interpretation will often lose all meaning and come out as nonsense.
3. **Expect medical interpreters to abide by a code of ethics.** A trained/certified medical interpreter will adhere to confidentiality, accuracy and impartiality. A qualified interpreter will know which ethical code(s) and standards he or she is required or expected to adhere to.
4. **Don't ask interpreters to be healthcare providers.** We hope to make your job easier, but we act only as the bridge to communication. We will interpret any message you wish to relay, but we are not the messenger.
5. **Clarify abbreviations and minimize medical jargon.** Medical acronyms, etc., will make no sense to the limited-English speaker since medical English is a language unto itself.
6. **Don't ask interpreters NOT to interpret something.** Part of our code of ethics says that we interpret everything that is said, as it is said. If you don't want it repeated, it is best not to say it in front of an interpreter.
7. **Address the patient, not the interpreter and maintain primary eye contact with your patient**. The role of the interpreter is essential, but is secondary to your relationship with the patient. Let us help you develop this trust by allowing the interpreter to not take center stage.
8. **Speak at a comfortable pace. *Consecutive* interpretation is the mode a medical interpreter will use most often.** Pause frequently. In order to allow for a complete *consecutive* interpretation, one or two sentences at a time are the most an interpreter can handle. The interpreter will let you know if you

are speaking too fast or too much at once. ***Simultaneous*** **interpretation is sometimes preferable.** In situations such as family conferences or for lengthy histories or declarations, simultaneous or "UN style" is best and allows for a more seamless conversational flow between patient and provider. With a proficient interpreter, simultaneous interpretation actually has a lower margin of error. Consult with all parties about their comfort level. Bilingual providers may be less comfortable if they are attempting to monitor the interpreter or improve language skills rather than concentrate on their role as practitioner.

9. **Don't ask the patient to bring their own interpreter; don't ask another patient to interpret for you; don't use a child as interpreter and don't use friends, family or nonqualified hospital staff as your first line of defense during medical encounters unless it is an emergency.** Our legal obligations make it imperative that qualified language services are utilized in each clinical encounter where the patient/ family members and their providers cannot communicate at the same level that two English speakers would be able to.
10. **Document the use of an interpreter. Document when it is not possible to use a qualified/certified interpreter. Be sure to document your attempts and the reason(s) why such an interpreter was not utilized.** Circumstances may make it impossible to utilize qualified language services in a timely manner. The medical record should reflect when an interpreter was used, who that interpreter was and any obstacles in using an interpreter. Know how to locate an interpreter, either over the phone or in person and return to using qualified language services as soon as possible.

Note: Number 8 in the original document was as follows and the version above is changed.

Speak at a comfortable pace and pause frequently to allow for the interpretation. In order to render a complete interpretation, one or two sentences are the most an interpreter can handle. The interpreter will let you know if you are speaking too fast or too much at once.

APPENDIX 2.2

General language access resources

Note: These resources were developed by Cross-Cultural Communications to support language access to healthcare in the United States and are used here by permission.

General resources

The Migration Policy Institute (MPI) Language Portal is a Translation and Interpretation Digital Library where anyone can search the database to find resources used to provide services to LEP individuals, including the following:

- Statistics and other information about LEP populations
- Language access plans
- Translated documents
- Interpreter/translator contracts
- Sample forms

The portal can be accessed at www.migrationpolicy.org

Resources for offices

Interpreter ID badges

Not every workplace needs badges for interpreters, but many interpreters find them helpful. For contract interpreters, they add a cachet of professionalism. For bilingual employees, putting on an interpreter badge helps to identify which role they are in. Various companies make such badges. For example, one used by interpreters is ID Matters at www.idmatters.biz

Multilingual "I speak" posters

For a federal document in 38 languages saying (for example), "Check here if you speak Arabic" in both English and Arabic, so that a client could point to his or her own language, go to www.lep.gov/ISpeakCards2004.pdf. The material can be downloaded at no cost, then printed and laminated to be used as posters.

The U.S. Social Security Administration has an attractive poster in color available in 20 languages on the Internet in a PDF that could be printed on large paper (20" × 32") and laminated. It reads: "We provide free interpreter services on request to conduct your Social Security business. Please call first so that someone who speaks your language will be available to help you." A list of this statement repeated in 20 languages follows on the website. The poster is available at www.ssa.gov/multilanguage/20x32Poster8_13_03.pdf

The Massachusetts Department of Public Health has similar "I Speak" sheets available on its website in 30 languages saying, "You have a right to a medical interpreter at no cost to you. Please point to your language. A medical interpreter will be called. Please wait."

To access the poster, go to www.mass.gov/eohhs/gov/departments/dph/programs/admin/health-equity/interpreter-services.html and click under the section titled "DPH Interpreter Services Poster."

APPENDIX 2.3

Sample "I speak" cards

Healthcare organizations can create their own "I speak" cards, which are interpreter request cards. Feel free to use the examples here. Copy, edit, laminate, cut, share and distribute this format, or simply design your own card!

Spanish

Yo hablo español. **Por favor, use un intérprete cualificado para hablar conmigo.** Yo tengo derecho a un intérprete de forma gratuita. Es la ley. —Gracias	**I speak Spanish.** **Please use a qualified interpreter to speak with me.** I have the right to an interpreter free of charge. It's the law. —Thank you
Yo hablo español. **Por favor, use un intérprete cualificado para hablar conmigo.** Yo tengo derecho a un intérprete de forma gratuita. Es la ley. —Gracias	**I speak Spanish.** **Please use a qualified interpreter to speak with me.** I have the right to an interpreter free of charge. It's the law. —Thank you
Yo hablo español. **Por favor, use un intérprete cualificado para hablar conmigo.** Yo tengo derecho a un intérprete de forma gratuita. Es la ley. —Gracias	**I speak Spanish.** **Please use a qualified interpreter to speak with me.** I have the right to an interpreter free of charge. It's the law. —Thank you

Cantonese, Mandarin (in traditional and modern script) and Russian

Я говорю по-русски. **Пожалуйста, мне необходима помощь квалифицированного переводчика.** По закону у меня есть право на бесплатные услуги переводчика.	I speak Russian. Please use a qualified interpreter to speak with me. I have the right to an interpreter free of charge. It's the law. —Thank you
我是說廣東話的。請使用一位有資格的翻譯員 與我對話。 在法律上我是有權免費使用翻譯員的。	**I speak Cantonese.** **Please use a qualified interpreter to speak with me.** I have the right to an interpreter free of charge. It's the law. —Thank you
我是普通话的。 请使用一位有资格的翻译员 与我对话。 在法律上我是有权免费使用翻译员的。	**I speak Mandarin.** **Please use a qualified interpreter to speak with me.** I have the right to an interpreter free of charge. It's the law. —Thank you

This sample does not specify the language. Simply write in the language needed. The blank format can be an especially valuable tool for LEP patients who speak less common languages.

I speak **Please use a qualified interpreter to speak with me.** I have the right to an interpreter free of charge. It's the law. Thank you.	I speak **Please use a qualified interpreter to speak with me.** I have the right to an interpreter free of charge. It's the law. Thank you.
I speak **Please use a qualified interpreter to speak with me.** I have the right to an interpreter free of charge. It's the law. Thank you.	I speak **Please use a qualified interpreter to speak with me.** I have the right to an interpreter free of charge. It's the law. Thank you.
I speak **Please use a qualified interpreter to speak with me.** I have the right to an interpreter free of charge. It's the law. Thank you.	I speak **Please use a qualified interpreter to speak with me.** I have the right to an interpreter free of charge. It's the law. Thank you.
I speak **Please use a qualified interpreter to speak with me.** I have the right to an interpreter free of charge. It's the law. Thank you.	I speak **Please use a qualified interpreter to speak with me.** I have the right to an interpreter free of charge. It's the law. Thank you.
I speak **Please use a qualified interpreter to speak with me.** I have the right to an interpreter free of charge. It's the law. Thank you.	I speak **Please use a qualified interpreter to speak with me.** I have the right to an interpreter free of charge. It's the law. Thank you.

APPENDIX 2.4

What you don't know might hurt you

Downing, B., and Roat, C.E. (2002). *Models for the provision of language access in health care settings*. Washington, DC: The National Council on Interpreting in Health Care. This paper was produced under a contract between Hablamos Juntos and the National Council on Interpreting in Health Care (NCIHC). Available at: www.hablamosjuntos.org/pdf_files/Models_for_the_Provision_of_Language_Access_final_.pdf

The following excerpt is taken from page 10 of this document.

Family and friends as interpreters

"Finally, the Office for Civil Rights (DHHS) has made it clear that the practice of 'requiring, suggesting, or encouraging' a patient to bring his or her friends, minor children, or family members to serve as interpreter infringes on the patient's civil rights under Title VI of the 1964 Civil Rights Act (see reference in fn. 15). This aspect of the Family and Friends model is simply illegal, at least when the provider institution is a recipient of federal funds.

The only circumstances under which the use of family or friends to interpret may be justified is at the direct request of the patient and only after it has been made clear to the patient that a professional interpreter is readily available at no cost. In many cases, healthcare institutions are requiring the patient to sign a waiver in these cases to release the institution from liability. Others will allow family and friends to interpret only if a professional interpreter is present in the room to assure accuracy in the communication. By and large, however, this model is not conducive to meaningful language access."

APPENDIX 2.5

Why do they wing it?

by Suzanna Reiss-Končar

Trade-offs between the perceived value of communication and patient health outcomes

A continuing challenge in healthcare is the provision of qualified language access for patients. Receiving healthcare in a language you don't understand is akin to not being there. Receiving healthcare in a language you partially don't understand is akin to being only partially there to receive it.

Some institutions may recognize this (they might need your help) and will set up programs to measure bilingual proficiency for healthcare providers. There is much debate about which of several provider exams are the most valid and reliable, what they should test and the need for a standard, generalizable measure. There is also discussion about what a "passing" mark is. For example, if passing is at 80 percent on a proficiency test, does that mean that patients will get 80 percent of a provider's expertise? Should insurance pay 80 percent of the bill? Which 80 percent of the visit will the patient miss, and how significant is that portion? Is medical vocabulary in another language sufficient without fluency, linguistic training or cultural competency? Will the missing pieces make the difference between adherence to the treatment plan or medical advice, or result in serious health consequences?

Evidence that the use of professional interpreters as compared to ad hoc interpreters results in improved health outcomes for LEP patients is now well established, yet underutilization continues. Even with proven economic benefits, a lack of language access services is widespread. Noncompliance with legal requirements for meaningful language access in healthcare continues to plague a significant part of the patient population.

Despite legal requirements, the absence of professionally trained, skilled interpreters is the norm in most clinical settings in the United States (Divi et al., 2007). Many health institutions do not actively foment or enforce language policies or follow legal guidelines. According to Leighton Ku, teacher of Health Policy at George Washington University, "Every day there are thousands of patients whose English is not very good who have a faltering ability to talk to their doctor or nurse...There's no serious monitoring or enforcement of the law" (Ludden, 2009).

Resistance to language proficiency testing from the medical community

Resistance from the medical community to language testing is well documented and takes many forms. Understanding the reasons can help inform ways to break down the barriers. Some institutions will focus on incentives for providers (gift certificates, money, salary increases, listing of privileges and competencies).

In the end, these incentives are encouragements to providers and the institutions they work for rather than directives to ensure compliance with federal and state laws. The reality is that when a measure of practitioner bilingual proficiency is a policy, enforcement is rare. Until the highest levels of an institution make reliable, valid verification of bilingual proficiency an enforced requirement, the situation is unlikely to change. Why does the practice of offering substandard care to LEP patients continue?

Why do providers wing it? Here are some possible explanations.

Despite the proven benefits, reasons for the continuing gulf between the need to provide professional medical interpreters and underutilization are many and should inform solutions. Practitioners' attitudes may contribute to use or underuse of professional interpreters. In a study by Diamond et al. (2009), many resident physicians admitted to regrettable underuse of interpreters while recognizing a resulting disparity of care. Their rationales included getting by, weighing the perceived value of communication against time constraints, convenience of asking family members or of using the physician's second language skills and normalization of underuse of trained interpreters.

In other studies, practitioners identified reasons for interpreter underuse, such as time constraints; scheduling problems; and limited availability of interpreters, even though interpreters were readily available (Lee, Winickoff, & Kim, 2006; Karliner, Perez-Stable, & Gildengorin, 2004; Schenker et al., 2008).

A study participant (Diamond et al., 2009) identifies a key point: that practitioners weigh *perceived value of communication* against other constraints. A nonproficient bilingual cannot, without specialized knowledge, adequately assess the value of communication that they don't understand. The participant's astute observation applies to the findings in studies that follow.

In one study, some physicians reported, "they preferred direct communication with the patient to working through an interpreter" (Karliner et al., 2007). In another study, some resident physicians reported perceptions of interpreters as "limiting"; only 33 percent of the provider participants felt that they had learned about another culture (Karliner et al., 2004, p. 178). One physician's assistant (PA) responded, "But how else will I get better if I don't practice my Spanish with my patients?" (Reiss-Končar, 2010). These statements might beg the questions of what, for each of these practitioners, was the *perceived value* and what was the *health outcomes value* in the communication. For this PA, it appears that time constraints, personal language learning opportunity and convenience held greater sway than the importance of accurate and complete communication, understanding, quality of participation and delivery of care.

In two studies with 24-hour interpreter availability, resident physicians chose to use their limited second-language skills, ad hoc interpreters or family members (Burbano et al., 2003; Yawman et al., 2006). In other studies physicians describe being unaware of the need for an interpreter, yet after the need was discovered, they often still elected to continue to deliver care without an interpreter (Burbano et al., 2003; Diamond et al., 2009; Narrigan, 2003; Schenker et al., 2008).

Practitioners may be unaware of the dangers of foregoing professional interpretation (Diamond et al., 2009). While several studies examine practitioners' subjective feelings about using interpreters, they do not look at the information most likely to influence their interpreter-use decisions: health outcomes.

Institutional level factors that influence use and underuse of interpreters

Institutions can do a great deal to remedy the situation. Training practitioners on how to work with professional interpreters appears to improve utilization (Karliner et al., 2004). Several excellent articles provide tips for providers on how to work with interpreters (Diamond & Jacobs, 2010). Training should involve consultation and collaboration with interpreters. Practitioner training regarding what is at stake medically in addition to legal obligations to meaningful language access is also promising and effective (Roat, 2010). An absence of information about legal assurances and patient's rights among both providers and patients exacerbates inequities. Adherence and compliance can be greatly improved through language access advocacy and education.

How the interpreter matters

The question of equal access to healthcare is where the medical interpreter enters the picture. All these challenges to equity in quality and delivery of care can be turned into tools. As pivotal, powerful members of healthcare teams, interpreters are in an advantageous position, poised to effect meaningful change to enhance health equity and support social justice through language access advocacy.

Think about the ways that you, as an interpreter, can influence health equity on different levels. Think about the individual health providers, managers, groups, committees and institutions where you work and the ways you can educate and contribute to the understanding of appropriate language services use.

Appendix 3

Spanish-English and English-Spanish medical glossaries

The following two glossaries are intended only as a guide for this textbook. They are in no way exhaustive or complete and should not be used by practicing interpreters as a substitute for a standard medical glossary, whether monolingual or bilingual.

Notes

1. Three-letter abbreviations are used for countries rather than standard international two-letter designations. The goal is to make the abbreviations easy to understand for a general reader.
2. Country abbreviations are in italics; abbreviations for diseases or disorders (e.g., HIV/AIDS) are not italicized.
3. References to Central America are noted as (*C.A.*) and to South America as (*S.A.*).
4. References to California are noted as (*Calif*).
5. Other countries noted in these glossaries include Colombia (*COL*), Cuba (*CUB*), México (*MEX*), Peru (*PER*), El Salvador (*SLV*), Spain (*ESP*), United States (*USA*) and Venezuela (*VEN*).
6. Most Spanish words noted only in masculine gender: e.g., *enfermero, feo, aguado*.
7. The letters *c* and *ch* are listed as separate letters in the Spanish-English glossary. In the English-Spanish glossary, words beginning with the letter *c* or *ch* are listed under the letter *c* only.
8. Parts of speech are noted occasionally and only to clarify instances of potential ambiguity.
9. The following notes are used.

    a. *reg.* refers to "regional."
    b. *vea* refers to "see."
    c. *n.* means "noun."
    d. *v.* means "verb."
    e. *adj.* means "adjective."

Spanish-English medical glossary

Glosario médico Español-Inglés

A

a salvo safe, out of danger
aborto miscarriage, abortion
  aborto espontáneo miscarriage, spontaneous abortion
  aborto médico medical abortion
  aborto provocado medical abortion
abrazar hug
absceso abscess
abuja (*reg.*, **aguja**) needle
ácaros dust mites
accidente cerebral stroke, cerebral accident
accidente cerebrovascular (embolia) cerebrovascular accident (stroke)
accidente cerebrovascular hemorrágico hemorrhagic stroke, hemorrhagic cerebrovascular accident
acidez acidity, heartburn, stomach acid
ácido desoxirribonucleico (ADN) deoxyribonucleic acid DNA
acogido, famila de foster family
acostado lying down, prostrate
acta de nacimiento birth certificate
ad hoc ad hoc
adenoides (*reg.*) adenoids, tonsils
adenoma adenoma
adherencia adhesion
adiposo adipose
ADN DNA
adrenoleucodistrofia (ALD) adrenoleukodystrophy (ALD)
afección preexistente preexisting condition
aféresis (plasmaféresis) apheresis (plasmapheresis)
agitado agitated, nervous, restless, anxious
agitar shake, agitate, stir
agriera (*COL*) heartburn
agruras (*MEX*) heartburn
aguadito floppy, lazy, week
aguja needle
alambre lead, wire, sensor, electrode
alcohol alcohol
ALD (adrenoleucodistrofia) ALD (adrenoleukodystrophy)
alergia allergy
alergias de la temporada seasonal allergies, hay fever
alfafetoproteína (AFP) alpha fetoprotein (AFP)
aliento breath
alimentación diet, food, feeding
  llevar un régimen de alimentación to be on a diet
  bolo alimenticio bolus feed
alimentación insuficiente malnutrition
alimento food, diet, feed
  alimento alto en fibra high-fiber diet
  alimento bajo en potasio low-potassium diet
  alimento balanceado balanced diet
  alimento blando soft diet
  alimento equilibrado balanced diet
  alimento libre de sodio sodium-free diet
  carencia alimenticia o nutritiva dietary deficiency
  deficiencia alimenticia o nutritiva dietary deficiency
aliviar relieve, alleviate
alivio relief
amamantar breastfeed
amígdala (brain structure; *vea* **amígdalas)** amygdala
amígdalas tonsils, adenoids
  amígdalas paletinas palatine tonsils
amigdalectomía tonsillectomy
amigdalitis tonsillitis
amigdaloadenoidectomía adenotonsillectomy
aminoácido amino acid
amniocentesis amniocentesis
amplitud width, range limit
amplitud de movimiento range of motion
ampolla blister
ampolleta vial
anafiláctico anaphylactic
  shock anafiláctico anaphylactic shock
anafilaxia anaphylaxis
análisis analysis, test
  análisis de laboratorio lab tests
andrógenos androgens
anemia anemia
  anemia aplásica aplastic anemia
  anemia de Fanconi (anemia aplásica) (aplastic anemia) Fanconi anemia
  anemia Diamond Blackfan Diamond Blackfan anemia
  anemia falciforme o de las células falciformes sickle cell anemia

anemia hipoplásica congénita congenital hypoplastic anemia
anemia megaloblástica anemia megoblastic
anemia perniciosa pernicious anemia
aneurisma aneurysm
aneurisma cerebral cerebral aneurysm
angina (*vea* **anginas**) angina
angina de pecho angina pectoris
anginas tonsils
inflamación de las anginas tonsillitis
angiografía coronaria coronary angiography, cardiac catheterization
angiograma coronario coronary angiogram, cardiac catheterization
ano anus
anteojos glasses (eye)
anticoagulantes anticoagulants, blood thinners
anticuerpo antibody
anticuerpos antiplaquetarios antiplatelet antibodies
antígeno antigen
antigüedad seniority
antiplaquetarios blood thinners, antiplatelet drugs
antirechazo antirejection
antiretroviral antiretroviral
antirreflujo antireflux
apapachar to hug, to cuddle
apapacho hug
apestar stink, smell bad
aplásica aplastic
aplastar smash, crush
apnea apnea
apóinmen (cita) (*reg.*) apoingmen
apoplejía apoplexy
apósito dressing, bandages
apretar squeeze
arrancar jump-start (heart), start
arrecho angry, rabidly angry (*VEN, C.A.*) horny (*PER*)
arriba de la boca above the mouth
arriesgar risk
arritmia arrhythmia
arrojar vomit, throw up, upchuck, spit up, yack
articulación joint
artritis arthritis
artritis reumatoide rheumatoid arthritis
artritis reumatoide juvenil juvenile rheumatoid arthritis
asistencia care, attention
asistencia deshumanizada inhumane care
asistente de médico physician's assistant (PA)
asistente médico medical assistant (MA)
asma asthma
ataque de asma asthma attack
aspiración aspiration
aspiración (biopsia, prueba) de médula ósea bone marrow biopsy (aspiration, test)
aspiración con aguja fina fine needle aspiration
aspirar to breathe in, to vacuum, to suction
ataque seizure, attack, convulsion
ataque al corazón heart attack
ataque cardíaco heart attack
ataque cerbrovascular, ACV brain attack cerebrovascular attack, stroke
ataque cerebral (*vea* **infarcto**) brain attack, seizure, brain seizure
ataque cerebral hemorrágico cerebrovascular hemorrhage, hemorrhagic brain attack
ataque cerebral isquemico transitorio transient ischemic brain attack (ministroke)
ataque de pánico panic attack
ataque isquémico transitorio (AIT) transient ischemic attacks (TIAs)
atarantado lightheaded, dizzy, out of it
atencíon attention, care
atención deshumanizada inhumane care
aterronado lumpy
atole atole (thick, corn-based drink of Mesoamerican origin)
atresia atresia
atresia pulmonar pulmonary atresia
atresia tricuspídea tricuspid atresia
atrofia atrophy
aturdido lightheaded, dizzy, out of it
audicón hearing
audiolología audiology
auditivo auditory
canal auditivo auditory canal
nervio auditivo auditory nerve
aurícula atrium
autismo autism
trastorno del espectro autista autism spectrum disorder
autorización authorization
autosoma autosome
autosómico autosomal
auxiliar de enfermería nursing assistant
axila axilla
axón axon
azucar sugar, glucose, blood sugar

B

baipás, derivación bypass
bajar poco a poco (la dosis de una medicina) taper, reduce
balance balance, balance sheet
balancearse to balance, to weigh
balanza (*vea* **báscula**) scale, scales
bálsamo balm
bálsamo labial lip balm
bálsamo para dermatitis de pañal butt balm, diaper rash cream or balm
báscula scale, scales

basófilo basophil
bata gown
bata quirúgica scrubs
bazo spleen
bebé prematuro premature baby, preemie
biliar biliary
  atresia biliar biliary atresia
  conductos biliares biliary ducts
  cálculo biliar gallstone
  tracto biliar biliary tract
  vías biliares biliary ducts
  vías biliares biliary tree
bilis bile
biopsia biopsy, sample
bipolar, trastorno afectivo bipolar affective disorder
bisbisear whoosh
blanca, sustancia o materia white matter
boca abajo face down, prone
boca abajo a boca arriba (voltearse) (roll over) back to front
boca arriba face up, supine
boca arriba a boca abajo (voltearse) (roll over) front to back
bocadillo snack
bochornos hot flashes
bola lump, bump
bolita little lump, little bump
bolo bolus
  bolo alimenticio bolus feed, nutritional bolus
bomba (*vea* ***bompa, pompa***) pump, bomb
bomba y sonda de alimentación de gastrostomía gastrostomy tube and pump, feeding tube and pump
bombita pump, little pump, inhaler, puffer
bompa **(bomba)** pump, bomb
bonbona (*VEN*) oxygen tank
borujoso lumpy
botón Bard (botón MIC-KEY) Bard Button (MIC-KEY)
bradicardia bradycardia
brazo arm (*"mano" is sometimes used in México to indicate "arm"*)
brote rash
bypass **(derivación)** bypass

C

caballo, irse de uno el, *modismo* to drop dead, kick the bucket, *idioms*
  se le fue el caballo, *modismo* he dropped dead, *idiom*
cabello hair (on head) (*vea* **pelo**)
cable lead, wire, sensor, electrode
cabrón fucker, fucked, fucked up, asshole, bastard, jerk, bad, tough, difficult
cada ocho días once a week
cada tercer día, *modismo* every other day
calabacita zucchini (*MEX*)
calabaza pumpkin, squash
calambres cramps
  calambres nocturnos en las piernas nocturnal leg cramps
calcomanías stickers
calentura fever
calenturas fevers, hot flashes
calorones hot flashes
cámara (para el inhalador) spacer, chamber
campo visual range of vision, visual field
canal canal
  canal auditivo auditory canal, ear canal
  canal de parto birth canal
  canales semicirculares semicircular canals
cáncer cancer
  cáncer colorrectal colorectal cancer
  cáncer colorrectal hereditario no asociado a poliposis, síndrome de Lynch hereditary nonpolyposis colorectal cancer, Lynch syndrome (HNPCC)
  cáncer de mama, seno o pecho breast cancer
  cáncer del colon y el recto colorectal cáncer
  exámen preliminar para el cáncer cancer screening test
cándida candida, yeast
candidiasis (hongos) candidasis (fungus) (fungus),
  candidasis bucal candidasis bucal
  candidiasis cutanea cutaneous candidasis
  candidiasis de la boca thrush, candidasis of the mouth
  candidiasis de la piel candidasis (yeast) infections of the skin
  candidiasis oral candidasis oral
cangrejos (*vea* **piojos del pubis, piojos púbicos**) crabs (*vea* **pubic lice**)
cantidad amount, volume
capa layer, cap
  capa de hielo polar polar ice cap
características characteristics
carajito (*VEN*) kid, child
cardiomiopatía cardiomyopathy
carencia deficiency, lack, scarcity, shortage
carga viral viral load
carraspear clear the throat
caspa dandruff
CAT **(tomografía axial computarizada),** escán *CAT* (*vea* **catescán, TAC, tacesán**) CAT scan (computer axial tomography scan)
catescán (tomografía axial computarizada, TAC) CAT scan (computer axial tomography scan)
catéter catheter, tube, line
  catéter Broviac Broviac catheter
  catéter de la vejiga urinary catheter
  catéter central central line
  catéter con acceso debajo de la piel *portacath, port*

catéter permanente permanent line
catéter venoso central subcutáneo (Port-a-Cath; InfusaPort, PassPort, Medi-port, port) subcutaneous central venous catheter, port
cateterismo catheterization
cateterismo cardíaco cardiac catheterization
cateterismo del corazón cardiac catheterization
cateterización catheterization
cateterización cardíaca cardiac catheterization
cateterización de la vejiga urinary catheterizat**ion**
causa subyacente underlying cause
ceco cecum
cefalorraquídeo brain and spine or spinal
líquido cefalorraquídeo brain and spinal fluid
ceguera blindness
ceguera nocturna night blindness
ceja eyebrow
CellCept (mycophenolate) CellCept (micofenolato)
célula (*vea* **glóbulo**) cell
células cells
células de base stem cells
células de sangre (*vea* **glóbulo**) blood cells
células de sangre de cordón cord blood cells
células linfocito-T T-lymphocyte cells
células madre hematopoyéticas hematopoietic stem cells
células madres stem cells
células progenitoras stem cells
células sanguíneas (*vea* **glóbulo**) blood cells
células Schwann Schwann cell
células-T T-cells
células tipo anillo signet-ring cell type
celulitis cellulitis
centro de cuidados paliativos hospice, center for palliative care
centro para cuidados de enfermos terminales hospice
cerebral cerebral
cerebro brain
certificado de defunción death certificate
cérvix (cerviz) cervix
cesárea Caesarean
parto por cesárea, nacimiento por cesárea Caesarean section, C-section
cetogénico ketogenic
ciego blind
punto ciego blind spot
agujero (ciego) blind spot
cigoto zygote
cintura waist, lower back
cirugía surgery
cirugía de Norwood Norwood surgery (primero de tres procedimientos denominados Fontan)
cirujano surgeon
cistitis cystitis
cistitis intersticial interstitial cystitis
cita appointment
cita de control follow-up visit, regular checkup
cita de seguimiento follow-up visit
cita subsecuente next visit, follow-up visit
citomegalovirus (CMV) cytomegalovirus (CMV)
citoplasma cytoplasm
citotóxico cytotoxic
clamidia chlamydia
claro clear, egg white
clítoris clitoris
clónico clonal
convulsión clónica clonal convulsion
coagulación coagulation
coágulo clot
coccidioidomicosis aguda (fiebre del Valle) coccidioidomycosis (Valley fever, San Joaquin Valley fever)
cóccix coccyx
cóclea cochlea
cola tail, butt, vagina (*MEX*)
hueso de la cola tailbone, coccyx
colgajo flap
cólico colic, cramps
colon (intestino grueso) colon (large intestine)
colon ascendente ascending colon
colon decendente descending colon
colon sigmoide sigmoid colon
colon transverso transverse colon
colonoscopia (colonoscopía) colonoscopy
colorrectal colorectal
colostomía colostomy
colposcopia (colposcopía) colposcopy
columna column, spine
columna cervical cervical spine
columna lumbar lumbar spine
columna torácica thoracic spine
columna vertebral vertebral column
comadre good friend, best bud, in-law, confidant, comrade, my child's godmother
comadrona midwife
comezón itch, itching
compadre good friend, best bud, in-law, confidant, comrade, my child's godfather
compresa poultice, compress
compresiones cardíacas chest compressions
común common
concuña sister of one's brother-in-law or sister-in-law; wife of one's brother-in-law
concuño brother of one's brother-in-law or sister-in-law; husband of one's sister-in-law
condición condition, disorder, problema
condón condom
conducto duct, conduct
conducto galactóforo milk duct
conducto radicular root canal
conductor conductor, cable, wire, sensor, electrode, shunt

congelación localizada frostbite
congestión congestion, engorgement
  congestión nasal nasal congestion
  congestión primaria primary congestion
  congestión primaria de los pechos engorged breasts
congestionado congested, engorged, swollen
  insuficiencia cardíaca congestive congestive heart failure
consanguíneo consanguinity
consaguinidad consanguinity
consejo sobre la genética genetic counseling
consentimiento consent, authorization
  dar contentimiento u autorización consent
consentir pamper, spoil, indulge
consulta sobre la genética genetic consultation
conteo absoluto de neutrófilos absolute neutrophil count (ANC)
conteo completo de células sanguineas (CSC) complete blood count (CBC)
conteo sanguineo completo (CSC) complete blood count (CBC)
convulsión convulsion, seizure
  convulsiones clónicas clonal convulsions
  convulsiones febriles febrile seizures or convulsions
copo flake
cordón (*vea* **médula**) cord
  cordón umbilical umbilical cord
  sangre de cordón cord blood
coriónico chorionic
coriza (*CUB*) runny nose, a cold
cornetas (nasales) turbinates (nasal)
corriente eléctrica electric current
corteza cerebral cerebral cortex
cortisol cortisol
costado side, flank
  dolor de costado flank pain, pain in the sides
  dolor de riñones flank pain, kidney pain
coxis coccyx
coyuntura joint
CPRE (colangiopancreatografía retrógrada endoscópica) ERCP (endoscopic retrograde cholangiopancreatography)
crecimiento growth
crema cream
  crema de hormonas hormone cream
  crema tópica topical cream
  crema vaginal vaginal cream
Creutzfeldt-Jakob, enfermedad de (EDJ) Creutzfeldt-Jakob disease (CJD)
Crohn, enfermedad de (*vea* **enfermedad inflamatoria intestinal)** Crohn's disease (*vea* **regional ileitis**)
cromosoma chromosome
crónico chronic
CSC (conteo sanguíneo completo) CBC (complete blood count)
CT, CTescán (tomografía computarizada) CT scan (computerized tomography scan)
cuadro chart, graph, file
  cuadro clínico clinical chart, medical chart
  cuadro médico medical chart, clinical chart
cuello de la matriz cervix (uterine)
cuello uterino cervix (uterine)
cuerpo body
  índice de masa corporal body mass index
  masa corporal body mass
cuidado care
  cuidado de niños child care
  cuidado infantil child care, infant care, nursery care
  cuidado legal temporal legal foster care
  cuidado temporal temporary care, foster care
cuidador del paciente (*vea* **persona que cuida al enfermo)** caregiver
cuidados care
  cuidados de acogido foster care
  cuidados de crianza foster care
  cuidados de crianza temporales temporary foster care
  cuidados de la salud healthcare
  cuidados de las heridas site care, wound care
  cuidados de tutela legal legal guardianship
  cuidados intensivos (terapia intensiva) intensive care
  cuidados paliativos palliative care
  cuidados temporales foster care
cuidar care
cuidar a care for, take care of
culebrilla (herpes zóster) shingles (herpes zoster)
culo (*ESP*) asshole, butt, bum
cultivar to culture, cultivate
cultivo culture (laboratory, agriculture)
  cultivo bacteriano bacterial culture
  cultivo de esputo sputum culture
  cultivo de orina urine culture
  cultivo endocerviccal endocervical culture
  cultivo mucoso mucosal culture
  hacer un cultivo grow out a culture
cultura culture
  cultura indígena indigenous culture
  cultura occidental Western culture
cuñada sister-in-law (*vea* **concuña**)
cuñado brother-in-law (*vea* **concuño**)
curación care, healing, site care, wound care
curación y cuidados de la herida o lesión wound site care
curita Band-Aid
custodia custody
  custodia legal temporal temporary legal custody
cutis cutis, skin

CH

chamo (*VEN*) kid, child
chavalo (*C.A.*) kid, child
chela, chelo (*C.A.*) (*vea* **güera**) light-skinned and/or light-haired person
chelita, chelito (*C.A.*) (*vea* **güera**) light-skinned and/or light-haired person
chicha (*S.A.*) fermented corn drink (*MEX*) breast, tit
chichi breast, tit
chichón lump, bump
chikungunya (virus) chikungunya (virus)
chingo de a lot, lots, a ton, hella (*Calif*), a shitload
chinguísimo a hell of a, very, really, super, hella (*Calif*)
chís (*MEX*) pee, piss
choclo (*S.A.*) corn
choque shock

D

dañar, hacer daño damage, hurt, cause pain, wound
daño harm
  daño cerebral brain damage
  reducción del daño harm reduction
dar de alta discharge
dar pecho breastfeed, put to breast
de la temporada seasonal
debajo de la boca below the mouth
debajo de la piel under the skin
debilidad weakness
dedo (de la mano) finger
  cuarto dedo fourth finger
  dedo anular ring finger
  dedo índice index finger
  dedo medio middle finger
  dedo meñique little finger
  dedo pulgar thumb
  primer dedo first finger
  pulgar thumb
  quinto dedo fifth finger
  segundo dedo second finger
  yema del dedo fingertip
defensas immunity, immunological system, defenses
deficiencia en la reparación del ADN mismatch repair deficiency
deficiencia inmunitaria combinada severa (DICS) severe combined immunodeficiency (SCID)
deglutir to swallow
dejar con hoyos to pit, pitting
dejar que crezca grow (something) out, let grow
deleción (genetica) deletion (genetic)
delgado thin, lean (body)
dendrita dendrite
densidad ósea bone density
derivación shunt, bypass
derivación de Glenn o hemi-fontan Glenn surgery (segunda parte de la cirugía cardiaca Fontan para tratar los defectos congénitos del corazón)
dermatofitosis (tiña) ringworm
dermatomiositis dermatomyositis
derrame hemorrhage, bleed
derrame cerebral brain hemorrhage, cerebral hemorrhage, brain bleed
desarrollo development
  desarrollo del feto fetal development
  desarrollo fetal fetal development
  trastorno generalizado del desarrollo general developmental disorder
descarga discharge
  descarga eléctrica electric shock
desequilibrado maladjusted, unbalanced
desesperado anxious, desperate
desecho discharge (from body)
desgaste wasting
  desgaste de SIDA AIDS wasting, wasting syndrome
desigualdad inequality, disparity, inequity
desmayarse faint, pass out, lose consciousness
desmayo fainting
  episodios de desmayo fainting spells
desnutrición malnutrition
desorden disorder, condition, problem
  desorden de las plaquetas platelet disorder
devolver return, vomit, throw up, upchuck, spit up, yack
diabetes diabetes
  diabetes gestacional gestational diabetes
  diabetes insípida diabetes insipidus (DI)
  diabetes insulinodependiente insulin dependent diabetes
  diabetes mellitus diabetes mellitus
  diabetes no insulinodependiente non-insulin dependent diabetes
  diabetes tipo 1 diabetes type 1
  diabetes tipo 2 diabetes type 2
diabético diabetic
diáfisis (del hueso) bone shaft
diagnosticar diagnose
diagnóstico diagnosis
  prueba diagnóstica diagnostic test
diálisis dialysis
  diálisis peritoneal peritoneal dialysis
  hemodiálisis hemodialysis
diámetro diameter
diarrea diarrhea
dieta (*vea* **alimentación, alimento**) diet
  dieta alta o rica en fibra high-fiber diet
  dieta baja en potasio low-potassium diet
  dieta balanceada balanced diet
  dieta blando soft diet
  dieta equilibrada balanced diet
  dieta especial special diet

dieta libre de sodio sodium-free diet
dieta relámpago crash diet
dieta saludable o sana healthy diet
pastillas para bajar de peso/adelgazar diet pills
estar en dieta to be on a diet
ponerse a dieta to go on a diet
restricciones en la dieta dietary restrictions
dietético dietician, nutritionist
dilitarse to become engorged
disco disc
disco abultado bulging disc
disco degenerado degenerative disc
disco deteriorado degenerative disc
disco herniado herniated disc
disco intervertebral intervertebral disc
disco sobresaliente bulging disc
disfagia dysphagia
disminuir taper, diminish, go down (on a dose) little by little
displasia dysplasia
displasia anal anal dysplasia
displasia cervical cervical dysplasia
displasia septo-óptica (síndrome de Morsier, síndrome del nervio óptico) septo-optic dysplasia (optic nerve hypoplasia, de Morsier syndrome)
distrofia muscular progresiva muscular dystrophy
disuria dysuria
doctor (*vea* **médico**) doctor, physician, medical doctor, PhD, MD
(*las siguientes demomnaciones varían entre países y sistemas, en el inglés y el español*)
doctor a cargo attending physician, head doctor, chief physician
doctor de cabecera attending physician, head doctor, chief physician
doctor de medicina doctor
doctor de medicina medical doctor, (medical) doctor, physician
doctor encargado attending physician, head doctor, chief physician
doctor jefe head doctor, chief doctor
doctor residente resident doctor
doctor responsable attending physician, head doctor, chief physician
doctor supervisor attending physician, supervising doctor
médico en el primer año de especialización intern (doctor)
médico en el segundo año de especialización resident (doctor)
médico en el tercer año de especialización resident (doctor)
médico internista intern (doctor)
médico pasante fellow (doctor)
médico residente resident (doctor)
médico residente auxiliar resident (doctor)
dolor pain
dolor agudo sharp pain
dolor como corriente eléctrica o descarga eléctrica electric shock pain
dolor constante constant pain
dolor de cabeza headache
dolor de cerebro headache
dolor embotado dull pain, aching pain
dolor insoportable unbearable pain
dolor intermitente intermittent pain
dolor palpitante throbbing pain
dolor punzante stabbing pain
dolor que se irradia shooting pain
dolor sordo dull pain, aching pain
donador donor
donante donor
drenaje drain
drenar drain
duodeno duodenum
duodenoyeyunal duodenojejunal

E

ébola Ebola
ECG (electrocardiograma) EKG (electrocardiogram)
echándole ganas keep trying, moving forward,
echarle ganas a algo keep going, try hard, have faith, give it a try, put your best foot forward, give it your best shot
edad fecunda childbearing age
edad fértil childbearing age
edema edema
edema con fóvea pitting edema
ELA ALS
electrocardiograma electrocardiogram
electrodo electrode, sensor, wire, cable
electroencefalograma electroencephalogram (EEG)
ELISA, prueba (enzimoinmunoanálisis de absorción) ELISA test (enzyme-linked immunoassay)
elote corn (*MEX*)
emaciación wasting
emaciación del rostro facial wasting
emaciación muscular muscular wasting, muscular emaciation
síndrome de emaciación por SIDA AIDS wasting síndrome
***emarrái* (MRI, imágenes de resonancia magnética)** MRI, magnetic resonance imaging
embarazada pregnant
embarazo pregnancy
embarazo a término full-term pregnancy
embarazo a término completo full-term pregnancy
embolia (*vea* **coágulo**, aneurisma, accident cerebrovascular) embolism, stroke
embolismo (*vea* **coágulo**, aneurisma, accident cerebrovascular) embolism

embolización embolization
empujar hacia afuera protrude, push out
encargado in charge, attending (doctor)
encefalopatía espongiforme bovina (EEB, enfermedad de Creutzfeldt-Jakob, ECJ enfermedad de las vacas locas) bovine spongiform encephalopathy (BSE, Creutzfeldt-Jakob disease, CJD, mad cow disease)
encefaloraquítico cerebrospinal
encías gums
endocrino endocrine
  sistema endocrino endocrine system
endocrinólogo endocrinologist
endometrio endometrium
  biopsia del endometrio endometrial biopsy
  cáncer del endometrio endometrial cancer
  del endométrio endometrial
  endometrio uterino uterine endometrium
enema enema
enfermedad disease, illness
  enfermedad de Creutzfeldt-Jakob (ECJ) (encefalopatía espongiforme bovina (EEB) enfermedad de la vaca loca) Creutzfeldt-Jakob disease, (CJD) (mad cow disease), bovine spongiform encephalopathy (BSE)
  enfermedad de Crohn (*vea* **enfermedad inflamatoria intestinal**) Crohn's disease (*vea* **regional ileitis**)
  enfermedad de Hirschsprung's Hirschsprung's disease
  enfermedad de injerto versus huésped graft versus host disease (GVHD)
  enfermedad de la neurona motora (ENM) motor neuron disease (MND)
  enfermedad de las arterias coronarias (EAC) coronary artery disease (CAD)
  enfermedad de transmisión sexual (ETS) sexually transmitted disease (STD)
  enfermedad inflamatoria intestinal (*vea* **enfermedad de Crohn**) regional enteritis, regional ileitis
  enfermedad por reflujo gastroesofágico (ERGE) gastroesophageal reflux disease (GERD)
  enfermedad reactiva de las vías respiratorias reactive airway disease
enfermería nursing
  asistente de enfermería nursing assistant
  auxiliar de enfermería nurse's aide, nursing assistant
  estudiante de enfermería nursing student
enfermero, enfermera nurse[49]
  enfermero auxiliar de médico nurse practitioner
  enfermero clínico especialista clinical nurse specialist
  enfermero de práctica avanzada advanced practice nurse
  enfermero de salud pública public health nurse
  enfermero de visita a domicilio home health nurse
  enfermero diplomado registered nurse
  enfermero especialista nurse practitioner, nurse specialist
  enfermero recibido registered nurse
  enfermero registrado registered nurse
enjuagar flush, rinse
enrojecer to turn red
enrojecido redness
enrojecimiento reddening
ensayo clínico clinical trial, clinical study, investigational study, research study, experimental study (*use caution with this last phrase as it may be misinterpreted*)
enterocolitis necrosante (ECN) necrotizing enterocolitis
entornar squint
entrecerrar squint, half close
entumecer numb
entumecido numb
entumecimiento numbness
eosinófilo eosinophil
epigenética epigenetics
episiotomía episiotomy
equidad equity
  equidad en la atención equity in care
  equidad en la salud health equity
  equidad sanitaria health equity
equilibrarse to balance, get one's balance
equilibrio equilibrium, balance
erección erection
eréctil erectile
  disfunción eréctil erectile dysfunction
eritrocito erythrocyte
eritrocitosis erythrocytosis
eritropoyetina erythropoietin
erupción rash
escama scale, flake
escamoso flaky, scaly, squamous
escán scan, tomography
escarlatina scarlet fever
esclerosis lateral amiotrófica (ELA) amyotrophic lateral sclerosis (ALS)
escotoma scotoma
escuincle, escuintle (*MEX*) kid, child, runt
eso es la talla, modismo that's it that's what I'm talking about
esofagrama (esofagrama con ingestión de barrio) swallow study (barium swallow study)
espalda back
  parte inferior de la espalda, cintura lower back
espasmos del sollozo breath-holding spells
especialista en lactación lactation specialist

49 Los títulos de enfermeros cambian de país en país y sistema en sistema; los títulos pueden tener diferentes significados. Nursing titles change from country to country and system to system; titles may not be equivalent.

espécimen specimen (sample, biopsy)
espéculo speculum
espejuelos glasses (eye)
espina spine, thorn
  espina bífida spina bifida
  espina bífida abierta open spina bifida
  espina bífida oculta spina bifida occulta
  espina cervical cervical spine
  espina dorsal spine, spinal column
  espina lumbar lumbar spine
  espina torácica thoracic spine
espora spores
esporas de moho mold spores
estándar standard
estandarizado standardized
  prácticas estandarizadas standard practices
estar tieso to be stiff, to have stiffness
estenosis arterial arterial stenosis
esteroides steroids
estíquers (*C.A.*, lcomanias, pegantines) stickers
estógamo (*reg., MEX, vea* **estómago**) stomach
estoma stoma
estómago stomach
estrabismo (ojos biscos) strabismus (crossed eyes)
estreptococo streptococcus, strep
estrés stress
estribo stapes
estribos stirrups
estrujar squeeze
estudiar study
  estudio del sueño sleep study
  estudio del tragar swallow study
  estudio del tragar (esofagrama con ingestion de barrio) swallow study (barium swallow study)
etapas en el desarrollo (*vea* **hitos de desarrollo**) developmental milestones
examen exam, evaluation, test
examen preliminar para el cáncer cancer screening test
excoriación excoriation
experimento experiment (*caution; vea* **ensayo clínico**)
extirpar remove
eyaculación ejaculation
  eyaculación prematura premature ejaculation
eyaculatorio ejaculatory
  líquido pre-eyaculatorio pre-ejaculatory fluid

F

facciones features, characteristics
  facciones identificadoras identifying features
factor de coaglación clotting factor
fagocitos phagocyte
falla glitch, failure, fault
fallo cardíaco (*vea* **insuficiencia cardíaca**) cardiac failure
familia family
  familia adoptiva adoptive family
  familia de acogida foster family
  familia de crianza temporal foster family, temporary foster family
  familia temporal foster family, temporary foster family
faringe pharynx
faringomalasia pharyngomalacia
farmacéutico pharmacist
farmacia pharmacy
farmacólogo pharmacologist
febril febrile
fecha date
  fecha prevista de parto due date
  fecha probable de parto due date
fenobarbital phenobarbital
fenotipo phenotype
feo ugly, difficult, really bad
fibrilación auricular atrial fibrillation
fibroide fibroid
  fibroide uterino (*vea* **mioma**) uterine fibroid
fibroma fibroma
fibroquístico fibrocystic
  enfermedad fibroquística fibrocystic disease
  mastopatía fibroquística fibrocystic breast disease
fibromialgia fibromyalgia
fibrosis fibrosis
  fibrosis pulmonar pulmonary fibrosis
  fibrosis quística cystic fibrosis
fiebre del Valle (fiebre del Valle San Joaquin, coccidioidomicosis aguda) Valley fever (San Joaquin Valley fever, acute coccidioidomicosis)
fisiología physiology
fisioterapeuta (*vea* **terapeuta, terapista**) physical therapist
fisioterapia physiotherapy
fístula fistula
flu (influenza) flu
flujo fluid, discharge, secretion, flow
Fontan procedimiento Fontan procedure (in black)
fontanela (*vea* **mollera**) fontanel, soft spot (on infant's head), pate
fórceps forceps
fórmula formula
formulario form, slip
  formulario u hoja para análisis de laboratorio lab slip
forro (*vea* **revestimiento**) lining
  forro de la matriz uterine lining
fosa pit
  fosa común common grave
fregar scrub, annoy, bother, mess with, fuck with (*C.A.*)
frialdad cold, a cold
frío cold
frotar rub, rub in

fuera de onda out of it, lightheaded
fuera de peligro out of danger, safe
fuerza muscular muscle strength
fundoplicatura fundoplication a laparascopic surgery to treat hiatal hernia

G

gafas de protección goggles
gammagrafía scan
  gammagrafía ósea bone scan
ganglio lymph node
  ganglio linfático lymph gland or lymph node
gangrena gangrene
garganta throat
  carraspear la garganta clear the throat
  dolor de garganta sore throat
gárgaras (hacer) to gargle
garrapata tick
gasa gauze
gastroesofágico gastroesophageal
  enfermedad por reflujo gastroesofágico (ERGE) gastroesophageal reflux disease (GERD)
  reflujo gastroesofágico gastroesophageal reflux
gastrostomía (sonda G) gastrostomy (G-tube)
  bomba y sonda de alimentación de gastrostomía gastrostomy feeding tube pump
gen gene
  gen causante causative gene
general general
  en general in general
  por lo general mainly, principally, generally
generalmente generally, in general, principally, mainly
genérico generic
genética (n.) genetics
genético (v.) genetic
genoma genome
genotipo genotype
gingivitis gingivitis
girando spinning
girar spin, spinning
glándula gland
  glándula mamaria mammary gland
  glándula pituitaria pituitary gland
  glándula suprarrenal adrenal gland
  glándula tiroidéa thyroid gland
glóbulo blood cell
  glóbulos blancos (leucocitos) white blood cells (leukocytes)
  glóbulos rojos (eritrocitos) red blood cells (erythrocytes)
glucosa glucose
golpe blow, shock, bump
  golpe eléctrico electric shock
golpearse hit, bump, bang
gomitar (*reg., MEX*) vomit, throw up, upchuck, spit up, yack
gónada gonad
gordo (adj.) fat
  cuerpo gordo fat body
  persona gorda fat person
grasa fat (noun)
  bajo en grasa low fat
  full fat grasa entera
  grasa animal animal fat
  grasa corporal body fat
  grasa vegetal vegetable fat
  libre de grasa fat free
  sin grasa fat free
gratis, gratuito free of charge, free, at no cost
grave grave, serious
gravemente enfermo gravely ill
gripa flu, cold
gripe (influenza) flu (influenza)
gruma en el pecho breast lump
guagua (*CUB*) bus
güera, güero (*MEX*) (*vea* **chela**) light-skinned and or light-haired person
güerita, güerito (*MEX*) (*vea* **chela**) light-skinned and or light-haired person
GVHD enfermedad de injerto versus huésped graft versus host disease

H

HAART (siglas en inglés que equivale a "terapia antiretroviral altamente activa") HAART (highly active antiretroviral therapy)
harina flour
  harina de maíz corn flour
  harina de trigo wheat flour
hacer to do, to make
  hacer del baño, *modismo* go to the bathroom, have a bowel movement, poop
  hacer del cuerpo, *modismo* go to the bathroom, have a bowel movement, poop
  hacer popó go poop
  hacer un cultivo to do a lab culture
  hacer una cita make an appointment schedule an appointment
hacérsele a uno un nudo en la garganta, *modismo* get a frog in one's throat, *idiom*
harto (*reg., MEX*) really, very, a lot of, hella, sick and tired of
hematocrito hematocrit
hematopoiesis hematopoiesis
hemodiálisis hemodialysis
hemopoyética hematopoietic
hemorragia hemorrhage, bleed
  hemorragia cerebral brain hemorrhage, brain bleed

hendido cleft
  paladar hendido cleft palate
  labio hendido cleft lip
hepático (del hígado) hepatic (pertaining to the liver)
hereditario hereditary
herida wound
herir hurt, injure, damage
hernia hernia
  hernia de hiato hiatal hernia
  hernia diafragmática congénita congenital diaphragmatic hernia
  hernia epigástrica epigastric hernia
  hernia femoral femoral hernia
  hernia inguinal inguinal hernia
  hernia umbilical umbilical hernia
herpes herpes
  herpes congénito congenital herpes
  herpes genital genital herpes
  herpes labial oral herpes
  herpes labialis herpes labial
  herpes oral oral herpes
  herpes orales oral herpes
  herpes simplex virus (HSV) virus herpes simplex (VHS)
  herpes tipo 1 (VHS-1) herpes type 1(VHS-1)
  herpes tipo 2 (VHS-2) herpes type 2 (HSV-2)
  herpes zóster (culebrilla) herpes zoster (shingles)
hidratación hydration
hidratante hydrating
  loción hidratante hydrating lotion
hidrocefalia hydrocephalus
  hidrocefalia de presión normal normal pressure hydrocephalus (NPH)
hidrocele hydrocele
hidrocortisol hydrocortisol
hinchado swollen
hincharse swell, to become engorged
hinchazón swelling, lump
hiper- hyper-
hiperpituitarismo hyperpituitarism
hipo hiccough, hiccup
hipo- hypo-
hipopituitarismo hypopituitarism
hiposepto óptico hypo septo-optic
hipospadias hypospadias
hipotálamo hypothalamus
Hirschsprung's, enfermedad de Hirschsprung's disease
hisopos swab, wipe
histerectomía hysterectomy
  histerectomía radical radical hysterectomy
histiocitos histiocytes
histocompatibilidad histocompatibility
histopatología histopathology
historia clínica clinical history, health history, medical history,
historia de la salud, health history, clinical history, medical history
historia médica medical history, health history, clinical history
hisutismo hirsutism
hitos del desarrollo developmental milestones
hogar home
  hogar de acogida foster home
  hogar de crianza foster home
  hogar temporal foster home
hojuelo flake
hombro shoulder
hongos fungus, candida, yeast
hormona hormone
hospicio hospice
huella digital fingerprint
huesero bonesetter, healer
hueso bone
  caña del hueso bone shaft
  hueso compacto compact bone
  hueso corto short bone
  hueso esponjoso spongy bone
  hueso largo long bone
  injerto de hueso u óseo bone transplant
  rastreo de los huesos bone scan
  tomografía de los huesos bone scan
humidificador humidifier

I

ibuprofeno ibuprofen
idiopático idiopathic
  púrpura trombocitopénica idiopática idiopathic thrombocytopenic purpura (ITP)
(IGIV) inmunoglobulina intravenosa IVIG (intravenous immunoglobulin)
íleon ileum
ilíaco iliac
imágenes de resonancia magnética (IRM) magnetic resonance imaging (MRI)
imán magnet
impétigo impetigo
importar to care about, to be important, to import
inadaptado maladjusted
incidencia incidence
incidente incident
inclinarse to lean, to lean toward
incontinencia incontinence
  incontinencia imperiosa urge incontinence
  incontinencia urinaria urinary incontinence
índice rate, speed
indiferenciado undifferentiated
indisposición malaise
indocumentado undocumented

inequidad inequity
  inequidades de salud health inequities, health disparities
  inequidades sanitarias health inequities, health disparities
infarto
  infarto cerebrovascular cardiovascular attack
  infarto de miocardio myocardial infarction
infección infection
  infección de hongos fungal infection, yeast infection, candidiasis
  infección de la orina urinary tract infection, urine infection
  infección de la vejiga urinaria bladder infection
  infección de las vías urinarias urinary tract infection
  infección necrosante de tejidos blandos necrotizing soft tissue infection
  infección neumocócica pneumococcal infection
  infección oportunista opportunistic infection
  infección por estreptococos de la garganta strep throat
  infeccion por neumococo pneumococcal infection
  infecciones de transmisión sexual sexually transmitted infections (STIs)
  infecciones neumocócicas pneumococcal infections
  infecciones por neumococo pneumococcal infection
  infecciones vaginales por vaginal yeast infections
inflamación inflammation, swelling
inflamado inflamed
influenza (gripe) influenza (flu)
  inyección contra la influenza o gripe flu shot
  vacuna contra la influenza flu vaccine
ingurgitación engorgement
ingurgitados engorged
ingurgitarse engorge
inhalador inhaler, puffer
inhibidores inhibitors
inhibidores de la proteasa protease inhibitors
inhibidores nucleósidos de la transcriptasa reversa nucleoside analog reverse transcriptase inhibitors
injerto graft
  enfermedad del injerto versus el huésped graft versus host disease
inmune immune
inmunidad immunity
  inmunidad adquirida acquired immunity
  inmunidad innata o inespecífica innate immunity
  inmunidad pasiva passive immunity
inmunitario immunological
  sistema inmunitario immunological system
inmunización immunization
inmunocompetente immunocompetent
inmunodeficiencia immunodeficiency
  inmunodeficiencia combinada severa severe combined immunodeficiency (SCID)
inmunodeficiente immunodeficient
inmunología immunology
inmunológico immunology
  sistema inmunológico immunological system
inmunosupresor immunosuppressant
inquieto restless
inspeccion de seguridad y sanidad a domicilio home safety check
insuficiencia insufficiency, failure
  insuficiencia cardíaca congestiva congestive heart failure (CHF)
internista intern
intravenoso intravenous, IV
  antibióticos por vía intravenosa intravenous antibiotics
  terapia por via intravenosa intravenous therapy
interpretación interpretation
intérprete interpreter
intervención intervention, surgery
  intervención temprana early intervention
intestine intestine
  intestino delgado small intestine
  intestino grueso (*vea* **colon**) large intestine
introducir (*vea* **presentar**) introduce (speculum, bacteria)
invasivo invasive
investigación investigation, research
  investigación clínica clinical trial, experimental study, research study
inyección injection, shot
  inyección en contra de la gripe flu shot
  inyección rápida bolus injection
irritación irritation
irse el caballo, *modismo* (*CUB*) kick the bucket, *idiom*
isquémico ischemic
  ataque cerebral isquémico ischemic brain attack (stroke)

J

jaqueca (*MEX*) headache
jarabe syrup
jengibre ginger
jeringa syringe
jitomate ***(MEX)*** tomato
jornalero day laborer

K

Kawasaki, endfermedad de Kawasaki disease

L

labia labia (vaginal)
labio (boca) lip
  labio lepoino cleft lip
laboratorio laboratory, lab
lactación lactation
lactulosa lactulose
ladillas (piojos del pubis, piojos púbicos) crabs (pubic lice)
lanolina lanolin
lastimar hurt, injure, damage, wound
lente lens
lentes glasses (eye)
lesión lesion, wound
lesionar wound, hurt, injure, damage
leucemia leukemia
  leucemia linfoblástica aguda (enfermedad de Hodgkin) acute lymphoblastic leukemia (Hodgkin disease)
leucocito leukocyte
leucopenia leukopenia
leucositosis leukocytosis
libre free
  libre de congestión free of congestion, clean, clear
ligadura de trompas tubal ligation, tie tubes
ligamento ligament
ligeramente lightly, quickly
ligerito quickly, right away
ligero light (weight)
límite limit, parameter, range
  límites de movimiento range of motion
limpiar to clean, to wipe
limpio clean, clear, free of congestion
línea line, catheter
  línea PIC, (catéter venoso central de inserción periférica) PICC line (percutaneously inserted central catheter)
  línea o catéter venoso central (*vea* **port**) central venous line
linfa lymph
linfectomía lymphectomy
linfocito lymphocyte
líquido liquid, fluid
  drenaje de líquido cefalorraquídeo cerebrospinal fluid drainage (CSFD)
  líquido cefalorraquídeo (LCR) cerebrospinal fluid (CSF)
loción humectante hydrating lotion
lumbar lumbar

M

mácula macula
  degeneración macular macular degeneration
madre soltera single mother
madreado, estar madreado to be fucked up, to be messed up, a mess, to be beat up, to be wrecked
madrear to fuck up, mess up, beat up, wreck up
magro lean (meat) (*vea* **delgado**)
magulladura bruise
mal ajustado maladjusted
mal de orín burning, frequency and or discomfort with urination, urinary tract infection, urine infection, bladder infection
mal de orina burning, frequency and or discomfort with urination, urinary tract infection, urine infection, bladder infection
mala o poca alimentación malnutrition
malestar malaise
malformación malformation, deformation
  malformación arteriovenosa cerebral (MAV) arteriovenous malformation (AVM)
malparto abortion, spontaneous abortion, stillbirth
mama breast, mammary
  cáncer del mama breast cancer
  dolor de mama breast pain
mamá mom, mother
mamila (*MEX*) bottle (baby)
mamografía mammogram, mammography
mancha spot, stain
manchar to spot or stain (uterus, menstruation)
manchas flotantes en la vista floaters
mandíbula jaw, mandible
manzana de Adán Adam's apple
marcador (de tumores, en la sangre) marker
marcar mark
  marcar con hoyos pitting
  marcar con fóvea pitting
mareado dizzy, lightheaded
mareo dizziness, lightheadedness
margen margin, range, parameter, limit
martillo malleus
masa mass, lump, bump, flour, dough
  excisión de una masa (*vea* tumorectomía) lumpectomy
  masa muscular muscle mass
mastalgia mastitis
mastopatía breast disease
materia blanca (*vea* **sustancia**) **white** matter
materia gris (*vea* **sustancia**) **grey** matter
maternidad maternity, childbearing
  sala de gineco maternity ward
  sala de maternidad maternity ward
  sala de partos maternity ward
materno maternal
  salud maternoinfantil maternal and child health
matriz uterus, womb
medicamentos medications, medicines, meds
medicina medicine, medications, meds

médico (*vea* **doctor**) (medical) doctor, medical doctor, physician, PhD, MD, medical
- **asunto médico** medical issue
- **médico a cargo** attending physician, head doctor, chief physician
- **médico de cabecera** attending physician, head doctor, chief physician
- **médico de cabezera** primary care doctor
- **médico de cuidados primarios** primary care doctor
- **médico en el primer año de especialización** intern (doctor)
- **médico en el segundo año de especialización** resident (doctor)
- **médico en el tercer año de especialización** resident (doctor)
- **médico encargado** attending physician, head doctor, chief physician
- **médico internista** intern (doctor)
- **médico jefe** head doctor, chief doctor
- **médico pasante** fellow (doctor)
- **médico residente** resident (doctor)
- **médico residente auxiliar** resident (doctor)
- **médico responsable** attending physician, head doctor, chief physician
- **médico supervisor** attending physician, supervising doctor

medio oído middle ear
médula marrow
- **médula espinal** spinal cord
- **médula espinal anclada** tethered cord
- **médula ósea** bone marrow

membrana membrane
- **membrana mucosa** mucous membrane
- **membrana timpánica** tympanic membrane

meningocele meningocele
menopausia menopause
menstruación menstruation, period
merienda snack
metotrexate methotrexate
MIC-KEY, botón Mic-Key (botón Bard) MIC-KEY (Bard Button)
microcefalia microcephaly
mielina myelin
- **vaina de mielina** myelin sheath

mieloma múltiple multiple myeloma
mielomeningocele myelomeningocele
mimar pamper, spoil
miocardio myocardium
miocarditis myocarditis
mioma (*vea* **fibroide**) myoma
- **mioma uterino** uterine myoma

miositis myositis
moco mucus, snot, runny nose
mocoso brat
- **mocoso malcriado** snot-nosed brat

modificado geneticamente genetically modified
molécula molecule
molecular molecular
mollera (*vea* fontanela) fontanel, pate, soft spot (on infant's head)
monitores monitors
monocito monocyte
morder bite
mordida bite, bribe
morete bruise
moretón bruise
mosaicismo mosaicismo
motoneurona **motor neuron**
motor motor
- **habilidades motoras** motor skills
- **motor fino** fine motor
- **motor grueso** gross motor
- **motricidad fina** fine motor movements
- **motricidad gruesa** gross motor movements
- **movimientos de motor fino** fine motor movements
- **movimientos de motor grueso** gross motor movements
- **neurona motora** motor neuron

mucosidad mucous, runny nose
mucositis mucositis
mucoso mucus
- **membrana mucosa** mucous membrane
- **tapón mucoso** mucus plug

mudar mutate, move, relocate
mudo mute
muerte death
muestra sample, specimen, biopsy
- **muestra de vellosidades coriónicas (MVC)** chorionic villus sampling (CVS)
- **muestra del vello coriónico** chorionic villus sampling, (CVS)

músculo muscle
muslo thigh
mutación mutation
MVC (muestra de vellosidades coriónicas) CVS (chorionic villus sampling)
myo- (musculo) mio- (músculo)

N

nalgas *butt, buns, bum, rear end*
nariz nose
- **nariz congestionada** stuffy nose, congested nose
- **nariz constipada** stuffy nose, congested nose
- **nariz mormada** stuffy nose

natural natural
- **desastre natural** natural disaster
- **parto natural** vaginal birth, natural childbirth
- **planificación familiar natural** natural family planning

neutrófilo neutrophil
nervio óptico optic nerve
nervioso nervous, anxious, restless, agitated
neumococo pneumococci
neumonía pneumonia
neuropatía neuropathy
  neuropatía diabética diabetic neuropathy
neutropenia neutropenia
ni madres, *modismo* nothing, shit, ain't shit, ain't got shit, no shit, *idioms*
ni modo oh, well, whatever
niño pequeño small child, toddler
nistagmus nystagmus
no riesgoso not risky, safe
Norwood surgery cirugía de Norwood; primero de tres procedimientos denominado Fontan
nódulo linfático lymph gland, lymph node
nota necrológica (obituario) obituary
nuez nut, prominence
  nuez de la garganta Adam's apple
  prominencia laríngea Adam's apple
nutrición nutrition
nutricionista *(vea* **nutriólogo)** nutritionist, dietician
nutriólogo nutritionist, dietician

O

obituario (nota necrológica) obituary
obrero laborer, worker
ocular ocular
  órbita ocular ocular orbit
oculista oculist
ocupar to need, to use, to occupy
odontología dentistry, odontology
odontólogo odontologist, dentist
oftalmólogo ophthalmologist
oído ear (inner; *vea* **oreja**)
  medio oído middle ear
  oído externo (oreja, auricular) outer ear (auricle, pinna)
  oído interno inner ear
  oído medio middle ear
oíme (*C.A.*) **óigame** listen, listen to me
ojo eye
  cejas del ojo eyebrows
  globo del ojo eyeball
  globo ocular eyeball
  gotas para los ojos eye drops
  mal de ojo evil eye
  niña del ojo pupil
  ojos bizcos crossed eyes
  ojos cruzados cross-eyed, crossed eyes
  párpado del ojo eyelid
  pestaña del ojo eyelash
  pupila del ojo pupil
oler smell
ombligo umbilicus, navel, belly button
óptico optic
optómetra optometrist
optometrista optometrist
órbita orbit
  órbita ocular ocular orbit
orden order
  orden fija standing order
  orden para análisis de laboratorio lab order, laboratory analysis order, lab slip
oreja ear (outer), auricle
orina urine
  infección de la orina urine infection, bladder infection
  mal de orina urine infection, bladder infection
  prueba de citología de la orina urine cytology test
osteogénesis imperfecta osteogenesis imperfecta
osteopenia (pérdida de densidad ósea) osteopenia (low bone density)
osteoporosis osteoporosis
ostomía ostomy
ovario ovary
óvulo ovum
oxitocina oxytocin

P

pabellón auricular pinna (auricle), external part of the ear
pacha (*C.A.*) bottle (baby)
padre soltero single father
padres solteros single parents
paladar palate
  paladar hendido cleft palate
paludismo (síntomas de malaria) paludism
pamper pamper
pañal diaper
  pañal desechable disposable diaper
pancita belly, tummy
páncreas pancreas
pañito towelette, wipe
panza belly, tummy, abdomen, pot belly
panzón fat, potbellied, pregnant (*derogatory*)
Papanicolau Pap smear, Papanikolaou test
parálisis cerebral cerebral palsy
parámetros parameters, limits, range
  parámetros de movimiento range of motion
parar stop
pararse stand, stand up
parejo even, same, match, equal
párpado eyelid
parte part, private part
  parte inferior de la espalda lower back
  parte privada private part

parto birth
  parto natural vaginal birth
  parto sin medicina para el dolor natural childbirth, childbirth without medicine for pain
pecho chest, breast
pedido order, request, requisition
pegamento paste, glue
  pegamento quirúrgico surgical glue
pegantines stickers
pegar hit, bang, bump
pelo hair (*vea* **vello**, **cabello**)
pelota bump, lump, ball
pelotita little lump, little bump, little ball
pélvico pelvic
pelvis pelvis
pene penis
percutáneo percutaneous
perder peso y masa muscular muscular wasting
periférico peripheral
período period, menstruation, menstrual period
perjudicar damage, compromise, put at risk, hurt
persona que cuida al enfermo caregiver
personal de salud healthcare provider, healthcare staff, healthcare personnel
peso seco dry weight (*i.e., weight in the morning after urinating and before eating or drinking*)
pestaña eyelash
peste stench, bad smell
petequia petechiae
petición request, petition, order
pezón nipple
  pezones agrietados cracked nipples
  pezones invertidos inverted nipples
picadura (de insecto) sting, stick, bite (insect)
picar stick, vaccinate, give an injection or shot, to itch, to snack, to sting
picazón itch, itching
PICC, línea PICC (catéter intervenoso central de inserción periférica) PICC, PICC line (percutaneously inserted central catheter)
pichi (PER) pee, piss
piojo louse
  piojos de la cabeza head lice
  piojos del cuerpo body lice
  piojos del pubis pubic lice
piojos lice
  piojos púbicos (del pubis) pubic lice
pipí pee, piss
piquete de aguja needle stick
pituitaria pituitary
  glándula pituitaria pituitary gland
placas (*MEX*) x-rays
placenta placenta, afterbirth
  placenta previa placenta previa
plan de educación personalizado individualized education program (IEP), *also called an individualized education plan*
plaqueta platelet
plata silver
  nitrato de plata silver nitrate
pleura pleura
pleuresía pleurisy
pleuritis pleurisy
polainas weights, balls (testicle, *C.A., MEX*), flip-flop, rubber thong
pólipo polyp
pompa (bomba) pump, bomb
pompas butt, buns, bum, rear end
pompis butt, buns, bum, rear end
poner una inyección give a shot
port (puerto, cateter con acceso debajo de la piel) port (catheter with access under the skin, portacath)
portador carrier
  portador genético genetic carrier
portar (en los genes) to carry (in one's genes)
posición position
postrado prostrate, lying face down
práctica rutinaria routine practice, standard practice
predisposición predisposition
  predisposición genética genetic predisposition
predispuesto prone, predisposed to, at risk for
prednisona prednisone
preeclampsia preeclampsia
prescripción (receta médica) prescription
presentación de nalgas breech
presentación fetal fetal presentation
presentarse (*vea* **introducir**) introduce register, show up, present
preservar conserve, preserve, save
preservativo condom, preservative
primario primary
  cuidados primarios primary care
  médico de cuidados primarios primary care doctor
principal main, principle, central
principalmente principally, mainly, in general
principio beginning, start; principle
  por principio on principle
prisa rush
  de prisa in a rush, quickly, rushing
problema problema, disorder, condition
  problema técnico technical problem, glitch
procedimiento procedure, process
  procedimiento Fontan (último paso de tres de la cirugía Fontan para tratar defectos congénitos del corazón) Fontan procedure
  procedimiento invasivo invasive procedure
profesional de la salud healthcare provider, healthcare professional
profilaxis prophylaxis
profundo deep
profundamente deeply

programar to schedule, to program
prolapso prolapse, descended
  prolapso de la pelvis pelvic organ prolapse
  prolapso de la válvula mitral mitral valve prolapse
  prolapso uterino uterine prolapse
prolongado prolonged, protracted
prominencia laríngea Adam's apple
promotora promoter, navigator
  promotora de salud community health worker, health navigator
prono prone
pronóstico prognosis
propenso prone, susceptible
próstata prostate
protuberancia protuberance, lump, bump
proveedor de atención al paciente healthcare provider, patient caregiver
proveedor de cuidados de salud healthcare provider
prueba test
  prueba clínica clinical trial, experimental study
  prueba confirmatoria western blot western blot test
  prueba de embarazo pregnancy test
  prueba de función de la vejiga urinaria urodynamics test
  prueba de gama genética genetic array test
  prueba de inmunoelectrotransferencia indirecta o western blot protein immunoblotting test or western blot test
  prueba de laboratorio lab test
  prueba de orina urine test
  prueba de Papanicolau Pap smear, Papanikolaou test
  prueba de paternidad paternity test
  prueba de tuberculina en la piel TB skin test
  prueba de Wada (técnica de la anestesia hemisférica para la evaluación de la lateralidad del lenguaje) Wada test (cerebral hemispheric dominance of language function)
  prueba ELISA (enzimoinmunoanálisis de absorción) ELISA test (enzyme-linked immunoassay)
  prueba inicial investigatoria screening test
  prueba para detección temprana y prevención cancer screening test
  prueba preliminar de detección screening test
  prueba rápida quick test
  prueba serológica serologic test
psicología psychology
psicosis maníaco-depresiva manic-depression, manic-depressive psychosis; bipolar disorder
psicosomático psychosomatic
psicoterapeuta psychotherapist
psicoterapia psychotherapy
psiquiatra psychiatrist
psiquiatría psychiatry
PSTD (trastorno de estrés postraumático) PTSD (post-traumatic stress disorder)
pubertad puberty
púbico pubic
  area del pubis pubic area
  area púbica pubic area
  picjos del pubis (ladillas) pubic lice (crabs)
  picjos púbicos pubic lice
  vellos del pubis pubic hair
  vello púbico pubic hair
pubis pubis, pubic area
pudrirse to spoil, to rot
puerto (port) (catéter con acceso debajo de la piel) port, catheter with access under the skin, portacath
  puerto subclavio subclavian port
pues well, ah, and
pulga fleas
pulgar (dedo) thumb
pulmonía pneumonia
puncíon puncture
  punción de la espina dorsal spinal tap
  punción lumbar lumbar puncture, spinal tap
pupila pupil (eye)
púrpura purpura
  purpura trombocitopénica idiopática idiopathic thrombocytopenic purpura (ITP)

Q

quedito softly, gently
queja complaint
  presentar una queja o demanda file a complaint
quejarse complain, whine, cry, moan
quemadura burn
  quemadura de primer grado first-degree burn
  quemadura de segundo grado second-degree burn
  quemadura de tercer grado third-degree burn
  quemaduras por frío frostbite
quijada jaw
químico chemical
quimioterapia chemotherapy
quirófano operating room
quiropráctico chiropractor
quirúrgicamente surgically
quirúrgico surgical
quiste cyst
  quiste benigno benign cyst
  quiste dermoide dermoid cyst
  quiste ováico ovarian cyst
  quiste sebáceo sebaceous cyst
quitar remove, take off, remove, take away

R

rabdomiosarcoma rhabdomyosarcoma
radiación radiation

radiografía radiography, x-ray
radiología radiology
radioterapia radiation therapy, radiotherapy
rápidamente rapidly, quickly, fast
rápido fast, quick, rapid
rascar to scratch
rasgo trait
raspado scrape, scraping
raspar scrape
rastreo scan
  rastreo de los huesos bone scan
raya stripe, line
rayar scratch, scrape, stripe, to draw (child), to scribble
rayos-x x-ray, radiography
razgos features
  razgos identificadores identifying features
razguño scratch
re really, very, super (*prefix to add emphasis*)
reacción reaction, response
recaer to relapse
recaída relapse
receta prescription, recipe
  receta médica prescription
rechazar reject
rechazo rejection
recomendación referral, recommendation
recto rectum
reevaluate volver a evaluar, evaluar de nuevo
refeo really ugly, super ugly, really bad
referencia referral, reference
refil, anglicisimo refill
reflejo reflex
  reflujo gastroesofágico gastroesophageal reflux
  reflujo urinario urinary reflux
registrarse register, sign up, check in
regla period, menstruation, time of the month
relaciones relations, relationships
  relaciones sexuales sexual relations
remal really bad
remover remove
renal renal
reparar el daño to repair damage
requisición pedido, petición, autorización, peticionar, pedir requisition
resaltar to protrude, to stick out
resecar to resect, to remove
resección resection
resfriado cold, chill
residente resident
  medico residente resident (doctor)
  residente legal (*estado inmigratorio*) residente legal
  residente legal permanente (*estado inmigratorio*) legal permanent resident
resistir to resist, to tolerate (treatment)
respirar to breathe
  respirar profundamente to breathe deeply
responder to respond, to answer
respuesta answer, response
  respuesta inmunitaria immune response
restricciones en la dieta dietary restrictions
  restricciones dietéticas dietary restrictions
resucitación cardio pulmonar (RCP) cardiopulmonary resuscitation (CPR)
resuello (*vea* **sibilancias**) wheezing, whistling
resultados de análisis de laboratorio laboratory analysis results, lab results, labs
resurtir to refill
  resurtido refill
retina retina
retinopatía retinopathy
  retinopatía diabética diabetic retinopathy
retorcijones abdominal cramps, menstrual cramps
reumatoide rheumatoid
revestimiento lining
  revestimiento del estómago stomach lining
  revestimiento uterino uterine lining
revivir to revive, to come back, to stay alive
riesgo risk
  en riesgo at risk
  poner en riesgo to risk, to put at risk
  riesgo de contagio risk of infection
riñón kidney
  dolor de riñones kidney pain, pain in the sides, flank pain
  trasplante de riñon kidney transplant
rinoplastia rhinoplasty
rinoscopia rhinoscopy
rinoscopio rhinoscope
rodilla knee
  reemplazo total de rodilla total knee replacement
rojizo redness
rojo red
  glóbulos rojos, eritrocitos red blood cells
  glóbulos rojos red cells
rosásea rosacea
rozadura chafing
rozar to rub against, to chafe
rubor blush, flush, glow
  rubor facial facial flushing
rubores hot flashes
ruborizarse to blush, to flush

S

saco vitelino yolk sac
sacro sacrum, sacral
  columna sacra sacral spine
  hueso sacro sacral bone
sacudir shake

sáculo saccule
sal (*vea* **sodio**) salt
  bajo en sal low-salt
  libre de sal salt-free
  sin sal salt-free
sala ward, room
  sala de gineco maternity ward
  sala de partos maternity ward
saliendo hacia afuera protruding
salpullido rash
salud health
  salud frágil fragile health
sample muestra
sanidad health
sangrado hemorrhage, bleed
sangre blood
  sangre oculta en heces (SOH) fecal occult blood test (FOBT)
sanguíneo sanguineous, blood
  flujo sanguíneo blood flow
  grupo sanguíneo blood type
  riego sanguíneo blood circulation
  torrente sanguíneo blood stream
sección transversal cross section
  secreción nasal nasal secretion
  tener secreción nasal have a runny nose
secreción secretion, flujo, discharge
sectiembre (*C.A., reg.*) September
seguimiento follow-up
según according to
  según las necesidades according to need
  según lo necesite as needed
seguro sure, safe
seguro, cierto sure
  absolutamente seguro absolutely sure
  casi seguro (de un resultado) almost sure (of a test result)
  muy seguro very sure, very safe
seguro social (*MEX*) general, state or public hospital; social security
  número de seguro social social security number
seno breast, sinus
sensor sensor, electrode, wires, cable
sepsis sepsis
septicemia septicemia
septo septum
séptico septic
  choque séptico septic shock
  shock séptico septic shock
sequedad vaginal vaginal dryness
seroconversión seroconversion
sexo sex
  sexo anal anal sex
  sexo oral oral sex
  sexo seguro safe sex
  sexo vaginal vaginal sex
sexual sexual
  práctica sexual segura safe sex
  práctica sexual más segura o menos riesgosa safer sex
  relaciones sexuales sex, sexual relations
  tener relaciones sexuales to have sex
shant shunt, canal, tube, conduct
shock (choque) shock
  shock anafiláctico anaphylactic shock
  shock cardiógeno cardiogenic shock
  shock hipovolémico hypovolemic shock
  shock séptico septic shock
  shock tóxico toxic shock
shunt (shant) shunt
  shunt de Glenn Glenn shunt (*vea* **derivación**)
sibilancias (*vea* **resuello**) wheezing
SIDA (síndrome de inmunodeficiencia adquirida) AIDS (acquired immunodeficiency syndrome)
SIDSC (síndrome de inmunodeficiencia severo combinada) SCID (severe combined immunodeficiency)
sigmoidoscopia sigmoidoscopy
  sigmoidoscopia flexible flexible sigmoidoscopy
síncope syncope
síndrome syndrome
  síndrome constitucional de deficiencia en la reparación del ADN (Síndrome de Lynch, cáncer colorrectal hereditario no asociado a poliposis) constitutional mismatch repair deficiency syndrome (Lynch syndrome, hereditary nonpolyposis colorectal cancer)
  síndrome de anticuerpos antifosfolípidos antiphospholipid antibody syndrome (APLS)
  síndrome de Guillain-Barré Guillain-Barré syndrome (GBS)
  síndrome de inmunodeficiencia adquirida (SIDA) acquired immunodeficiency syndrome (AIDS)
  síndrome de inmunodeficiencia severo combinada (SIDSC) severe combined immunodeficiency (SCID)
  síndrome de las piernas inquietas restless legs syndrome (RLS)
  síndrome de Lynch (cáncer colorrectal hereditario no asociado a poliposis) Lynch síndrome (hereditary nonpolyposis colorectal cancer)
  síndrome de Marfan Marfan syndrome
  síndrome de muerte infantil súbita (SMIS) sudden infant death syndrome (SIDS)
  síndrome de muerte súbita del lactante (SMSL) sudden infant death syndrome (SIDS)
  síndrome de nystagmu infantil (SNI) infantile nystagmus syndrome (INS)
  síndrome de Prader-Willi Prader-Willi syndrome
  síndrome de Tourette Tourette syndrome
  síndrome de Turner Turner's syndrome

síndrome del bebé sacudido shaken baby syndrome
síndrome del corazón derecho hipoplásico hypoplastic right heart syndrome
síndrome del corazón izquierdo hipoplásico hypoplastic left heart syndrome
síndrome del cromosoma X frágil fragile X syndrome
síndrome del ovario poliquístico polycystic ovary syndrome
síndrome del shock tóxico toxic shock syndrome
síndrome del túnel carpiano carpal tunnel syndrome
síndrome hereditario de deficiencia en la reparación del ADN syndrome hereditary mismatch repair deficiency syndrome (HMRDS)
síndrome nefrótico congénito de tipo finlandés congenital nephrotic syndrome of the Finnish type
síndrome premenstrual (SPM) premenstrual syndrome (PMS)
síndrome x frágil fragile X syndrome
sinovial synovial
membrana sinovial synovial membrane
líquido sinovial synovial fluid
sinusitis sinusitis
sistema system
sistema inmunitario immunological system, immune system
sistema linfático lymphatic system
sitio site
SMIS (síndrome de muerte infantil súbita) SIDS
SMLS (síndrome de muerte súbita del lactante) SIDS
sobar rub
sodio (*vea* **sal**) sodium
alimento bajo en sodio low-sodium diet
bicarbonato de sodio sodium bicarbonate
bicarbonato sódico sodium bicarbonate
sofoco hot flashes
som- (cuerpo) som- (body)
sonda catheter, tube, probe
sonda de alimentación nasogástrica nasogastric feeding tube
sonda gástrica gastrostomy tube, G-tube
sonda nasogástrica (sonda NG) nasogastric tube (NG tube)
sonda nasogástrico nasogastric tube
sopesar (*vea* **balancearse**) weigh the difference, consider the difference
soplar blow
soplo murmur
soplo cardíaco (**ruido chirriante o sivilante del corazón**) heart murmur (whooshing or blowing sound from the heart)
soplo del corazón heart murmur
soportar tolerate, put up with, stand
SPM (síndrome premenstrual) PMS (premenstrual syndrome)
subcutáneo subcutaneous
subyacente underlying
causa subyacente underlying cause
suceptible susceptible, prone
sudar to sweat, to perspire
sudor sweat
sudor excesivo excessive sweat
sudores nocturnos night sweats
sudoración nocturna night sweats
sufrir suffer
sufrir mutación mutate
supino supine, face up
surtir (medicina) refill, stock
volver a surtir refill, reorder, restock
suspender suspend, stop
suspender la medicina stop medication
sustancia blanca (*vea* **materia blanca**) white matter
sustancia gris (*vea* **materia gris**) grey matter

T

tabique septum
tabique desviado deviated septum
tabique nasal nasal septum
TAC, escán TAC, (tomografía axial computada), (*vea* **catescán, escán CAT**) CAT scan (computer axial tomography scan)
tacescán (tomografía axial computarizada, TAC) CAT scan (computer axial tomography scan)
tálamo thalamus
talasemia thalassemia
talla size, stem
tanque tank
taquicardia tachycardia
tasa rate, speed
técnico technician, tech, technical
técnico de radiología radiology technician
Tegaderm Tegaderm (artificial skin to cover wounds)
tejido tissue
tejido adiposa adipose tissue
temporada season, seasonal
temporal temporary, temporal
lóbulo temporal temporal lobe
tendón tendon
tener la nariz chorreando have a runny nose
tener mal olor to have a bad smell
tener manchas (menstruación) spot
tener moco have a runny nose
tentempié snack
terapeuta therapist
terapéutico therapeutic
terapia therapy
terapia de radiación, radioterapia radiation therapy
terapia física, fisioterapia physical therapy

terapia intensiva intensive care, intensive therapy
terapia quimioterapia chemotherapy
terapias therapies
terapista (*vea* **terapeuta**) therapist
testículo testicle
testosterona testosterone
teta tit, teat, breast, boob, nipple, nipple (for baby bottle)
tierno sensible, tender
tieso stiff
tímpano tympanic membrane, eardrum, tympani
tin a bit
tiña (dermatofitosis) ringworm
tincito a little bit (*CUB*)
tipificación typing
tipificación confirmatoria confirmatory typing
tipificación de tejido (examen de antígeno de histocompatibilidad) tissue typing (histocompatibility antigen test)
tipo type, guy
tiroides thyroid
glandula tiroidea thyroid gland
toallitas towelettes, wipes
toallitas empapadas en alcohol alcohol wipe
tomar sangre take blood
tomate tomato
tomografía tomography, scan
tomografía de los huesos bone scan
toñeco (*VEN*) **(consentido)** spoiled
tónico-clónica clonic tonic
tono muscular muscle tone
torácica thoracic
columna torácica thoracic spine
tórax thorax
torrente sanguíneo bloodstream
toxoplasmosis toxoplasmosis
traducción translation
traducir to translate
traductor translator
tragar swallow
estudio del tragar swallow study (barium swallow study)
transfundir transfuse
transfusión transfuse, give a transfusion
transparente transparent, clear
transpirar perspire, sweat
tráquea trachea
traqueostomía tracheostomy
traqueotomía tracheotomy
trasero butt, buns, bum, rear end
trasplantar, **transplantar** transplant
trastorno disorder, condition, problem
PSTD crónico chronic PTSD
trastorno afectivo bipolar bipolar affective disorder
trastorno autoinmunitario autoimmune disorders
trastorno de estrés postraumático (PSTD) post-traumatic stress disorder (PTSD
trastorno generalizado del desarrollo pervasive developmental disorder
trastorno hereditario autosómico recesivo hereditary autosomal recessive disorder
traumatismo cerebral traumatic brain injury
tricomoniasis trichomoniasis
trisomía trisomy
trisomía 18 (síndrome de Edwards) trisomy 18 (Edwards syndrome)
trisomía 21 (síndrome de Down) trisomy 21 (Down syndrome)
trombocito thrombocyte
trompa tubes, trunk (elephant)
trompa de eustaquio eustachian tubes
trompas de Falopio Fallopian tubes
tronco trunk
tronco pulmonar pulmonary trunk
tubo tube, catheter, shunt
tumor tumor
efecto injerto contra tumor tumor versus host effect
excisión de un tumor, masa o bola tumorectomy, lumpectomy
tumor maligno de la vaina de un nervio periférico malignant peripheral nerve sheath tumor
tumorectomía tumorectomy, lumpectomy
turbinas nasales turbinates (nasales)
tutela legal legal guardianship
tutor guardian, tutor
tutor legal legal guardian

U

uretra urethra
uréter ureter
uterino uterine
utrículo utricle
útero uterus (*vea* **matríz**)

V

vacuna vaccine, shot
vacunar to vaccinate
vagina vagina
vaginal vaginal
anillo vaginal vaginal ring
examen vaginal pelvic exam, vaginal exam
fluido vaginal vaginal fluid
flujo vaginal vaginal discharge
infección vaginal de hongos o de candidiasis vaginal yeast infection
parto vaginal (parto natural) vaginal birth
sangrado vaginal vaginal bleeding
sequedad vaginal vaginal dryness

valores inciales baseline
válvula de derivación ventrículo-peritoneal ventriculoperitoneal shunting (VP shunt)
vapué (*SLV, C.A.*) ok, all right, there you go
varicela varicella (chickenpox)
varicela-zóster virus varicella-zoster virus
váscula *(vea* **balanza)** scale, balance
veá (*reg., C.A.*) **(verdad)** right, true
vejiga bladder
  infección de la vejiga bladder infection
  vejiga urinaria urinary bladder
vello (*vea* **pelo, cabello**) hair
  muestreo del vello coriónico chorionic villus sampling (CVS)
  vello de las axilas underarm hair
  vello de los brazos arm hair
  vello del pecho chest hair
  vellos de las piernas leg hair
  vellos del pubis pubic hair(s)
  vello facial facial hair
  vello púbico pubic hair
velocidad speed, rate
vena vein
vendar to bandage, to dress a wound
vendas bandages, dressing
venipuntura venipuncture
ventrículo ventricle
ver cómo se encuentra to see how one is doing, to check in, to touch base
ver cómo sigue see how one is doing, check in, touch base
vértebra vertebra
  columna vertebral vertebral column, spinal column
  disco intervertebral intervertebral disc
vértebras vertebrae
  vértebras cervicales cervical vertebrae
  vértebras del sacro sacral vertebrae
  vértebras lumbares lumbar vertebrae
  vértebras torácicas thoracic vertebrae
vértigo vertigo
  vértigo postural paroxístico benigno (VPPB) benign paroxysmal positional vertigo (BPPV)
vesícula gallbladder
  vesícula biliar gallbladder
vía respiratoria airway
  enfermedad reactiva de las vías respiratorias reactive airway disease
  vía respiratoria obstruida obstructed airway
vigilante o portero caretaker
VIH (virus de inmunodeficiencia humana) HIV (human immunodeficiency virus)
violación rape, violation
violar rape, violate
virus virus
  virus de herpes simplex (VHS) herpes simplex virus (HSV)
  virus del Nilo occidental West Nile virus
  virus sincicial respiratorio respiratory syncytial virus (RSV)
visita a domicilio house call
vista vision, view, eyesight
  manchas, puntos o moscas volantes flotantes en la vista floaters
visual visual
  campo visual visual field
voltearse roll over, turn over
  voltearse boca abajo a boca arriba roll over back to front
  voltearse boca arriba a boca abajo roll over front to back
volumen volume, amount
vomitar vomit, throw up, upchuck, spit up, yack (*USA*)
vulva vulva

W

Wada, prueba de (técnica de la anestesia hemisférica para la evaluación de la lateralidad del lenguaje) Wada test (cerebral hemispheric dominance of language function)
western blot test (prueba de inmunoelectrotransferencia indirecta western blot) western blot test (protein immunoblotting test)

X

Y

yema del dedo fingertip
yeyuno jejunum
yunque incus

Z

Zika Zika
  virus del Zika Zika virus

English-Spanish medical glossary

A

abortion aborto, aborto médico, aborto terapéutico (*see* **miscarriage**)
abscess absceso
absolute neutrophil count (ANC) conteo absoluto de neutrófilos
absolutely definitivamente, claro que sí
according (to) según
  according to need según las necesidades
acid ácido, agruras, acidez, indigestión
  acid indigestion agruras, acidez
  acid reflux reflujo
acidity acidez, agruras, indigestión, reflujo
acoustic acústico
acquired immunity inmunidad adquirida
acquired immunodeficiency syndrome (AIDS) síndrome de inmunodeficiencia adquirida (SIDA)
acute immunity inmunidad agudo
acute lymphoblastic leukemia (Hodgkin disease) leucemia linfoblástica aguda (enfermedad de Hodgkin)
ad hoc ad hoc
Adam's apple nuez, nuez de la garganta, manzana de Adán, prominencia laríngea
adenoids adenoides, amígdalas (*see* **tonsils**)
adenoma adenoma
adenotonsillectomy amigdaloadenoidectomía
adhesion adherencia
adhesive adhesivo, pegamento
adipose adiposo
  adipose tissue tejido adiposo
adoptive family familia adoptiva
adrenal gland glándula suprarrenal, glándula adrenal
adrenoleukodystrophy (ALD) ALD (adrenoleucodistrofia)
advanced practice nurse enfermero de práctica avanzada
AFP (alpha fetoprotein) AFP (alfafetoproteína)
AIDS (acquired immunodeficiency syndrome) SIDA (síndrome de inmunodeficiencia adquirida)
  AIDS wasting syndrome síndrome de emaciacón por SIDA
airway vía respiratoria
  obstructed airway vía respiratoria obstruida
alcohol alcohol
  alcohol wipe toallita empapada en alcohol
ALD (adrenoleukodystrophy) ALD (adrenoleucodistrofia)
alleviate aliviar
alpha fetoprotein (AFP) alfafetoproteína (AFP)
ALS (amyotrophic lateral sclerosis) ELA (esclerosis lateral amiotrófica)
ambiguous genitalia genitales ambiguos
amino acid amino ácido
amniocentesis amniocentesis
amount cantidad
amygdala (structure in brain) amígdala
amyotrophic lateral sclerosis (ALS) esclerosis lateral amiotrófica (ELA)
analysis análisis
anaphylactic shock shock anafiláctico
anaphylaxis anafilaxia
androgens andrógenos
anemia anemia
  aplastic anemia anemia aplásica
  Diamond Blackfan anemia (congenital hypoplastic anemia) anemia Diamond Blackfan (anémia hipoplásica congénita)
  Fanconi anemia (aplastic anemia) anemia de Fanconi (anemia aplásica)
  megaloblastic anemia anemia megaloblástica
  sickle cell anemia anemia falciforme o de las células falciformes
aneurysm aneurisma
angina angina de pecho
angioplasty angioplastía
antibody anticuerpo
anticoagulants anticoagulantes
antigen antígeno
antiphospholipid antibody syndrome (APLS) síndrome de anticuerpos antifosfolípidos
antiplatelet antibodies anticuerpos antiplaquetario
antiplatelet drugs antiplaquetarios
antireflux antirreflujo
antirejection antirechazo
antiretroviral antiretroviral
anus ano, *culo* (considered vulgar in Latin America, can be *butt* in Spain) (*see* **butt**)
apheresis (plasmapheresis) aféresis (plasmaféresis)
aplastic anemia anemia aplásica
APLS (antiphospholipid antibody syndrome) síndrome de anticuerpos antifosfolípidos
apnea apnea

apoplexy apoplejía
appointment cita, apóinmen
arm brazo (*mano* is sometimes used in to indicate *brazo MEX*)
  arm hair vello del brazo
arrhythmia arritmia
arterial stenosis estenosis arterial
arteriosclerosis (*see* **atherosclerosis**)
arteriovenous malformation (AVM) malformación arteriovenosa cerebral (MAV)
artery arteria
arthritis artritis
  juvenile rheumatoid arthritis artritis reumatoide juvenil
  rheumatoid arthritis artritis reumatoide
as needed según lo necesite
aspiration aspiración
  bone marrow aspiration aspiración de médula osea
  fine needle aspiration aspiración con aguja fina
asshole (*see* ***butt***) culo, ano, pendejo (pubic hair), comemierda
asthma asma
  asthma attack ataque de asma
at risk en riesgo, de riesgo, vulnerable, expuesto al peligro, comprometido, predispuesto a
atherosclerosis (hardening of or accumulation of plaque in the arteries, *see* **arteriosclerosis)** ateroesclerosis (endurecimiento de o acumulación de placa en las arterias)
atria aurículo
atrium aurículos
atrophy atrofia
attack (*see accident, seizure, stroke*) ataque
  brain attack (*see seizure*) ataque cerebral
  cerebrovascular attack (*see stroke*) ataque cerebrovascular, ACV
  heart attack ataque al corazón, ataque cardiaco
  panic attack ataque de pánico
  transient ischemic attack (TIA) ataque isquémico transitorio (AIT)
attending asistiendo; médico encargado
attending physician doctor encargado, doctor supervisor, doctor jefe
audiology audiolología
auditory canal canal auditivo
auditory nerve nervio auditivo
authorization autorización, consentimiento
autism autismo
  autism spectrum disorder trastorno del espectro autista
autoimmune disorders trastorno autoinmunitario
autosomal autosómico
autosome autosoma
axilla axila
axon axón

B

babysitter niñera, *beibisida* (*USA*)
back espalda
  lower back cintura, parte inferior de la espalda
back to front (roll over) (voltearse) boca abajo a boca arriba
bacteria bacteria
balance (n.) balance, equilibrio; **(v.)** equilibrar, sopesar
balm bálsamo, pomada, crema
  butt balm bálsamo para dermatitis de pañal
  diaper rash cream or balm bálsamo o crema para dermatitis de pañal
  lip balm bálsamo labial
bandages vendas, vendaje, gasas, apósito
  to bandage vendar
Band-Aid curita
bang golpear, golpearse, topar, pegar
Bard Button (MIC-KEY) botón Bard (botón MIC-KEY)
barium bario
  barium enema enema de bario
baseline valores inciales, base
basophil basófilo
belladonna belladona
belly panza, pancita, barriga, barriguita
belly button ombligo tuch (yuc)
benign paroxysmal positional vertigo (BPPV) vértigo posicional paroxístico benigno
bifida bífida
bifurcation bifurcación
bilateral bilateral
bile bilis
biliary biliar
  biliary atresia atresia biliar
  biliary ducts conductos biliares, vías biliares
  biliary tract tracto biliar, vías biliares
  biliary tree vías biliares, tracto biliar
bilirubin bilirubina
biopsy biopsia
bipolar affective disorder trastorno afectivo bipolar
birth parto, nacimiento
  birth by Caesarean section cesárea, nacimiento por cesárea
  birth canal canal de parto
  birth certificate acta de nacimiento
  stillbirth parto de un feto muerto, malparto, aborto
  vaginal birth parto natural, parto vaginal
bite morder, picadura (insecto), mordida persona (animal)
bladder vejiga
  bladder infection infección de la vejiga, infección de la orina, mal de orina
  gallbladder vesícula biliar
  urinary bladder vejiga urinaria
bleed sangrar, sangrado, derrame, hemorragia

bleeding sangrado, sangrando
  bleeding disorder desórden de la sangre, desórden de sangrado, trastorno de la sangre
blind ciego
  blind spot punto ciego
blindness ceguera
  night blindness ceguera nocturna
blister ampolla
blood sangre
  blood brother hermano consanguíneo
  blood cell glóbulo
  blood cells glóbulos, glóbulos de sangre, células de sangre, células sanguíneas
  blood clotting factor factor de coaglación
  blood count conteo de células sanguíneas, conteo sanguíneo
  blood disorder problema, trastorn, desorden o condición de la sangre
  blood draw toma de sangre
  blood factor factor
  blood levels niveles (de sustancias, glóbulos, virus) en la sangre
  blood relative pariente consanguíneo **blood serum** suero sanguíneo
  blood test prueba de sangre, análisis de sangre
  blood thinners anticoagulantes, antiplaquetarios
  blood type grupo sanguíneo
  blood work pruebas o análisis de sangre
bloodstream torrente sanguíneo
blow golpe, soplar
blush ruborizarse
body cuerpo
  body mass masa corporal
  body mass index índice de masa corporal
bolt perno
bolus bolo
  bolus feed bolo alimenticio
  bolus injection inyección rápida
  nutritional bolus bolo alimenticio
bone density densidad ósea
bone hueso
  bone marrow médula ósea
  bone marrow biopsy (aspiration, test) aspiración (biopsia, prueba) de médula ósea
  bone mineral density (BMD) test
  bone shaft caña del hueso, diáfisis
  compact bone hueso compacto
  long bone hueso largo
  short bone hueso largo
  spongy bone hueso esponjoso
bonesetter huesero
bottle (baby) mamila (*MEX*), pacha (*S.A.*), teta, botella
bovine spongiform encephalopathy (BSE) encefalopatía espongiforme bovina (EEB) **(mad cow disease, Creutzfeldt-Jakob disease, CJD)** (enfermedad de la vaca loca, enfermedad de Creutzfeldt-Jakob)
brain cerebro, cerebral
  brain and spinal fluid líquido cefalorraquídeo
  brain attack (*see* **seizure**) ataque cerebral, ataque cerebrovascular, ACV
  brain damage daño cerebral
  brain hemorrhage hemorragia cerebral, derrame cerebral
  brain seizure ataque cerebral
brat mocoso, malcriado, engreído
  snot-nosed brat mocoso malcriado
breast pecho, mama, seno, chichi, chicha
  breast cancer cáncer de la mama
  breast disease mastopatía
  breast lump grumo en el pecho
  breast tenderness dolor o irritación de los pechos
  breast tenderness or sensitivity (to have) tener los pechos adoloridos o sensibles, o dolor en los pechos o senos o mamas
  breastfeed amamantar, dar pecho, lactar
  breastfeeding lactancia
  put to breast dar pecho, amamantar, lactar
breath aliento
  breath-holding spells espasmos del sollozo
  take a deep breath respire profundamente
breathe respirar, inhalar
  breathe deeply respirar profundamente
breech (birth) presentación de nalgas
bronchoscopy broncoscopia
brother-in-law cuñado
Broviac catheter catéter Broviac
bruise morete, moretón, magulladura
bum nalgas, pompas (*MEX*), pompis (*PER*), trasero, culo (*ESP*)
buns nalgas (*MEX*), pompis (*PER*), trasero, culo (*ESP*) (*see* **asshole**)
burn quemar, arder, quemadura
  first-degree burn quemadura de primer grado
  second-degree burn quemadura de segundo grado
  third-degree burn quemadura de tercer grado
burning ardor, ardiendo, quemando
bus bus, autobús, camion (*MEX*), gua gua (*CUB*)
butt nalgas (*MEX*), pompis (*PER*), trasero, culo (*ESP*), *see* ***asshole***)
bypass derivación, baipas, baipás

C

cabbage repollo (*MEX*) col (*C.A., other*)
cables (wires) alambres, cables, sensores, conductores
cactus fruit (prickly pear) tuna
Caesarean cesárea
  Caesarean section parto por cesárea
canal canal
  auditory canal canal auditivo
  birth canal canal de parto
  ear canal canal auditivo
  semicircular canals canales semicirculares

cancer cáncer
- **cancer screening test** examen preliminar para el cáncer; prueba para detección temprana y prevención

candida cándida, hongos

candidiasis candidiasis
- **candidiasis of the mouth** candidiasis de la boca, candidiasis bucal, candidiasis oral
- **candidiasis of the skin** candidiasis de la piel
- **oral candidiasis (oral thrush)** candidiasis oral

cardiac cardíaco
- **cardiac catheterization** cateterismo cardéaco, angiografía coronaria, arteriografía coronaria, angiograma coronario
- **cardiac failure** insuficiencia cardíaca, fallo cardíaco
- **cardiac stent** dispositivo intracoronario; dispositivo intravascular

cardiomyopathy cardiomiopatía

cardiopulmonary resuscitation (CPR) resusitación cardio pulmonar

care atención, asistencia, importar, prestar importancia, cuidar, cuidado, cuidados
- **care for** cuidar a
- **child care** cuidado de niños, cuidado infantil
- **foster care** cuidados de crianza, cuidados temporales, cuidados de acogido
- **inhumane care** asistencia o atención deshumanizada
- **legal foster care** cuidado legal temporal
- **palliative care** cuidados paliativos
- **site care (wound)** curación o cuidados del sitio
- **take care of** cuidar a
- **temporary care** cuidado temporal
- **temporary foster care** cuidados de crianza temporales
- **wound care** curación
- **wound site care** curación y cuidados de la herida o lesión

caregiver proveedores de atención al paciente, cuidador del paciente, persona que cuida al enfermo

caretaker vigilante, portero

carpal tunnel syndrome síndrome del túnel carpiano

carrier portador

CAT scan (computer axial tomography scan) TAC escán (tomografía axial computada)

catheter (*see* **port**) catéter, sonda, línea
- **Broviac catheter** catéter Broviac
- **urinary catheter** catéter de la vejiga
- **permanent or semi-permanent catéter** (*see* **port, central line**) catéter con acceso debajo de la piel

catheterization cateterismo, cateterización
- **cardiac catheterization** cateterismo cardíaco
- **cardiac catheterization** cateterismo del corazón, cateterización cardíaca
- **urinary catheterization** cateterización de la vejiga

causative gene gen causante

CBC complete blood count (CSC) conteo sanguíneo completo

cecum ceco

cell célula (*see* **blood cell**)
- **blood cell** glóbulo, célula sanguínea, célula de sangre
- **cord blood cell** célula de sangre de cordón
- **hematopoietic stem cell** célula madre hematopoyética
- **red cell** glóbulo rojo
- **Schwann cell** célula Schwann
- **signet-ring cell type** célula tipo anillo
- **stem cell** célula de base, célula madre, célula progenitora
- **T-cell** célula-T
- **T-lymphocyte cell célula linfocito-T**
- **white cell** glóbulo blanco

Cellcept (mycophenolate) CellCept (micofenolato)

cellulitis celulitis

central line (permanent catheter) catéter central, catéter permanente

cerebral cerebral
- **cerebral aneurysm (stroke)** aneurisma cerebral
- **cerebral cortex** corteza cerebral
- **cerebral hemorrhage** hemorragia cerebral
- **cerebral palsy** páralisis cerebral

cerebrospinal fluid (CSF) líquido cefalorraquídeo

cerebrovascular accident (stroke) accidente cerebrovascular

cervical cervical
- **cervical dysplasia** displasia cervical
- **cervical spine** espina cervical

cervix cérvix,
- **cervix (uterine)** cérvix, cuello uterino, cuello de la matriz

chafe rozarse

chafing rozadura

chamber (heart) cámara

characteristics características, facciones, rasgos

chart cuadro
- **clinical chart** cuadro clínico, cuadro médico
- **medical chart** cuadro médico, cuadro clínico

check in presentarse, registrarse, ver cómo sigue, ver cómo se encuentra

chemical químico

chemotherapy quimioterapia

chest compressions compresiones cardíacas

CHF (congestive heart failure) insuficiencia cardíaca congestiva

chickenpox varicela

Chikungunya virus virus chikungunya

child niño, chavalo (*C.A.*), escuincle (*MEX*), chamo (*VEN*), carajito (*VEN*)

child care cuidado infantil, cuidado de niños

childbearing maternidad

childbearing age edad fértil, edad fecunda

Children's Protective Services (CPS) Servicios de Protección para los Niños
chiropractor quiropráctico
chlamydia clamidia
chorionic villus sampling (CVS) muestra de vellosidades coriónicas (MVC)
chromosome cromosoma
chronic crónico
clear claro, transparente, limpio, libre de congenstión
clear the throat carraspear
cleft
  cleft lip labio leporino
  cleft palate paladar hendido
clinical nurse specialist (CNS) enfermero clínico especialista
clinical study ensayo clínico, investigación clínica, prueba clínica
clinical trial prueba clínica, prueba de investigación clínica, ensayo clínico
clitoris clítoris
clonal clónico
  clonal convulsion convulsión clónica
clonic tonic tónico-clónica
clot coágulo, coagular
cloudy turbio, nublado
  cloudy urine orina turbia
  cloudy vision vista nublada
coagulation coagulación
coccidioidomycosis (Valley fever, San Joaquin Valley fever) coccidioidomicosis aguda (fiebre del Valle)
coccyx cóccix
cochlea cóclea
cold frío, resfriado, (coger) frialdad (*CUB*)
colic cólico
colon (large intestine) colon (intestino grueso)
  ascending colon colon ascendente
  descending colon colon decendente
  sigmoid colon colon sigmoide
  transverse colon transverso colon
colonoscopy colonoscopia (colonoscopía)
colorectal colorrectal
  colorectal adenoma adenoma colorrectal
  colorectal cancer cáncer colorrectal, cáncer del colon y el recto
colostomy colostomía
colposcopy colposcopía
common común
  common grave fosa común
complain quejarse
complaint queja
  file a complaint presentar una queja o demanda
complete blood count (CBC) conteo sanguíneo completo (CSC), conteo completo de células sanguíneas (CSC)
compress compresa
condition condición, trastorno, problema
condom condón
conductors conductores, cables, alambres, sensores, electrodos
congenital congénito
  congenital defect defecto de nacimiento, defecto congénito
  congenital hypoplastic anemia (Diamond Blackfan anemia) anémia hipoplásica congénita
  congenital nephrotic syndrome of the Finnish type síndrome nefrótico congénito de tipo finlandés
congestive heart failure (CHF) insuficiencia cardíaca congestiva
consanguineous consanguíneo
  consanguineous marriage matrimonio consanguíneo
consanguinity consanguinidad
consent dar consentimiento, autorizar
consenter persona que consigue el consentmiento
convulsion convulsión, ataque
cord cordón, médula
  spinal cord médula espinal
  tethered cord médula espinal anclada
  umbilical cord cordón umbilical
corn
  corn dough masa
  corn flour harina de maíz
  corn syrup jarabe de maíz
  cornmeal harina de maíz
  cornstarch maicena
coronary artery disease (CAD) enfermedad de las arterias coronarias (EAC)
coronary artery stent intraluminal, dispositivo o stent coronario, stent de la arteria coronaria
coronary coronario
cortisol cortisol
  cortisol level nivel de cortisol
CPR (cardiopulmonary resuscitation) resusitación cardio pulmonar
CPS (Children's Protective Services) Servicios de Protección para los Niños
crabs (pubic lice) cangrejos, ladillas (piojos del pubis, piojos púbicos)
crack (bones) tronar (huesos)
cramp calambre, retorcijón, cólico
cream crema
  hormone cream crema de hormonas
  topical cream crema tópica
  vaginal cream crema vaginal
creatnine creatinina
Crohn's disease (*see* **regional ileitis**) enfermedad de Crohn (*see* **enfermedad inflamatoria intestinal**)
cross section sección transversal
crouch down (squat) ponerse en cuclillas
crush aplastar
CT scan (computerized tomography scan) CT escán (tomografía computarizada)

culture cultivo (laboratorio), cultura (personas)
- **bacterial culture** cultivo bacteriano
- **endocervical culture** cultivo endocervical
- **grow out a culture** hacer un cultivo
- **indigenous culture** cultura indígena
- **mucosal culture** cultivo mucoso
- **sputum culture** cultivo de esputo
- **urine culture** cultivo de la orina
- **western culture** cultura occidental

custody custodia
- **temporary legal custody** custodia legal temporal

cutaneous cutánea
- **cutaneous candidiasis** candidiasis cutánea

cutis cutis, skin
CVS (chorionic villus sampling) MVC (muestra de vellosidades coriónicas)
cyst quiste
- **benign cyst** quiste benigno
- **dermoid cyst** quiste dermoide
- **ovarian cyst** quiste ováico
- **sebaceous cyst** quiste sebáceo

cystic fibrosis fibrosis quística
cytomegalovirus (CMV) citomegalovirus (CMV)
cytoplasm citoplasma
cytotoxic citotóxico

D

daily a diario, cada día, todos los días
dandruff caspa
day laborer jornalero
death certificate certificado de defunción, acta de defunción
deep profundo
deeply profundamente
deficiency deficiencia, carencia
deletion (genetic) deleción (genetica)
dendrite dendrita
dentist odontólogo, dentista
deoxyribonucleic acid (DNA) ácido desoxirribonucleico (ADN)
dermatitis dermatitis
dermatomyositis dermatomiositis
development desarrollo
developmental del desarrollo
- **developmental milestones** etapas en el desarrollo, hitos del desarrollo
- **pervasive developmental disorder (PDD)** trastorno generalizado del desarrollo

diabetes diabetes
- **diabetes insipidus (DI)** diabetes insípida

diabetes mellitus diabetes mellitus
- **diabetes type 1** diabetes tipo 1
- **diabetes type 2** diabetes tipo 2
- **non-insulin dependent diabetes** diabetes no insulinodependiente

diabetic diabético
- **diabetic neuropathy** neuropatía diabética
- **diabetic retinopathy** retinopatía diabética

diagnose diagnosticar
diagnosis diagnóstico
diagnostic test prueba diagnóstica
dialysis diálisis
diaper pañal, Pampers
diaphragm diafragma
- **congenital diaphragmatic hernia** hernia diafragmática congénita
- **diaphragmatic hernia** hernia diafragmática

diarrhea diarrea
diastolic diastólico
diet (n.) dieta, alimentación. alimento; **(v.)** ponerse a dieta, estar en dieta, llevar un régimen de alimentación
- **balanced diet** dieta balanceada, dieta equilibrada
- **crash diet** dieta relámpago
- **diet pills** pastillas para bajar de peso o adelgazar
- **healthy diet** dieta saludable o sana
- **high-fiber diet** dieta altao rica en fibra
- **low-potassium diet** dieta baja en potasio
- **sodium-free diet** dieta libre de sodio
- **soft diet** dieta blanda
- **special diet** dieta especial

dietary deficiency deficiencia nutritiva, carencia nutritiva
dietary restrictions restricciones en la dieta, restricciones diatéticas
dietician dietético, nutriólogo, nutricionista
disc disco
- **bulging disc** disco abultado, disco sobresaliente
- **degenerative disc** disco deteriorado disco degenerado
- **herniated disc** disco herniado
- **intervertebral disc** disco intervertebral

discharge (from hospital) dar de alta, el alta **(from body)** flujo, secreción, desecho, descarga, supuración, escurrimiento
discontinue suspender, descontniuar
disease enfermedad, malestar
disorder desorden, problema, trastorno, condición
- **autoimmune disorders** trastorno autoinmunitario
- **bipolar affective disorder** trastorno afectivo bipolar
- **chronic PTSD** PSTD crónico
- **hereditary autosomal recessive disorder** trastorno hereditario autosómico recesivo
- **immunodeficiency disorder** trastornos por inmunodeficiencia
- **pervasive developmental disorder** trastorno generalizado del desarrollo
- **post-traumatic stress disorder (PTSD)** trastorno de estrés postraumático (PSTD)

disparity desigualdad, inequidad

disposable desechable
  disposable diaper pañal desechable
dizziness mareo
dizzy mareado, atarantado
DNA ADN
doctor (physician, medical) médico, doctor (*the following terms vary between countries and systems in English and Spanish*)
  attending doctor médico a cargo, médico de cabecera, médico encargado, médico jefe, médico supervisor, medico responsable
  fellow (doctor) médico pasante
  intern (doctor) médico internista, médico en el primer año de especialización
  medical doctor médico, doctor de medicina
  resident (doctor) médico residente, médico
  residente auxiliar médico en segundo el año de especialización médico en el tercer año de especialización
donor donador, donante
dose dosis
  doses dosis
Down syndrome síndrome de Down
drain drenaje, drenar
dressing vendas, gasas, curas, apósito
  dressing change cambio de vendas
dry weight peso seco (lo que pesa a primera hora de la mañana después de orinar y antes de comer o beber)
due date fecha prevista de parto, fecha probable de parto
dull sordo, no afilado, aburrido
  dull pain dolor sordo
duodenojejunal duodenoyeyunal
duodenum duodeno
dust mites ácaros
dysphagia disfagia
dysplasia displasia
  anal dysplasia displasia anal
  cervical dysplasia displasia cervical
  septo-optic dysplasia (optic nerve hypoplasia, de Morsier syndrome) displasia septo-óptica (síndrome de Morsier, síndrome del nervio óptico)
dysuria disuria

E

each day cada día, todos los días, a diario
ear (internal) oído **(auricle, outer)** oreja
  ear canal canal auditivo
  ear drum membrana timpánica, tímpano
  inner ear oído interno
  middle ear oído medio
  outer ear oreja
early intervention intervención temprana
Ebola Ebola
ECJ (Creutzfeldt-Jakob disease, mad cow disease) CJD (enfermedad de Creutzfeldt-Jakob, de las vacas locas)
edema edema
  pitting edema edema con fóvea
EEG (electroencephalogram) electroencefalograma
effort esfuerzo, trabajo
  make your best effort hacer su major esfuerzo, hecharle ganas
ejaculation eyaculación
  premature ejaculation eyaculación prematura
ejaculatory eyaculatorio
  EKG (electrocardiogram) ECG electrocardiograma
  pre-ejaculatory fluid líquido pre-eyaculatorio
electric current corriente eléctrica
electric shock choque eléctrico
electrocardiogram electrocardiograma
electrode eléctrodo, sensor, alambre, cable
electroencephalogram (EEG) electroencefalograma
ELISA test (enzyme-linked immunoassay) prueba ELISA (enzimoinmunoanálisis de adsorción)
embolism embolismo, stroke (*see* **cerebrovascular accident, clot, hemmorhage, bleed, aneurisma**)
embolization embolización
emesis emesis, vómitos
endocrine endocrino
  endocrine system sistema endocrina
endocrinologist endocrinólogo
endometrial del endométrio
  endometrial biopsy biopsia del endometrio
  endometrial cancer cáncer del endométrio
endometrium endometrio
  uterine endometrium endometrio uterino
endoscopic retrograde cholangiopancreatography (ERCP) olangiopancreatografía retrógrada endoscópica (CPRE)
endoscopy endoscopia
enema enema
engorge ingurgitarse, hincharse, dilitarse
engorged congestionado, ingurgitados
engorgement ingurgitación
eosinophil eosinófilo
epigenetics epigenética
episiotomy episiotomía
equal igual, los mismo
equally likely igualmente propenso, igualmente probable
equilibrium equilibrio, balance
equity equidad
  equity in care equidad en la atención
  health equity equidad sanitaria, equidad en la salud
ERCP (endoscopic retrograde cholangiopancreatography) CPRE (olangiopancreatografía retrógrada endoscópica)
erectile eréctil
  erectile dysfunction disfunción eréctil

erection erección
erythrocyte eritrocito
erythrocytosis eritrocitosis
erythropoietin eritropoyetina
even parejo
every cloud has a silver lining no hay mal que por bien no venga
every day todos los días, cada día, a diario
every other day cada tercer día, un día sí un día no
every two weeks cada tercera semana, cada dos semanas, cada quincena
excessive excesivo
  excessive sweat sudor excesivo
excoriation escoriación
experiment (*see* **clinical trial**) experimento
experimental study ensayo clínico, investigación clínica, prueba clínica[50]
eye ojos
  cross-eyed con los ojos cruzados, bizco
  crossed eyes ojos cruzados, ojos bizcos, estrabismo, bizquera
  evil eye mal de ojo
  eye drops gotas para los ojos
  eye wash solución oftálmica
  eyeball globo del ojo, globo ocular
  eyebrow ceja
  eyelash pestaña
  eyelid párpado
  eyesight vista

F

face down boca abajo
face up boca arriba
facial hair vello facial
faint (v.) desmayarse **(adj.)** débil
fainting spells episodios de desmayo
Fallopian tubes trompas de Falopio
familial adenomatous polyposis poliposis familiar adenomatuo
Fanconi anemia (aplastic anemia) anemia de Fanconia (anemia aplásica)
fat (n.) grasa **(adj.)** gordo
  animal fat grasa animal
  body fat grasa corporal
  fat body cuerpo gordo
  fat free libre de grasa, sin grasa, descremada (milk)
  fat person persona gorda
  full fat grasa entera
  low fat bajo en grasa
  vegetable fat grasa vegetal
fatty acid ácido grasoso

50 Note that this usage is uncommon in English. Such an investigation is usually referred to as a clinical trial or research study; "experiment" might be interpreted as *experimenting on a person.*

FDA Food and Drug Administration Administración de Drogas y Alimentos
features facciones, características, rasgos
febrile febril
  febrile seizures convulsiones o ataques febriles
fecal occult blood test (FOBT) sangre oculta en heces (SOH)
feces heces
feeding tube sonda de alimentación
fellow (doctor)
fetal fetal
  fetal alcohol spectrum disorders (**FASDs)** trastornos del espectro alcohólico fetal (TEAF)
  fetal alcohol syndrome síndrome de alcoholismo fetal
  fetal development desarrollo fetal
  fetal presentation presentación fetal
  fetal ultrasound ultrasonido del feto, sonograma del feto
fetus (foetus) feto
fibrocystic fibroquística
  fibrocystic breast disease mastopatía fibroquística
  fibrocystic disease enfermedad fibroquística
fibroid fibroide
  uterine fibroid fibroide uterino
fibroma fibroma
fibromyalgia fibromialgia
fibrosis fibrosis
  cystic fibrosis fibrosis quística
  pulmonary fibrosis fibrosis pulmonar
finding hallazgo
finger dedo (*de la mano, see* **toe**)
  fingerprint huella digital
  fingertip yema del dedo
  fifth finger quinto dedo
  first finger primer dedo
  fourth finger cuarto dedo
  index finger dedo índice
  little finger dedo meñique
  middle finger dedo medio
  ring finger dedo anular
  second finger segundo dedo
  third finger tercer dedo
  thumb dedo pulgar
first-degree burn quemadura de primer grado
first-degree relative pariente inmediato
fissure fisura, surco
  anal fissure fisura anal
  cerebral fissure surco o hendidura cerebral
fistula fístula
flake hojuelo, copo, escama
flaky escamoso
flank costado
  flank pain dolor de costado, dolor de riñones
flap colgajo
flexible sigmoidoscopy sigmoidoscopía flexible
floaters manchas o puntos flotantes o moscas volantes

flu (influenza) gripe, gripa, flu
  flu shot inyección contra la gripe
  flu vaccine vacuna contra la influenza
flush enjuagar, ruborizarse
  facial flushing rubor facial
  flush a line enjuagar una linea intravenosa
folic acid ácido fólico
follow-up dar seguimiento, vigilar, vigilancia, monitoréo
follow-up visit cita de seguimiento, cita subsecuente, cita de control
Fontan procedure procedimiento Fontan; último paso de tres de la cirugía Fontan para tratar defectos congénitos del corazón
fontanel mollera, fontanela
foot pie (pie is sometimes used for the entire leg, *MEX*)
forceps fórceps
form formulario
formula fórmula
foster acogido, de crianza, temporal
  foster care cuidados temporales
  foster family familia de acogido
  foster family familia de crianza temporal
  foster home hogar de acogida, hogar de cuidados temporales
  medical foster care cuidados medicos por una familia de acogido
fragile frágil
  fragile health salud frágil
  fragile X syndrome síndrome x frágil, síndrome del cromosoma x frágil
free (from) libre, libre de
  fat free (milk) libre de grasa, descremada products
  free interpreting services servicios de intérprete libres de costo
  free of congestion libre de congenstión
free (no cost) gratis, gratuito, libre de costo, sin pagar
front to back (roll over) voltearse de boca arriba a boca abajo
frostbite congelación localizada, quemaduras por frío
full-term pregnancy embarazo a término
fundoplication fundoplicatura, a laparascopic surgery to treat hiatal hernia
fungal infection infección de hongos
fungus (*see* **yeast**) hongos, cándid

G

gallbladder vesícula, vesícula biliar
gallstones calculós o piedras bilares o en la vesícula
gangrene gangrena
gargle hacer gárgaras
gastric tube tubo gástrico
gastroesophageal gastroesofágico
  gastroesophageal reflux disease (GERD) enfermedad por reflujo gastroesofágico (ERGE)
  gastroesophageal reflux reflujo gastroesofágico
gastrostomy (G-tube) gastrostomía
gastrostomy feeding tube pump bomba y sonda de alimentación de gastrostomía
gauze gasa, gasas
gene gen
  gene alteration alteración de un gen
  gene mutation mutación de un gen
  gene translocation translocación genética
general general
  generally por lo general, generalmente
  in general en general
generic genérico
genetic genético
  genetic array test prueba de gama genética
  genetic consultation consulta sobre la genética
  genetic counseling consejo sobre la genética
  genetic predisposition predisposición genetica
genetically modified modificado geneticamente
genetics la genética
genital genital
  genital herpes herpes genital
  genital warts verrugas genitales
genitalia genitalia
genitals genitales
genome genoma
genotype genotipo
gently suavemente, mansamente, quedito, poco a poco, despacito
gestational diabetes diabetes gestacional
get a lump in one's throat hacérsele a uno un nudo en la garganta
gingivitis gingivitis
give a shot poner una inyección, picar
give an injection poner una inyección, picar
give it a shot hacer el intetno, intentar, tratar
give it a try intentar, probar, hacer un esfuerzo, echarle ganas a algo
gland glándula
gland mammary gland glándula mamaria, mamas
glasses (eye) espejuelos, anteojos, lentes
Glenn shunt (*see* **Glenn surgery**)
Glenn surgery derivación de Glenn o hemi-Fontan, segunda parte de la cirugía cardíaca Fontan para tratar el defectos congénitos del corazón
glitch problema técnico, falla
glucose glucosa
glue pegamento
  surgical glue pegamento quirúrgico
goggles gafas de protección
gonad gónada
gown bata
G-tube gastrostomia, tubo-g, sonda gástrica, tubo gástrico
graft injerto
graft versus host disease enfermedad de injerto versus huésped enfermedad de injerto contra huésped (EICH)

grave grave, serio, seriamente enfermo, gravemente enfermo
 common grave fosa común
grey matter materia gris, sustancia gris
grow (something) out cultivar, dejar que crezca
growth crecimiento
guardian tutor legal, guardián
 legal guardian tutor legal
 legal guardianship tutela legal
guidelines normas, reglas
Guillain-Barré syndrome (GBS) síndrome de Guillain-Barré
gums encías
GVHD graft versus host disease EICH enfermedad de injerto versus huésped

H

HAART (highly active antiretroviral therapy) HAART (siglas en inglés que equivale a "terapia antiretroviral altamente activa")
hair pelo, cabello, vello
 arm hair vello de los brazos
 chest hair vellos del pecho
 hair on the head cabello, pelo
 leg hair vellos de las piernas
 pubic hair vello púbico
 scalp hair cabello, pelo
 underarm hair vello de las axilas
hand mano, (brazo sometimes used for hand, *MEX*)
harm daño
 harm reduction reducción del daño
hay fever alergia, alergia al polen, alergia de la temporada, alergia de la estación
head cabeza
headache dolor de cabeza, dolor de cerebro, jaqueca (*MEX*)
health salud, sanidad
 community health worker promotora de salud
 health history historia clínica, historia de la salud, historia médica, cuadro clínico
 healthcare provider personal de salud, proveedor de cuidados de salud
heart corazón
 heart attack (*see* **myocardial infarction**) ataque al corazón, ataque cardíaco
 heart failure insuficiencia cardíaca
 heart murmur soplo cardíaco, soplo del corazón
heartburn agriera (*COL*), agruras (*MEX*), acidez
hella (a hell of a, very) (*reg., Calif*) muchísimo, re, muy, un chingo de, chinguísimo, de puta madre
hematocrit hematocrito
hematopoiesis hematopoyesis
hematopoietic stem cell célula madre hemopoyética
hemodialysis hemodiálisis
hemoglobin hemoglobina
hemorrhage hemorragia, derrame, sangrado
hemorrhagic brain attack (stroke) ataque cerebral hemorrágico (embolia)
hepatic hepático
hepatobiliary tract vía hepatobiliaria
hereditary autosomal recessive disorder trastorno hereditario autosómico recesivo
hereditary nonpolyposis colorectal cancer cáncer colorrectal hereditario no asociado a poliposis
hernia hernia
 congenital diaphragmatic hernia hernia diafragmática congénita
 epigastric hernia hernia epigástrica
 femoral hernia hernia femoral
 hiatal hernia hernia de hiato
 inguinal hernia hernia inguinal
 umbilical hernia hernia umbilical
herpes herpes
 congenital herpes herpes congénito
 genital herpes herpes genital
 herpes labialis herpes labial
 herpes simplex virus (HSV) virus herpes simplex (VHS)
 herpes type 1 (HSV-1) herpes tipo 1 (VHS-1)
 herpes type 2 (HSV-2) herpes tipo 2 (VHS-2)
 herpes zoster (shingles) herpes zóster (culebrilla)
 oral herpes herpes oral
hiccough (hiccup) hipo
hiccup (hiccough) hipo
Hirschsprung's disease enfermedad de Hirschsprung's
hirsutism hisutismo
histiocytes histiocitos
histocompatibility histocompatibilidad
histopathology histopaología
hit golpearse, golpear, pegar
HIV (human immunodeficiency virus) VIH (virus de inmunodeficiencia humana)
HNPCC (hereditary nonpolyposis colorectal cancer, Lynch syndrome) cáncer colorrectal hereditario no asociado a poliposis, síndrome de Lynch)
hormone hormonas
hospice hospicio, centro de cuidados paliativos, centro para cuidados de enfermos terminales
hospital hospital
 general, state or public hospital hospital general or público, seguro social (*MEX*)
hot flashes bochorno, calorones, sofoco, rubores
house call visita a domicilio
HPV (human papillomavirus) VPH (virus del papiloma humano)
hug abrazar, apapachar, apapacho
human papillomavirus (HPV) virus del papiloma humano (VPH)
humidifier humidificador
hurt lastimar, herir, lesionar, dañar, hacer daño, perjudicar

hydrating hidratante
  hydrating lotion loción hidratante
hydration hidratación
hydrocele hidrocele
hydrocephalus hidrocefalia
hydrocephaly normal pressure hydrocephaly (NPH) hidrocefalia de presión normal
hydrocortisol hidrocortisol
hyper- hiper-
hyperpituitarism hiperpituitarismo
hypo- hipo-
hypo-septo-optic hiposeptoóptico
hypopituitarism hipopituitarismo
hypoplastic left heart syndrome síndrome del corazón izquierdo hipoplásico
hypospadias hipospadias
hypothalamus hipotálamo
hysterectomy histerectomía
hysterotomy histerotomía

I

IC (intensive care) cuidados intensivos, terapia intensiva
ICU (intensive care unit) unidad de cuidados intensivos o terapia intensiva
identifying features características, facciones o rasgos identificadores
idiopathic thrombocytopenic purpura (ITP) púrpura trombocitopénica idiopática (PTI)
IEP (individualized education plan) plan de educación personalizado
ileum íleon
iliac ilíaco
immune inmune
  immune system sistema inmunitario, sistema inmunológico, sistema inmune
immunity inmunidad
immunization inmunización
immunocompetent inmunocompetente
immunodeficiency inmunodeficiencia
  acquired immunodeficiency syndrome (AIDS) síndrome de inmunodeficiencia adquirida (SIDA)
immunological response respuesta inmunológica
immunological system sistema inmunológico, sistema inmunitario
immunology inmunología
immunosuppressant inmunosupresor
impetigo impétigo
in utero en el utero
incidence incidencia
incident incidente
incontinence incontinencia
incus yunque
individualized education program, individualized education plan (IEP) plan de educación personalizado
induced labor parto provocado
inequality desigualdad
inequity inequidad, desigualdad
  health inequity inequidad sanitaria, inequidad en la salud
infantile nystagmus syndrome (INS) síndrome de nistagmo infantil (SNI)
infection infección
  candidiasis infection infección por candidasis
  fungal infection infección de hongos
  necrotizing soft tissue infection infección necrosante de tejidos blandos
  opportunistic infection infección oportunista
  pneumococcal infection infección neumocócica
  sexually transmitted infection (STI) infecciones de transmissión sexual (ITS)
  strep throat infection infección por estreptococos de la garganta
  urinary tract infection infección de las vías urinarias
  urine infection infección de la orina
  yeast infection infección de hongos
inflamed inflamado
inflammation inflamación
inflammatory bowel disease (IBD) enfermedad inflamatoria intestinal
influenza (flu) influenza
informed consent consentimiento informado
inguinal hernia hernia inguinal
inhaler inhalador, bombita
inhibitors inhibidores
  nucleoside analog reverse transcriptase inhibitors inhibidores nucleósidos de la transcriptasa reversa
  protease inhibitors inhibidores de la proteasa
injection inyección
injure lastimar, herir, lesionar, hacer daño, dañar, perjudicar
innate immunity inmunidad innata o inespecífica
inner ear oído interno
innocent murmur soplo inocente
insulin dependent diabetes diabetes insulinodependiente
intermittent intermitente
intern (doctor, student) interno
interpretation interpretación
interpreter intérprete
intestine intestino
  large intestine (*see* **colon**) intestino grueso
  small intestine intestino delgado
intramuscular intramuscular
intravenous intravenoso
intravenous line (IV) línea intravenosa
introduce introducir, presentarse
  introduce (people) presentarse
  introduce (a speculum) introducir

intubate intubar, introducir un tubo por la vía respiratoria
intubation intubación
invasive invasivo
  invasive procedure procedimiento invasivo
irritation irritación
ischemic brain attack (stroke) ataque cerebral isquémico
itch comezón, picar, picazón,
itching comezón, picazón, picando
ITP (idiopathic thrombocytopenic purpura) (PTI) púrpura trombocitopénica idiopática
IV (intravenous) por vía intravenosa
  IV antibiotics antibióticos por vía intravenosa
IVIG (intravenous immunoglobulin) (IGIV) inmunoglobulina intravenosa

J

jaundice ictericia
jaw mandíbula, quijada
jejunum yeyuno
joint articulación, coyuntura
jump-start (heart, monitor) arrancar

K

karyotype cariotipo
Kawasaki disease enfermedad de Kawasaki
ketogenic cetogénico
kick the bucket irse el caballo (*CUB*)
kid chavalo (*C.A.*), escuincle (*MEX*), chamo (*VEN*), carajito (*VEN*)
kidney riñón
  flank pain dolor de costado, dolor de riñones
  kidney pain dolor de riñones, dolor de costado
knee rodilla

L

lab laboratorio
  get labs hacerse análisis de laboratorio
  lab results resultados de los análisis de laboratorio
  lab slip hoja para análisis de laboratorio, orden para análisis de laboratorio
  lab tests análisis de laboratorio
  labs resultados de los análisis de laboratorio
labia labia
laboratory laboratorio
lactation lactación
  lactation specialist especialista en lactancia
lactate lactar, amamantar, dar pecho
lactic acid ácido láctico
lactulose lactulosa
lanolin lanolina
laryngomalacia faringomalasia
layer capa
lead (wire) cable, alambre, sensor
lean magro, delgado, apoyarse, inclinarse sobre
  lean meat carne magra
  lean body cuerpo delgado
leg pierna ("pie" is sometimes used to refer to leg, *MEX*)
  leg cramps calambres en las piernas
  leg hair vellos en las piernas
legal permanent resident residente legal permanente
legal temporary resident residente legal temporal
legitimate child hijo legítimo
lens lente
leukemia leucemia
leukocyte leucocito
leukocytosis leucositosis
leukopenia leucopenia
lice piojos
ligament ligamento
lightheaded aturdido, atarantado, estar con una pérdida de equilibrio, fuera de onda (*MEX*), mareado, darle a uno yeyo (*VEN*), dar le a uno yuyo (*ESP*)
likely probable
limits límites
line (intravenous) línea intravenosa
  central venous line catéter venoso central
  PICC line (percutaneously inserted central catheter) línea PICC (catéter venoso central de inserción periférica)
lining forro, revestimiento
  silver lining algo positivo, forro plateado
  stomach lining revestimiento del estómago
  uterine lining forro de la matríz o útero
lip (mouth) labio
  cleft lip labio leporino
louse piojo
low inferior, bajo
  low back pain dolor en la parte inferior de la espalda, dolor lumbar, dolor de cintura
lower back (*see* **waist**) parte inferior de la espalda, cintura
  lower back pain dolor lumbar, dolor de cintura, dolor en la parte inferior de la espalda
lumbar puncture punción lumbar
  lumbar spine espina lumbar
lump protuberancia, masa, bulto, bola, bolita, pelotita, chichón, hinchazón
lumpectomy tumorectomía, excisión de una protuberancia, tumor o masa
lumpy aterronado, borujoso, lleno de bolitas
lymph linfático
  lymph gland ganglio linfático, nódulo linfático
  lymph node ganglio linfático, nódulo linfático, gánglio

lymphatic system sistema linfático
lymphectomy linfectomía
lymphocyte linfocito

M

MA (medical assistant, *see also* **PA)** asistente médico
macula mácula
macular degeneration degeneración macular
magnet imán
magnetic magnético
magnetic resonance imaging (MRI) imágenes de resonancia magnética, emarrai (*USA*)
main principal, mayor, central
mainly principalmente, generalmente
maladjusted mal ajustado, inadaptado, desequilibrado
malaise malestar, indisposición
malignant peripheral nerve sheath tumor tumor maligno de la vaina de un nervio periférico
malleus martillo
malnutrition desnutrición, alimentación insuficiente, mala o poca alimentación
mammary gland glándula mamaria, mamas
mammogram mamografía, mamograma
mark marcar, rayar, indicar
marker (tumor, blood) marcador
marrow médula
bone marrow médula ósea
mash hacer puré, aplastar, mezclar
mastitis mastalgia
match, to estar parejo
maternal materno
maternal and child health salud materno infantil
maternity maternidad
maternity ward sala de maternidad, sala de partos, sala de gineco
medical abortion aborto médico terapéutico
medical assistant (MA, *see PA*) asistente médico
meds medicinas, medicamentos
megaloblastic anemia anemia megaloblástica
membrane membrana
meningocele meningocele
menopause menopausia
menstrual cramps calambres menstruales, retorcijones abdominales
menstruation menstruación, período, regla
methotrexate metotrexate
MIC-KEY (Bard Button) MIC-KEY, botón Mic-Key, botón miqui (botón Bard), tubo gástrico
microcephaly microcefalia
middle ear oído medio
midwife partera, concuña
milk duct conducto galactóforo
miscarriage aborto, aborto espontáneo, malparto
mismatch repair deficiency deficiencia en la reparación del ADN
molecular molecular
molecule molécula
mongolism mongolismo (termino de preferencia en inglés: síndrome de Down)
monitor monitor, monitorear, vigilar, dar seguimiento
monocyte monocito
mosaicism mosaicismo
motor motor
fine motor motor fino
fine motor movements movimientos de motor fino, moticidad fina
gross motor motor grueso
gross motor movements movimientos de motor grueso, moticidad gruesa
motor neuron neurona motora
motor skills habilidades motoras
MRI (magnetic resonance imaging) imágenes de resonancia magnética, IRM, emarrai (*USA*)
mucositis mucositis
mucous membrane membrana mucosa
mucus mucoso
mucus plug tapón mucoso
multiple myeloma mieloma múltiple
muscle músculo
muscle cramps calambres musculares
muscle mass masa muscular
muscle strength fuerza muscular
muscle tone tono muscular
muscular dystrophy distrofia muscular progresiva
mutate mudar, sufrir mutación
mutation mutación
mute mudo
myelin mielina
myelin sheath vaina de mielina
myelomeningocele mielomeningocele
myo- (muscle) mio- (músculo)
myocardial infarction infarto de miocardio
myocarditis miocarditis
myocardium miocardio
myositis miositis

N

nasogastric nasogástrico
nasogastric feeding tube (NG tube) sonda de alimentación nasogástrica (sonda NG)
nasolabial philtrum filtro, surco nasolabial
natural natural
natural childbirth (*see* **vaginal birth**) parto sin medicamentos para el dolor
natural disaster desastre natural
natural family planning planificación familiar natural, anticonceptivos naturales

navel ombligo, belly button
navigator navegador promotor
  health navigator promotor de salud
necrotizing enterocolitis necrosante (*ECN*)
necrotizing soft tissue infection infección necrosante de tejidos blandos
needle aguja, *abjua* (*reg., MEX*)
  needle stick piquete de aguja
neonatal neonato
neotrophil neutrófilo
neuron neurona
neutropenia neutropenia
NG tube sonda nasogástrica
night sweats sudoración nocturna, sudores nocturnos
nipple pezón
  cracked nipples pezones agrietados
  inverted nipples pezones invertidos
nocturnal leg cramps calambres nocturnos en las piernas
noise ruido, bulla
Norwood surgery cirugía de Norwood; primero de tres procedimientos denominado Fontan
nucleoside analog reverse transcriptase inhibitors inhibidores nucleósidos de la transcriptasa reversa
numb entumecido, entumido, entumecer
numbness entumecimiento
nurse enfermero (*nursing titles change between countries and programs: titles may not be equivalent*)
  clinical nurse specialist enfermero clinico especialista
  home health nurse enfermero de visita a domicilio
  nurse practitioner enfermero auxiliar de médico, enfermero especialista, enfermero practicante
  nurse specialist enfermero especialista
  public health nurse enfermero de salud pública
  registered nurse enfermero diplomado, enfermero registrado, enfermero recibido
nursing enfermería
  nurse's aide auxiliar de enfermería
  nursing assistant asistente de enfermería
  nursing assistant auxiliar de enfermería
  nursing student estudiante de enfermería
nutrients nutrientes
nutritionist nutricionista, nutriólogo, dietético
nutritious nutritivo
nystagmus nistagmo

O

obituary obituario, nota necrológica
occult blood test examen de guaycol oculto en heces
odontologist odontólogo
odontology dentistry odontología
oh, well ni modo, whatever
ok bien, oka, va pues (*SAL*)
once a week cada ocho días, una vez por semana
once every two weeks cada quince días, cada quincena, una vez cada dos semanas
once in a blue moon cada muerte de obispo, muy de vez en cuando, muy rara vez
operating room quirófano
ophthalmologist oftalmólogo
optic óptico
  optic nerve nervio óptico
optometrist optometrista optómetra
oral candidiasis (thrush) candidiasis oral candidasis de la boca, candidiasis bucal, hongos en la boca
oral herpes herpes oral, herpes bucal, herpes labiales
order (n.) orden, **(v.)** ordenar
osteogenesis imperfecta osteogénesis imperfect
osteopenia (low bone density) osteopenia (pérdida de densidad ósea)
osteoporosis osteoporosis
ostomy ostomía
out of it atarantado, aturdido, fuera de onda, confundido, raro, extraño
outer ear (auricle) oreja
ovary ovario
ovum óvulo
oxytocin oxitosina

P

PA (**physician's assistant**, *see MA*) auxiliar al médico, médico asociado
page (n.) pagina, **(v.)** localizar
  to be on the same page coincidir, entendernos, tener la misma información, enfocarnos en lo mismo, estar de acuerdo
pain dolor
  aching pain dolor sordo, dolor embotado
  constant pain dolor constante
  dull pain dolor sordo, dolor embotado
  electric shock pain dolor como corriente eléctrica o descarga eléctrica
  intermittent pain dolor intermitente
  sharp pain dolor agudo
  shooting pain dolor que se irradia
  stabbing pain dolor punzante
  throbbing pain dolor palpitante
palate paladar
  cleft palate paladar hendido
paludism (malaria symptoms) paludismo
pamper (v.) mimar, consentir, atender
Pampers (n.) pamper, pañal ("Pampers" is often used to refer to diaper just as "Kleenex" is often used to refer to facial tissue)
pancreas pancreas
Pap smear prueba de Papanicolaou

Papanikolaou test (Pap smear) prueba de Papanicolau
parameters parámetros
partial androgen receptor insensitivity insensibilidad parcial del receptor de andrógenos
passive pasiva
paste pegamento, pasta
pee pipí, orina, chis (*MEX*), pichi (*PER*)
pelvic pélvico
  pelvic exam examen vaginal, examen del pelvis
pelvis pelvis
penis pene
percutaneous percutaneo
period periódo, menstruación, regla
peripheral periférico
peritoneal dialysis diálisis peritoneal
permanent catheter (central line) catéter permanente
permanent legal resident (immigration status) residente legal permanente
pernicious anemia anemia perniciosa
pervasive developmental disorders trastornos generalizados del desarrollo
petechiae petequias
phagocyte fagocitos
pharmacist farmacéutico
pharmacologist farmacólogo
pharmacy farmacia
pharynx faringe
phenobarbital fenobarbital
phenotype fenotipo
phenylketonuria (PKU) fenilcetonuria
philtrum surco
  nasolabial philtrum surco nasolabial
physical therapist fisioterapeuta, fisioterapista
physical therapy fisioterapia, terapia física
physician médico, doctor de medicina, doctor
physician's assistant (*see* **medical assistant**) asistente del médico
physiology fisiología
physiotherapy fisioterapia
PICC line (percutaneously inserted central catheter) línea PICC (catéter venoso central de inserción periférica)
pinna (auricle) oreja, pabellón externo del oído (pabellón auricular)
pitting dejar con hoyos, marcar con hoyos o fovea
  pitting edema edema con fovea
pituitary pituitaria
  pituitary gland glándula pituitaria
placenta placenta
  placenta previa placenta previa
plasma plasma
platelet plaqueta
  platelet disorder desorden de las plaquetas
  platelet problems problemas plaquetarios
pleura pleura
pleurisy pleuritis, pleuresía
PMS (premenstrual syndrome) SPM (síndrome premenstrual)
pneumococcal infection infección neumocócica, infecciones por neumococo
pneumococci neumococo
pneumonia neumonía, pulmonía
polycystic ovary syndrome síndrome del ovario poliquístico
polyp pólipo
port (catheter) puerto, catéter puerto, puerto para vía venosa central
  Infusaport port (catheter) puerto
  Medi-port port (catheter) puerto
  Port-A-Cath port (catheter) puerto
  subclavian port puerto subclavio
  subcutaneous central venous catheter port catéter venoso central subcutáneo
  subcutaneous port catéter con acceso debajo de la piel, catéter venoso central subcutáneo
possible posible
postpartum depression depresión posparto
post-traumatic stress disorder (PTSD) trastorno por estres postraumático (PSTD)
  chronic PTSD PSTD crónico
  secondary PTSD tensión traumática secundaria, estres traumático secundario
poultice compresa
predisposed propenso
predisposition predisposisión
prednisone prednisona
preeclampsia preeclampsia
preemie bebé prematuro
preexisting condition afección preexistente
pregnancy embarazo
pregnant embarazada
premature baby bebé prematuro
premenstrual syndrome (PMS) síndrome premenstrual (SPM)
prescription receta, receta médica, prescripción
preservative preservativo, condón
primary care cuidados primarios
primary care doctor médico decuidados primarios, médico de cabezera
primary congestion congestión primaria
principal director, jefe
principally por lo general
principle principio
  on principle por principio
probable probable
probe sonda
problem problema, trastorno, condición, desorden
procedure procedimiento, intervención, proceso
prognosis prognosis, pronóstico
prolapse prolapso, caída, descenso
  mitral valve prolapse prolapso de la válvula mitral
  pelvic organ prolapse prolapso de la pelvis
  uterine prolapse prolapso uterino

prolonged prolongado
promoter (community health worker or navigator) promotor de salud
prone prono, boca abajo, prostrato, propenso, susceptible, predispuesto
prophylaxis profilaxis
prostate próstata
prostrate postrado, acostado
protease inhibitors inhibidores de la proteasa
protracted prolongado
protrude resaltar, empujar o salir hacía afuera
protruding saliente, resaltante, saliendo hacía afuera
provider profesional de la salud
psoriasis psoriasis
psychiatrist psiquiatra
psychiatry psiquiatría
psychology psicología
psychosis psicosis
  manic-depressive psychosis psicosis maníaco-depresiva
psychosomatic psicosomático
psychotherapist psicoterapeuta
psychotherapy psicoterapia
PTSD (post-traumatic stress disorder) PSTD (trastorno de estrés postraumático)
puberty pubertad
pubic púbico
  pubic area área del pubis, área púbica
  pubic hair vello púbico, vellos del pubis
  pubic lice piojos púbicos, piojos del pubis, ladillas
pubis pubis, área púbica
puffer inhalador, bombita
pulga flea
pulmonary atresia (*see* **tricuspid atresia**) atresia pulmonar
pulmonary trunk tronco pulmonar
pump bomba, *bompa, pompa*
puncture punción, perforación
  lumbar puncture punción lumbar, punción espinal
pupil (eye) pupila, niña del ojo
purpura púrpura
push out resaltar, empujar o salir hacia afuera
put up with tolerar, soportar

Q

quickly rápidamente, velozmente, a prisa, ligeramente, ligerito
quietly calladamente, silenciosamente, despacio, lentamente

R

radiation radiación
  radiation therapy radioterapia, terapia de radiación
radical hysterectomy histerectomía radical
radiography radiografía, rayos x
radiology radiología
radiology technician técnico de radiología
range límites, parámetros, márgen, amplitud
  range of motion parámetros de movimiento, amplitud de movimiento, límites de movimiento
  range of vision límites del campo visual
rape violar, violación
rash sarpullido
rate tasa, velocidad
reaction reacción
reactive airway disease enfermedad reactiva de las vías respiratorias
rectum recto
red rojo
  red blood cells (erythrocytes) glóbulos rojos (eritrocitos)
  red cells glóbulos rojos
  to turn red enrojecer
reddening enrojecimiento
redness rojo, rojizo, enrojecido, rubor
reevaluate volver a evaluar, evaluar de nuevo
referral recomendación, referencia
refill surtir, volver a surtir, resurtir, resurtido surtido, rebastecimiento, refil
reflux reflujo
  gastroesophageal reflux reflujo gastroesofágico
  urinary reflux reflujo urinario
regional ileitis (*see* **Crohn's disease, inflammatory bowel disease**) ileitis (see **enfermedad de Crohn, enfermedad inflamatoria intestinal**)
reject rechazar
rejection rechazo
relapse recaída
relations relaciones, parientes
  sexual relations relaciones sexuales
relationship relación
relief alivio
relieve aliviar
remove remover, quitar, extirpar, resecar
renal renal
repair damage reparar el daño
requisition pedido, petición, requisición, autorización
research investigación
  clinical research ensayo clínico, investigación clínica
  research study ensayo clínico, investigación clínica
resect resecar
resection resección
resident residente
  legal permanent resident (immigration) residente legal permanente
  legal resident (immigration) residente legal
resident doctor
respiratory syncytial virus (RSV) virus sincicial respiratorio

respond responder
response respuesta
restless inquieto
restless legs syndrome (RLS) síndrome de las piernas inquietas
retina retina
retinopathy retinopatía
  diabetic retinopathy retinopatía diabética
revive revivir
rhabdomyosarcoma rabdomiosarcoma
rhinoplasty rinoplastia
rhinoscope rinoscopio
rhinoscopy rinoscopia
ringworm tiña, dermatofitosis
risk riesgo, arriesgar
  risk of infection riesgo de infección o contagio
  to put at risk poner en riesgo
  to risk poner en riesgo, arriesgar
rod perno
roll rodar
  roll over voltearse, darse la vuelta
  roll over back to front voltearse boca abajo a boca arriba
  roll over front to back voltearse boca arriba a boca abajo
root canal conducto radicular
rosacea rosásea
RSV (respiratory syncytial virus) virus sincicial respiratorio
rub sobar, frotar
  rub in frotar
runny nose mucosidad, tener la nariz chorreándose, tener secreción nasal, tener moco

S

saccule sáculo
sacral sacro
  sacral spine columna sacra
  sacral bone hueso sacroa
sacrum sacro
safe seguro, a salvo, fuera de peligro, no riesgoso
salt (see **sodium**) sal
  low-salt bajo en sal
  salt-free libre de sal, sin sal
same igual, parejo
sample muestra, espécimen
scabies sarna
scale báscula, balanza, escama
scalp cuero cabelludo
scalp hair cabello
scan escanear, escán, tomografía, exploración, gammagrafía
scarlet fever fiebre escarlatina
schedule an appointment hacer una cita, programar una cita, hacer un apoinmen
SCID (severe combined immunodeficiency) deficiencia inmunitaria combinada severa (DICS)
scotoma escotoma
scrape raspar
scraping raspado, raspar para obtener una muestra
scratch (v.) rascar, rayar; **(n.)** rasguño
screening (test) prueba preliminaria de detección, prueba inicial investigatoria, averiguación
screw tornillo
scrub lavar detalladamente, fregar
scrubs bata quirúgica
season temporada
seasonal de la temporada
seborrheic dermatitis dermatitis seborreica
secondary PTSD secundario
seizure ataque, convulsión
semicircular canals canales semicirculares
seniority antigüedad
sensor sensor, electrodo, cable
sepsis sepsis
septic séptico
  septic shock choque séptico, shock séptico
septicemia septicemia
septo-optic dysplasia (optic nerve hypoplasia, de Morsier syndrome) displasia septo-óptica (síndrome de Morsier, síndrome del nervio óptico)
septum septo, tabique
  deviated septum tabique desviado
  nasal septum tabique nasal
seroconversion seroconversión
serum suero, whey
severe acute respiratory syndrome (SARS) síndrome respiratorio agudo y grave (SARS)
severe combined immunodeficiency (SCID) deficiencia inmunitaria combinada severa (DICS) inmunodeficiencia combinada grave
sex sexo
  anal sex sexo anal
  oral sex sexo oral
  safe sex sexo seguro, práctica sexual segura
  safer sex práctica sexual más segura o menos riesgoso
  to have sex tener relaciones sexuales
  vaginal sex sexo vaginal
sexual sexual
  sexual relations relaciones sexuales
sexually sexualmente, sexual
  sexually transmitted disease enfermedades de transmisión sexual
  sexually transmitted infection infección de transmisión sexual
shake agitar, sacudir
shaken baby syndrome síndrome del bebé sacudido
sharp pain dolor agudo
shingles (herpes zoster) culebrilla (herpes zóster)

shock choque, shock, descarga
- **anaphylactic shock** shock anafiláctico
- **cardiogenic shock** shock cardiógeno
- **electric shock** descarga eléctrica
- **hypovolemic shock** shock hipovolémico
- **septic shock** shock séptico
- **toxic shock** shock tóxico

shooting pain dolor punzante
shot inyección, vacuna
shoulder hombre
shunt derivación, conducto, vía, shant (*USA*)
sickle cell anemia anemia de las células falsiformes
SIDS (sudden infant death syndrome síndrome de muerte infantil repentina, síndrome de muerte infantile súbita (SMIS), síndrome de muerte súbita del lactante (SMSL)
sigmoidoscopy sigmoidoscopía
signet-ring cell type célula tipo anillo
silver plata
- **silver lining** algo positivo, revestimiento plateado
- **silver nitrate** nitrato de plata

single father padre soltero
single mother madre soltera
single parent padre soltero, padres solteros, padre o madre soltero
sinus senos
sinusitis sinusitis
sister-in-law cuñada
site sitio, lugar
sleep dormir, sueño
sleep apnea apnea del sueño
sleep study estudio del sueño
slip formulario, resbalarse, hoja, faldilla
slow despacio
slowly despacio, ligerito, despacito, quedito, poco a poco, calladito
small intestine (ileum) intestino delgado (ileon)
smash aplastar, machucar
smell (v.) oleer
- **smell (bad)** (**v.**) apestar, (**n.**) la peste

snack (n.) bocadillo, merienda, tentempié
snack (v.) merendar, picar
social security seguro social
- **número de seguro social** social security number

sodium (*see* **salt**) sodio
- **low-sodium diet** alimento bajo en sodio
- **sodium bicarbonate** bicarbonato de sodio, bicarbonato sódico

softly calladito, quedito
som- (body) som- (cuerpo)
spacer (for inhaler) cámara (para el inhalador)
specific inherited gene alterations alteración o mutación heredada de un gen
specimen espécimen (muestra, biopsia)
spectrum espectro
speculum espéculo
speed velocidad, índice, tasa
spin girar, dar vueltas, estar mareada
spina bifida espina bífida
- **open spina bifida** espina bífida abierta
- **spina bifida occulta** espina bífida oculta

spinal column espina dorsal, columna vertebral
spinal cord médula espinal
spinal tap punción de la espina dorsal, punción lumbar
spine espina dorsal, columna vertebral
spinning girando, girar, mareo, vertigo
spit up vomitar, arrojar (*reg., MEX*), devolver
spleen bazo
spoil (pamper, indulge) consentir, mimar;
- **(rot)** pudrirse, arruinarse

spoiled (food) podrida (child) consentido, mimado, toñeco (*VEN*)
spontaneous abortion aborto espontáneo, malparto
spores espora
- **mold spores** esporas de moho

spot mancha, manchar
spotting tener manchas (de sangre de la menstruacíon)
squamous escamoso
squat (crouch down) ponerse en cuclillas
squeeze apretar, estrujar
squint entrecerrar, entornar
stabbing pain dolor punzante
stand pararse
- **stand up** pararse

standard estándar
standard practice práticas estandarizadas, práticas rutinarias
standardized estandarizado
standing order orden fija
stapes estribo
STD (sexually transmitted disease) ETS (enfermedad de transmisión sexual)
stem cell célula madre, célula de base
stent stent; estént; resorte, tubo expansible, intraluminal, dispositivo (maya o sonda usada para facilitar comunicación entre estructuras vasculares, hecha por una materia descubierta por Charles Stent, odontólogo inglés)
steroids esteroides
STI (sexually transmitted infection) (infección de transmisión sexual)
stick picar (con una aguja hipodérmica)
stickers calcomanías, pegantinas, estiquers
stiff tieso
stiffness (to have) estar tieso
still quieto, estar sin mover
stillbirth parto de un feto muerto, malparto, aborto
sting picar, arder
stink apestar
stirrups estribos
stoma estoma
stomach estómago, *estógamo* (*MEX*)

stop parar
  stop medication suspender la medicina
strabismus (crossed eyes) estrabismo (ojos biscos)
strep estreptococo
strep throat infección por estreptococos de la garganta, anginas
streptococcus estreptococo
stress estrés
stripe raya, rayar
stroke ataque cerebral, ataque cerebrovascular, embolia (*MEX*)
study estudiar, estudio, investigación clínica
stuffy nose nariz constipada, nariz congestionada, nariz mormada, nariz tupida
subcutaneous subcutáneo, debajo de la piel
supine supino, boca arriba
sure seguro, cierto
  absolutely sure absolutamente seguro
  almost sure (of a test result) casi seguro (de un resultado)
  very sure muy seguro
surgeon cirujano
surgery cirugía
surgical quirúrgico
  surgical gown (scrubs) bata quirúrgica
surgically quirúrgicamente
swallow tragar, deglutir
  swallow study (barium swallow study) esofagrama (esofagrama con ingestion de barrio), estudio del tragar
sweat transpirar, sudar
sweat test prueba del sudo, prueba de electrolitos del sudor
swell hincharse
swelling hinchazón, hinchándose, inflamación, inflamándose
swollen hinchado
syncope síncope
syndrome síndrome
  acquired immunodeficiency syndrome (AIDS) síndrome de inmunodeficiencia adquirida (SIDA)
  antiphospholipid antibody syndrome (APLS) síndrome de anticuerpos antifosfolípidos
  carpal tunnel syndrome síndrome del túnel carpiano
  congenital nephrotic syndrome of Finnish type síndrome nefrótico congénito de tipo finlandés
  constitutional mismatch repair deficiency syndrome síndrome constitucional de deficiencia en la reparación del ADN
  fragile X syndrome síndrome x frágil
  Guillain-Barré syndrome (GBS) síndrome de Guillain-Barré
  hereditary mismatch repair deficiency syndrome (HMRDS) síndrome herditario de deficiencia en la reparación del ADN
  hereditary nonpolyposis colon cancer syndrome (HNPCC, Lynch syndrome) síndrome de cáncer no poliposo rectal hereditario (síndrome de Lynch)
  hypoplastic left heart syndrome síndrome del corazón izquierdo hipoplásico
  hypoplastic right heart syndrome síndrome del corazón derecho hipoplásico
  infantile nystagmus syndrome (INS) síndrome de nistagmo infantil (SNI)
  Lynch syndrome (hereditary nonpolyposis colorectal cancer) síndrome de Lynch (cáncer colorrectal hereditario no asociado a poliposis)
  Marfan syndrome síndrome de Marfan
  polycystic ovary syndrome síndrome del ovario poliquístico
  Prader-Willi syndrome síndrome de Prader-Willi
  restless legs syndrome (RLS) síndrome de las piernas inquietas
  shaken baby syndrome síndrome del bebé sacudido
  sudden infant death syndrome (SIDS) síndrome de muerte infantil súbita (SMIS), síndrome de muerte súbita del lactante (SMSL)
  Tourette syndrome síndrome de Tourette
  toxic shock syndrome síndrome del shock tóxico
  Turner syndrome síndrome de Turner
synovial sinovial, sinovio
  synovial membrane membrana sinovial
syringe jeringa
syrup jarabe
systolic sistólico

T

tailbone cóccix, hueso de la cola
take blood tomar sangre, tomar muestras o especímenes de sangre, extraer sangre
tank tanque, bombona (*VEN*)
taper bajar (la dosis de una medicina) poco a poco, disminuir, reducir
taper schedule horario o instrucciones para bajar la dosis de una medicina poco a poco sobre un período de tiempo
T-cells células-T
tech técnico
technician técnico
Tegaderm Tegaderm (venda de piel artificial para curar o cubrir heridas)
temporary temporal
temporary foster care cuidados de tutor legal temporal o cutodia legal temporal
tender sensible, tierno
tenderness, to have estar sensible o irritado
tendon tendón

test prueba, análisis, examen
- **cancer screening test** prueba para detección temprana y prevención de cáncer
- **ELISA test (enzyme-linked immunoassay)** prueba ELISA (enzimoinmunoanálisis de absorción)
- **genetic array test** prueba de gama genética
- **lab test** análisis de laboratorio, prueba de laboratorio
- **pap smear test** prueba de Papanicolau
- **Papanicolaou test** prueba de Papanicolau
- **paternity test** prueba de paternidad
- **pregnancy test** pueba de embarazo
- **protein immunoblotting test (western blot test)** prueba de inmunoelectrotransferencia indirecta
- **quick test** prueba rápida
- **screening test** prueba preliminar de detección, prueba inicial investigatoria
- **serologic test** prueba serológica
- **TB skin test** prueba de tuberculina en la piel
- **urine test** prueba de orina
- **Wada test (cerebral hemispheric dominance of language function)** prueba de Wada (técnica de la anestesia hemisférica para la evaluación de la lateralidad del lenguaje)
- **western blot** test prueba confirmatoria western blot

testicle testículo
testosterone testosterona
thalamus tálamo
thalassemia talasemia
that's it eso es la talla
the jury is still out no estamos seguros todavía, no tenemos los resultados todavía, no hemos tomado una decisión todavía
therapeutic terapéutico
therapist terapeuta, terapista
therapy terapia
- **chemotherapy** quimioterapia
- **intensive care therapy** terapia de cuidados intensivos
- **intensive therapy** terapia intensiva
- **physical therapy** terapia física, fisioterapia
- **radiation therapy** radioterapia, terapia de radiación

thoracic spine espina torácica
throat garganta
- **clear the throat** carraspear
- **sore throat** dolor de garganta

throbbing pain dolor palpitante
thrombocyte trombocito
throw up vomitar, arrojar, devolver (*MEX*)
thrush (oral candidiasis) candidiasis bucal, candidiasis oral, infección de hongos en la boca
thyroid tiroides
- **thyroid gland** glándula tiroidéa

tie tubes ligar las trompas de Falopio
tingling hormigueo
tissue tejido
tit chichi, chicha, teta
toddler niño pequeño
tolerate tolerar (cantidad de fórmula, dolor), soportar, aguantar (la presencia de alguien) resistir, sobrevivir (anestesia, quimioterapia)
tomography tomografía
tonsillectomy amigdalectomía
tonsillitis amigdalitis
tonsils anginas (*MEX*), amígdalas, amígdalas palatinas, adenoides
- **palatine tonsil** amígdala paletina

touch base ver como uno sigue, averiguar que opina, averiguar cómo uno se siente, averiguar que piensa
toxic shock shock tóxico
toxic shock syndrome síndrome del shock tóxico
toxoplasmosis toxoplasmosis
trach (abreviación para traqueostomía o traqueotomía)
trachea traquea
tracheostomy traqueostomía
tracheotomy traqueotomía
trait rasgo
transfuse dar una transfusión
transient ischemic brain attack (mini stroke) ataque cerebral isquémico transitorio (mini ataque)
translate traducir (escrito)
translation traducción (escrito)
translator traductor, traductora
transparent transparente
transplant trasplantar, transplantar
traumatic brain injury taumatismo cerebral
trichomoniasis tricomoniasis
tricuspid atresia atresia tricuspídea
trisomy trisomía
trisomy 18 (Edwards syndrome) trisomía 18 (syndrome de Edwards)
trisomy 21 (Down syndrome) trisomía 21 (syndrome de Down)
try intentar, probar, hacer un esfuerzo, tratar
- **really try** hecharle ganas, hacer un gran esfuerzo

tubal ligation ligadura de trompas
tube tubo, sonda, catéter, conducto, trompa
- **eustachian tubes** trompa de esustachio
- **Fallopian tubes** trompas de Falopio

tummy panza, pancita, barriga, barriguita
tumor versus host effect efecto injerto contra tumor
tuna atún
turbinates (nasal) cornetas o turbinas nasales
tympanic membrane membrana timpánico, tímpano
type tipo, grupo (sangre)
typing tipificación
- **confirmatory typing** tipificación confirmatoria
- **tissue typing (histocompatibility antigen test)** tipificación de tejido (examen de antígeno de histocompatibilidad)

U

umbilical hernia hernia umbilical
umbilicus ombligo
underlying subyacente
    underlying cause causa subyacente
undifferentiated pattern patrón no diferenciado
undocumented ("illegal") indocumentado
upchuck vomitar, arrojar (*reg., MEX*), devolver
ureter uréter
urethra uretra
urge incontinence incontinencia imperiosa
uric acid ácido úrico
urinary urinaria
    urinary bladder vejiga uriaria
    urinary incontinence incontinencia urinaria
    urinary reflux reflujo urinario
    urinary tract infection infección de las vías urinarias, infección de la orina, mal de orín (*MEX*)
urine orina
    urine cytology test prueba de citología de la orina
    urine infection infeción de la orina, mal de orín
urodynamics test prueba de la función de la vejiga urinaria
uterine uterino
    uterine cervix cuello de la matriz
    uterine lining revestimiento de la matriz o del útero, forro de la matriz
    uterine myoma mioma uterino
    uterine prolapse prolapso del útero, prolapso uterino
uterus útero, matriz
UTI (urinary tract infection) infección de las vías urinarias
utricle utrículo

V

vaccinate vacunar, picar
vaccine vacuna
vagina vagina **Note:** Some Spanish-speaking patients or parents might instead use slang or euphemistic terms such as cola, cosita or parte.
vaginal vaginal
    vaginal birth parto natural, parto vaginal
    vaginal bleeding sangrado vaginal
    vaginal discharge flujo vaginal
    vaginal dryness sequedad vaginal
    vaginal fluid fluido vaginal
    vaginal ring anillo vaginal
    vaginal yeast infection infección vaginal de hongos o de candidiasis
Valley fever (San Joaquin Valley fever, coccidioidomycosis) fiebre del Valle coccidioidomicosis aguda
varicella varicela
varicella-zoster virus virus varicela-zoster
vein vena
venipuncture venipuntura
ventricle ventrículo
ventriculoperitoneal shunt (VP shunt) derivación ventriculoperitoneal (shunt VP), válvula de derivación ventrículoperitoneal, shant
vertebra vértebra
vertebrae vértebras
    cervical vertebrae vértebras cervicales
    lumbar vertebrae vértebras lumbar
    sacral vertebrae sacro, vértebras sacras
    thoracic vertebrae vértebras torácicas
vertebral column columna vertebral
vertigo vértigo benign paroxysmal positional vertigo (BPPV) vértigo postural paroxístico benigno (VPPB)
vial ampolleta
vicarious PTSD PSTD secundario, tensión traumática secundaria, estrés traumático secundario
villus vello
    chorionic villus sampling muestreo del vello coriónico
viral load carga viral
virus virus
    herpes simplex virus (HSV) virus de herpes simplex (VHS)
    respiratory syncytial virus (RSV) virus sincicial respiratorio (VSR)
    West Nile virus virus del Nilo occidental
visual field campo visual
volume volumen, cantidad
vomit vomitar, arrojar, gomitar (*reg., MEX*), devolver
VP shunt, válvula de derivación ventrículo-peritoneal, *shant*
vulva vulva

W

Wada test (cerebral hemispheric dominance of language function) prueba de Wada (técnica de la anestesia hemisférica para la evaluación de la lateralidad del lenguaje)
waist cintura (*see* **lower back**)
wart verruga
wasting degaste, perder peso y masa muscular, atrofia, emaciación
    AIDS wasting syndrome síndrome de emaciacón por SIDA
    facial wasting pérdida de grasa en el rosto
weakness debilidad
weigh pesar, sopezar
West Nile virus virus del Nilo occidental
whatever ni modo, no importa, lo que sea

wheezing respiración silbante, silbancias, resuello
  wheezing noise ruido silbante, ruido chirriante
whistling chirriante, charriando, silbante, silbando
  whistling noise ruido chirriante, ruido silbante
white blood cells (leukocytes) glóbulos blancos (leucocitos)
white matter material blanca, sustancia blanca
whoosh bisbisear, silbar, chillar
whooshing bisbisea, bisbiseando
  whooshing noise ruido silbante
wipe limpiar
wipes toallitas pañitos
  alcohol wipe toallitas empapadas en alcohol, pañito con alcohol
wire alambre, cable, eléctrodo, sensor
womb matríz, útero, abdomen
worker trabajador, jornalero, obrereo
wound herida, lesión
wound site care curación y cuidados de la herida o lesión

X

x-ray rayos-x, radiografía, placa (*MEX*)

Y

yack (USA) arrojar, gomitar (*reg., MEX*), devolver, vomitar
yeast hongos, cándida, candidiasis (skin, mouth, vagina, newborn), levadura (bread)
  yeast infection infección de hongos, candidiasis
yolk (egg) yema
yolk sac saco vitelino

Z

Zika virus virus del Zika
zucchini calabacita (*MEX*)
zygote cigoto

Appendix 4

Medical terms: A study guide

Note: Most interpreters in hospitals should be prepared to interpret the terms in the following list. The purpose of the list is twofold. Interpreters can test themselves to see if they know the terms in their other working language(s). Interpreters can also, if they are not Spanish-speaking, research and write down the translation of each term in their non-English working language(s).

A

abortion
abscess
absolute neutrophil count (ANC)
absolutely
accuracy
acid
    acid indigestion
    acid reflux
acidity
acoustic
acquired immunity
acquired immunodeficiency syndrome (AIDS)
acute immunity
acute lymphoblastic leukemia (Hodgkin disease)
ad hoc
Adam's apple
adenoids (*see tonsils*)
adenoma
adenotonsillectomy
adhesion
adhesive
adipose
    adipose tissue
adoptive family
adrenal gland
adrenoleukodystrophy (ALD)
advanced practice nurse
aerosol
AFP (alpha fetoprotein)
AIDS (acquired immunodeficiency syndrome)
airborne
    airborne disease
    airborne precaution
airway
    obstructed airway
alcohol
    alcohol wipe
    alcoholic
    alcoholism
    fetal alcohol syndrome
ALD (adrenoleukodystrophy)
alleviate
almost sure (of a test result)
alopecia
alpha fetoprotein (AFP)
ALS (amyotrophic lateral sclerosis)
ambiguous genitalia
amino acid
amniocentesis
amoeba
amount
amygdala (structure in brain)
amyotrophic lateral sclerosis (ALS)
anal sex
analysis
anaphylactic shock
anaphylaxis
androgens
anemia
    aplastic anemia
    Diamond Blackfan anemia (congenital hypoplastic anemia)
    Fanconi anemia (aplastic anemia)
    megaloblastic anemia
    sickle cell anemia
aneurysm
anger
angina
angioplasty anguish
antibacterial
antibody
anticoagulants
antifungal
antigen
antiphospholipid antibody syndrome (APLS)
antiplatelet antibodies
antiplatelet drugs
antireflux
antirejection
antiretroviral
anus
anxiety
anxious
Apgar test
apheresis (plasmapheresis)
aplastic anemia
APLS (antiphospholipid antibody syndrome)
apnea
apoplexy
appointment
arm
armpit
arrhythmia
arterial stenosis
arteriosclerosis (*see atherosclerosis*)
arteriovenous malformation (AVM)
artery
arthritis
    juvenile rheumatoid arthritis
    rheumatoid arthritis
aspiration
    bone marrow aspiration
    fine needle aspiration assault
asshole (*see butt*)
asthma
    asthma attack
astigmatism
at risk
atherosclerosis (*see arteriosclerosis*)
athlete's foot (tinea)
atria
atrium

B

C

cabbage
cables (wires)
Caesarian
calf
canal
    auditory canal
    birth canal
    ear canal
    semicircular canals
cancer
    cancer screening test
candida
candidiasis
    candidiasis of the mouth
    candidiasis of the skin
    oral candidiasis (oral thrush)
cardiac
cardiac catheterization
    cardiac failure
cardiac stent
cardiomyopathy
cardiopulmonary resuscitation (CPR)
care
    care for
    child care
    foster care
    inhumane care
    legal foster care
    palliative care
    site care (wound)
    take care of
    temporary care
    temporary foster care
    wound care
    wound site care
caregiver
caretaker
carpal tunnel syndrome
carrier
CAT scan (computer axial tomography scan)
catheter (*see port*)
    Broviac catheter
    permanent or semi-permanent catheter (*see port, central line*)
    urinary catheter
catheterization
    cardiac catheterization
    urinary catheterization
causative gene
CBC complete blood count
cecum
cell
    blood cell
    cord blood cell
    hematopoietic stem cell
    red cell
    Schwann cell
    signet-ring cell type
    stem cell
    T-cell
    T-lymphocyte cell
    white cell
CellCept (mycophenolate)
cellulitis
central line (permanent catheter)
cerebral
    cerebral aneurysm (stroke)
    cerebral cortex
    cerebral hemorrhage
    cerebral palsy
cerebrospinal fluid (CSF)
cerebrovascular accident (stroke)
cervical
cervical dysplasia
    cervical spine
cervix
cervix (uterine)
chafe
chamber (heart)
    holding chamber (spacer)
characteristics
chart
    clinical chart
    medical chart
check in
chest compressions
CHF (congestive heart failure)
chickenpox
chikungunya virus
chilblain
child
child care
child care center
childbearing
childbearing age
Children's Protective Services (CPS)
chiropractor
chlamydia
choke
chorionic villus sampling (CVS)
chromosome
chronic
clear
    clear lungs
    clear the throat
    clear x-ray
cleft
    cleft lip
    cleft palate
clinical nurse specialist (CNS)
clinical study
clinical trial
clitoris
clonal
    clonal convulsion
clonic tonic
close, close friend
clot
cloudy
    cloudy urine
    cloudy vision
cluster
coagulation
coccidioidomycosis (Valley fever, San Joaquin Valley fever)
coccyx
cochlea
cold (adj.)
cold (n.)
colic
colon (large intestine)
colon ascending
colon descending
colon sigmoid
colon transverse
colonoscopy
color blind
colorectal
    colorectal adenoma
    colorectal cancer
colostomy
colostrum
colposcopy
complete blood count (CBC)
compress
condition
condom
conductors
congenital
    congenital defect
    congenital hypoplastic anemia (Diamond Blackfan anemia)
    congenital nephrotic syndrome of the Finnish type
congestive heart failure (CHF)
consanguinity
consent
consenter
convulsion
cord
    spinal cord
    tethered cord
    umbilical cord

D

duodenojejunal
duodenum dust mites
dysphagia
dysplasia
- anal dysplasia
- cervical dysplasia
- septo-optic dysplasia (optic nerve hypoplasia, de Morsier syndrome)

dysuria

E

each day
ear (internal) (auricle, outer)
- ear canal
- ear drum
- ear plugs
- inner ear
- middle ear
- outer ear

earache
early intervention
Ebola
ECJ (Creutzfeldt-Jakob disease, mad cow disease, CJD)
edema
- pitting edema

EEG (electroencephalogram)
effort
- make your best effort

ejaculation
- premature ejaculation

ejaculatory
- EKG (electrocardiogram) ECG
- pre-ejaculatory fluid

electric current
electric shock
electrocardiogram
electrode
electroencephalogram (EEG)
ELISA test (enzyme-linked immunoassay)
embolism
embolization
emesis
endocrine
- endocrine system

endocrinologist
endometrial
- endometrial biopsy
- endometrial cancer

endometrium
- uterine endometrium

endoscopic retrograde cholangiopancreatography (ERCP)
endoscopy
enema
engorge
engorged
engorgement
eosinophil
epigenetics
episiotomy
equal
equally likely
equilibrium
equity
- equity in care
- health equity

ERCP (endoscopic retrograde cholangiopancreatography)
erectile
erectile dysfunction
erection
erythrocyte
erythrocytosis
erythropoietineven
every cloud has a silver lining
every day
every other day
every two weeks
excessive
- excessive sweat

excoriation
exhaustion
experiment
experimental study (use caution as it may be misinterpreted; this is unusual in English and is usually referred to as a clinical trial or research study; "experiment" may be interpreted as *experimenting on a person*)
eye
- cross-eyed
- crossed eyes
- evil eye

eye drops
eye wash
eyeball
eyebrow
eyelash
eyelid
eyesight vista

F

face down
face up
facial hair
faint
Fallopian tubes
familial adenomatous polyposis
- Fanconi anemia (aplastic anemia)

fat (n.) (adj.)
- animal fat
- body fat
- fat body
- fat free
- fat person
- full fat
- low fat
- vegetable fat

fatigue
fatty acid
FDA Food and Drug Administration
febrile
- febrile seizures

fecal occult blood test (FOBT)
feces
feeding
- feeding tube
- intravenous feeding tube
- nasogastric feeding tube

fellow (doctor)
fetal
- fetal development
- fetal presentation
- fetal ultrasound

fetal alcohol spectrum disorders (FASDs)
- fetal alcohol syndrome

fetus (foetus)
fibrocystic
- fibrocystic breast disease
- fibrocystic disease

fibroid
- uterine fibroid

fibroma
fibromyalgia
fibrosis
- cystic fibrosis
- pulmonary fibrosis

file (medical, clinical)
file a complaint
finding
finger
- fingerprint
- fingertip
- first finger
- fifth finger
- fourth finger
- index finger
- little finger

- middle finger
- ring finger
- second finger
- third finger
- thumb

first aid
first aid kit
first-degree burn
first-degree relative
fissure
- anal fissure
- cerebral fissure

fistula
flake
flaky
flank
- flank pain

flap
flexible sigmoidoscopy
floaters (in eye)
flu (influenza)
- flu shot
- flu vaccine

flush
- facial flushing
- flush a line

folic acid
follow-up
follow-up visit
Fontan procedure
fontanel
foot
forceps
form
formula
foster
- foster care
- foster family
- foster home
- medical foster care

fragile
- fragile health
- fragile X syndrome

free (no cost)
- free interpreting services

free (from)
- fat free
- free of congestion

front to back (roll over)
frostbite
full-term pregnancy
fundoplication
fungal infection
fungus (*see yeast*)

G

gag
gallbladder
gallstones
gangrene
gargle
gastric tube
gastroesophageal
- gastroesophageal reflux

gastroesophageal reflux disease (GERD)
gastrostomy (G-tube)
gastrostomy feeding tube pump
gauze
gene
- gene alteration
- gene mutation
- gene translocation

general
- in general

generally
generic
genetic
genetic array test
genetic consultation
genetic counseling
genetic predisposition
genetically modified organism (GMO)
genital
genital herpes
genital warts
genitalia
genitals
genome
genotype
gently
gestational diabetes
get a lump in one's throat
ginger
gingivitis
give
give a shot
give an injection
give it a shot
give it a try
gland
- mammary gland

glasses (eye)
Glenn shunt (*see Glenn surgery*)
Glenn surgery
glitch
glue
- surgical glue

glucose
goggles
goiter
gonad
gown
graft
graft versus host disease (GVHD)
grave (adj.)
- common grave

grave (n.)
grey matter
grow (something) out
growth
G-tube
guardian
- legal guardian
- legal guardianship

guidelines
Guillain-Barré syndrome (GBS)
gums
GVHD graft versus host disease

H

HAART (highly active antiretroviral therapy)
hair
- arm hair
- chest hair
- hair on the head
- leg hair
- pubic hair
- scalp hair
- underarm hair

hand
harm
- harm reduction

hay fever
head
headache
healer
health
- community health worker

healthcare provider
heart
heart attack (*see myocardial infarction*)
- heart failure

heart murmur
heartburn
hella (a hell of a, very)
hematocrit
hematopoiesis
hematopoietic stem cell
hemodialysis
hemoglobin

hemorrhagic brain attack (stroke)
    hemorrhage
hepatic
hepatobiliary tract
hereditary autosomal recessive
    disorder
hereditary nonpolyposis colorectal
    cancer
hernia
    congenital diaphragmatic hernia
    epigastric hernia
    femoral hernia
    hiatal hernia
    inguinal hernia
    umbilical hernia
herpes
    congenital herpes
    genital herpes
    herpes labialis
    herpes simplex virus (HSV)
    herpes type 1 (HSV-1)
    herpes type 2 (HSV-2
    herpes zoster (shingles)
    oral herpes
hiccough (hiccup)
hiccup (hiccough)
Hirschsprung's disease
hirsutism
histiocytes
histocompatibility histopathology
hit
HIV (human immunodeficiency
    virus)
HNPCC (hereditary nonpolyposis
    colorectal cancer, Lynch
    syndrome)
home health nurse
home safety check
hormone
hormone cream
hospice
hot flashes
house call
HPV (human papillomavirus)
hug
human papillomavirus (HPV)
humidifier
hurt
hydrating
    hydrating lotion
hydration
hydrocele
hydrocephalus
hydrocephaly
hymen
hyper-
hyperpituitarism
hypo-
hypopituitarism
hypoplastic left heart syndrome
hypo-septo-optic
hypospadias
hypothalamus
hysterectomy
hysterotomy

I

IC (intensive care)
ICU (intensive care unit)
identifying features
idiopathic thrombocytopenic
    purpura (ITP)
IEP (individualized education plan)
ileum
iliac
illegitimate child
immune
    immune system
immunity
    innate immunity
immunization
immunocompetent
immunodeficiency
    acquired immunodeficiency
    syndrome (AIDS)
immunological response
immunological system
immunology
immunosuppressant
impetigo
in utero
incidence
incident
incontinence
incus
individualized education plan (IEP)
induced labor
inequality
inequity
    health inequity
infantile nystagmus syndrome (INS)
infection
    candidiasis infection
    fungal infection
    necrotizing soft tissue infection
    opportunistic infection
    pneumococcal infection
    sexually transmitted infection
    (STI)
    strep throat infection
    urinary tract infection
    urine infection
    yeast infection
inflamed
inflammation
influenza (flu)
informed consent
inguinal hernia
inhaler
inhibitors
    nucleoside analog reverse
    protease inhibitors
    transcriptase inhibitors
injection
injure
innate immunity
inner ear
innocent murmur
insulin dependent diabetes
intermittent
intern (doctor, student)
    intern doctor interpretation
interpreter
intestine
    large intestine (*see colon*)
    small intestine
intoxication
intramuscular
intravenous
intravenous line (IV)
introduce
    introduce (a speculum)
    introduce (people)
intubate
intubation
invasive
    invasive procedure
irrigation (cleaning)
irritation
ischemic brain attack (stroke)
itch
itching
ITP (idiopathic thrombocytopenic
    purpura
IV (intravenous)
    IV antibiotics
IVIG (intervenous immunoglobulin)

J

jaundice
jaw
jejunum
jock itch (tinea)
joint

mute
myelin
    myelin sheath
myelomeningocele
myo- (muscle)
myocardial infarction
myocarditis
myocardium
myositis

N

nasogastric
nasogastric feeding tube (NG tube)
nasolabial philtrum
natural
natural disaster
natural childbirth
natural family planning
navel
navigator
    health navigator
necrotizing soft tissue
    necrotizing enterocolitis
needle
    needle stick
neonatal
neotrophil
neuron
neutropenia
NG tube
night sweats
nipple
    cracked nipples
    inverted nipples
nocturnal leg cramps
noise
Norwood surgery
nucleoside analog reverse
    transcriptase inhibitors
numb
numbness
nurse (n.)
    clinical nurse specialist
    home health nurse
    nurse practitioner
    nurse specialist
    public health nurse
    registered nurse
nurse (v.)
nursing
    nurse's aide nursing assistant
    nursing assistant
    nursing student
nutrients
nutritionist
nutritious
nystagmus

O

obituary
obsessive-compulsive disorder
occult blood test odontologist
odontology
oh, well
ok
once a week
once every two weeks
once in a blue moon
operating room
ophthalmologist
optic
    optic nerve
optometrist
oral candidiasis (thrush)
oral herpes
order
osteogenesis imperfecta
osteopenia (low bone density)
osteoporosis
ostomy
out of it
outer ear
ovary
overindulge
ovum
oxytocin

P

PA (physician's assistant, *see MA*)
page (n.)
page (v.)
    to be on the same page
pain
    aching pain
    constant pain
    dull pain
    electric shock pain
    intermittent pain
    sharp pain
    shooting pain
    stabbing pain
    throbbing pain
palate
    cleft palate
paludism (malaria symptoms)
pamper (v.)
Pampers (n.)
pancreas
Pap smear
Papanikolaou test (Pap smear)
papule
parameters
partial androgen receptor
    insensitivity
passive
paste
pee
PEG tube
pelvic
    pelvic exam
pelvis
penis
percutaneous
perinatal
perinatal transmission
peripheral
period
periodontal disease
peritoneal dialysis
permanent catheter (central line)
permanent legal resident
    (immigration status)
pernicious anemia
pertussis (whooping cough)
pervasive developmental disorders
petechiae
phagocyte
pharmacist
pharmacologist
pharmacy
pharyngomalacia
pharynx
phenobarbital
phenotype
phenylketonuria (PKU)
philtrum
    nasolabial philtrum
phosphorus
physical therapist
physical therapy
physician
physician's assistant
physiology
physiotherapy
PICC line (percutaneously inserted
    central catheter)
pimple
pinna
pitting
    pitting edema
pituitary
pituitary gland
placenta
    placenta previa
plasma

platelet
  platelet disorder
  platelet problems
pleura
pleurisy
PMS (premenstrual syndrome)
pneumococcal infection
pneumococci
pneumonia
poison
poisoning
  blood poisoning
  food poisoning
polycystic ovary syndrome
polyp
port (catheter)
  InfusaPort
  Medi-port
  Port-a-Cathsubclavian port
  subcutaneous central venous catheter
  subcutaneous port
possible
postpartum depression
post-traumatic stress disorder (PTSD)
  chronic PTSD
  secondary PTSD
potassium
poultice
precision
predisposed
predisposition
prednisone
preeclampsia
preemie
preexisting condition
pregnancy
pregnant
premature baby
premenstrual syndrome (PMS)
prescription
preservative
preserve
primary care
primary care doctor
primary congestion
principal
principally
principle
  on principle
probable
probe
problem
procedure
prognosis
prolapse
  mitral valve prolapse
  pelvic organ prolapse
  uterine prolapse
prolonged
promoter (community health worker or navigator)
prone
prophylaxis
prostate
prostrate
protease inhibitors
protracted
protrude
protruding
provider
psoriasis
psychiatrist
psychiatry
psychology
psychosis
  manic-depressive psychosis
psychosomatic
psychotherapist
psychotherapy
PTSD (post-traumatic stress disorder)
puberty
pubic
  pubic area
pubic hair
pubic lice
pubis
puffer
pulmonary atresia (*see tricuspid atresia*)
pulmonary trunk
pump
pumpkin
puncture
  lumbar puncture
pupil (eye)
purpura
push out
put up with

Q

Q-tip
quickly
quietly

R

radiation
  radiation therapy
radical hysterectomy
radiography
radiology
radiology technician
range
range of motion
range of vision
rape
rash
rate
reaction
reactive airway disease
rectum
red
red blood cells (erythrocytes)
red cells
  to turn red
reddening
redness
reevaluate
referral
refill
reflux
  gastroesophageal reflux
  urinary reflux
regional ileitis (*Crohn's disease*)
reject
rejection
relapse
relations
  sexual relations
relationship
relief
relieve
remove
renal
repair damage
requisition
research
  clinical research
  research study
resect
resection
resident
  legal permanent resident
  legal resident
resident doctor
respiratory syncytial virus (RSV)
respond
response
restless
restless legs syndrome (RLS)
retina
  detached retina
retinal detachment

retinopathy
    diabetic retinopathy
revive
rhabdomyosarcoma
rhinoplasty
rhinoscope
rhinoscopy
rhythm
    rhythm method
ringworm (tinea)
risk
    risk factor
    risk of infection
    to put at risk
    to risk
rod
roll
roll over
roll over back to front
roll over front to back
root canal
rosacea
RSV (respiratory syncytial virus)
rub
    rub in
runny nose

S

saccule
sacral
sacral bone
sacral spine
sacrum
safe
salt (*see sodium*)
    low-salt
    salt-free
same
sample
scabies
scale
scalp
scalp hair
scan
scarlet fever
schedule an appointment
SCID (severe combined immunodeficiency)
sclera
scrape
scraping
scratch
screening (test)
screw
scribble
scrub
scrubs
season
seasonal
seborrheic dermatitis
secondary PTSD
seizure
semicircular canals
seniority
sensor
sepsis
septic
septic shock
septicemia
septo-optic dysplasia (optic nerve hypoplasia, de Morsier syndrome)
septum
    deviated septum
    nasal septum
seroconversion
serum
severe acute respiratory syndrome (SARS)
severe combined immunodeficiency (SCID)
sex
    anal sex
    oral sex
    safe sex
    safer sex
    to have sex
    vaginal sex
sexual
sexual relations
sexually
sexually transmitted disease
sexually transmitted infection
shake
shaken baby syndrome
sharp pain
shingles (herpes zoster)
shock
    anaphylactic shock
    cardiogenic shock
    electric shock
    hypovolemic shock
    septic shock
    toxic shock
shooting pain
shot
shoulder
shunt
sickle cell anemia
SIDS (sudden infant death syndrome)
sigmoidoscopy
signet-ring cell type
silver
    silver lining
    silver nitrate
single father
single mother
single parent
sinus
sinusitis
sister-in-law
site
sleep
sleep apnea
sleep study
slip
slow
slowly
small intestine (ileum)
smash
smell (bad)
smell (v.)
snack (n.)
snack (v.)
soda (pop)
sodium (*see salt*)
    low-sodium diet
sodium bicarbonate
soft
soft drink
softly
spacer (for inhaler)
    specific inherited gene alterations
specimen
spectrum
speculum
speed
spin
spina bifida
    open spina bifida
    spina bifida occulta
spinal column
spinal cord
spinal tap
spine
spinning
spit up
spleen
splint
spoil (pamper, indulge, rot)
spoiled child
spoiled food
spontaneous abortion
spores
    mold spores

spot
spotting
squamous
squat (crouch down)
squeeze
squint
stabbing pain
stand
stand (tolerate)
stand for
stand up
standard
standard practice
standardized
standing order
stapes
STD (sexually transmitted disease)
stem cell
stent
steroids
STI (sexually transmitted infection)
stick (v.)
stickers
stiff
stiffness (to have)
still
stillbirth
sting
stink
stirrups
stoma
stomach
stop
stop medication
strabismus (crossed eyes)
strep
strep throat
streptococcus
stress
stridor
stripe
stroke
study
- bone study
- clinical study

stuffy nose
subcutaneous
supine
sure
surgeon
surgery
surgical
- surgical gown (scrubs)

surgically
swab
swallow
swallow study (barium swallow study)
sweat
sweat test
swell
swelling
swollen
syncope
syndrome
- acquired immunodeficiency syndrome (AIDS)
- antiphospholipid antibody syndrome (APLS)
- carpal tunnel syndrome
- congenital nephrotic syndrome of Finnish type
- constitutional mismatch repair deficiency syndrome
- fragile X syndrome
- Guillain-Barré syndrome (GBS)
- hereditary mismatch repair deficiency syndrome (HMRDS)
- hereditary nonpolyposis colon cancer syndrome (HNPCC, Lynch syndrome)
- hypoplastic left heart syndrome
- hypoplastic right heart syndrome
- infantile nystagmus syndrome (INS)
- Lynch syndrome
- Marfan syndrome
- polycystic ovary syndrome
- Prader-Willi syndrome
- restless legs syndrome (RLS)
- shaken baby syndrome
- sudden infant death syndrome (SIDS)
- Tourette syndrome
- toxic shock syndrome
- Turner syndrome

synovial
- synovial membrane

syringe
syrup
systolic

T

tachycardia
tailbone
take blood
tank
taper
taper schedule
T-cells
tech
technician
teeth
Tegaderm
temporary
temporary foster care
tender
tenderness, to have
tendon
test
- cancer screening test
- ELISA test (enzyme-linked immunoassay)
- genetic array test
- lab test
- Pap smear test
- Papanikolaou test
- paternity test
- pregnancy test
- protein immunoblotting test (western blot test)
- quick test
- serologic test
- screening test
- TB skin test
- urine test
- Wada test (cerebral hemispheric dominance of language function)

testicle
testosterone
thalamus
thalassemia
that's it
the jury is still out
therapeutic
therapist
therapy
- chemotherapy
- intensive care therapy
- intensive therapy
- physical therapy
- radiation therapy

thoracic spine
throat
- clear the throat
- sore throat

throbbing pain
thrombocyte
throw up
thrush (oral candidiasis)
thyroid
- thyroid gland

tie tubes
tinea

tingling
tissue
tit
toddler
tolerate
tomography
tonsillectomy
tonsillitis
tonsils
    palatine tonsil
tooth
toothless
touch base
toxic shock
toxic shock syndrome
toxoplasmosis
trach
trachea
tracheostomy
tracheotomy
trait
transfuse
transient ischemic brain attack (mini stroke)
translate
translation
translator
transparent
transplant
traumatic brain injury
trichomoniasis
tricuspid atresia
trisomy
trisomy 18 (Edwards syndrome)
trisomy 21 (Down syndrome)
try
    really try
tubal ligation
tube
    eustachian tubes
    Fallopian tubes
tummy
tumor versus host effect
turbinates (nasal)
tympanic membrane
type
typing
    confirmatory typing
    tissue typing (histocompatibility antigen test)

U

umbilical hernia
umbilicus
underlying
underlying cause
undescended testes
undifferentiated pattern
undocumented ("illegal")
upchuck
urea
ureter
urethra
urge incontinence
uric acid
urinalysis
urinary
    urinary bladder
    urinary incontinence
    urinary reflux
urinary tract infection
urine
urine cytology test
urine infection
urodynamics test
uterine
    uterine cervix
    uterine lining
    uterine myoma
    uterine prolapse
uterus
UTI (urinary tract infection)
utricle

V

vaccinate
vaccine
vacuum
vagina
vaginal
vaginal birth
vaginal bleeding
    vaginal discharge
vaginal dryness
vaginal fluid
vaginal ring
vaginal yeast infection
Valley fever (San Joaquin Valley fever, coccidioidomycosis)
varicella
varicella-zoster virus
vasoconstrictor
vasodilator
vein
venipuncture
venom
ventricle
ventriculoperitoneal shunt (VP shunt)
vertebra
vertebrae
    cervical vertebrae
    lumbar vertebrae
    sacral vertebrae
    thoracic vertebrae
vertebral column
vertigo
    benign paroxysmal positional vertigo (BPPV)
vial
vicarious PTSD
villus
    chorionic villus sampling
viral load
virus
    herpes simplex virus (HSV)
    respiratory syncytial virus (RSV)
    West Nile virus
visual field
vomit
VP shunt
vulva

W

Wada test (cerebral hemispheric dominance of language function)
waist
wart
wasting
    AIDS wasting syndrome
    facial wasting
water pill (diuretic)
weakness
weigh
West Nile virus
whatever
wheal
wheezing
    wheezing noise
whistling
    whistling noise
white blood cells (leucocytes)
white matter
whoosh
whooshing
    whooshing noise
wipe
wipes
    alcohol wipe
wire

X

Y

Z

Bibliography

Bancroft, M.A. (2005). The interpreter's world tour: An environmental scan of standards of practice for interpreters. Menlo Park, California: The California Endowment. Available at www.ncihc.org.

Bancroft, M.A., Allen, K., Green, C., & Feuerle, L. (2016). *Breaking Silence: Interpreting for Victim Services.* Washington, DC: Ayuda.

Bancroft, M.A., García-Beyaert, S., Allen, K., Carriero-Contreras, G., & Socarrás-Estrada, D. (2015). *The Community Interpreter®: An International Textbook.* (M. A. Bancroft, Ed.). Columbia, Maryland: Culture & Language Press.

Bancroft, M.A., García-Beyaert, S., Allen, K., Carriero-Contreras, G., & Socarrás-Estrada, D. (2016). *The Medical Interpreter®: A Foundation Textbook for Medical Interpreting.* (M. A. Bancroft, Ed.). Columbia, Maryland: Culture & Language Press.

Bernstein, J., Bernstein, E., Dave, A., Hardt, E., James, T., Linden, J., Mitchell, P., Oishi, T., & Safi, C. (2002). Trained interpreters in the emergency department: Effects on services, subsequent charges, and follow-up. *Journal of Immigrant Health*, *4*(4), 171-176.

Bowen, S. (2015). *The Impact of Language Barriers on Patient Safety and Quality of Care.* Ottawa, Canada: Société Santé en français.

Burbano O'Leary, S.C., Federico, S., & Hampers, L.C. (2003). The truth about language barriers: One residency program's experience. *Pediatrics, 111*(5 Pt 1), e569-573.

Carrasquillo, O., Orav, E.J., Brennan, T.A., & Burstin, H.R. (1999). Impact of language barriers on patient satisfaction in an emergency department. *Journal of General Internal Medicine, 14,* 82-87.

CHIA (2002). *California standards for healthcare interpreters.* Sacramento, California: California Healthcare Interpreting Association. Available at www.chiaonline.org.

Crane, J.A. (1997). Patient comprehension of doctor-patient communication on discharge from the emergency department. *Journal of Emergency Medicine, 15*(1), 1-7.

Diamond, L.C., & Jacobs, E.A. (2010). Let's not contribute to disparities: The best methods for teaching clinicians how to overcome language barriers to healthcare. *Journal of General Internal Medicine*, *25*(2), 189-193.

Diamond, L.C., Schenker, Y., Bradley, E., Curry, L., & Fernandez, A. (2009). Getting by: Underuse of interpreters by resident physicians. *Journal of General Internal Medicine, 24*(2), 256-262.

Diamond, L.C., Wilson-Stronks A., & Jacobs, E.A. (2010). Do hospitals measure up to the national culturally and linguistically appropriate services standards? *Medical Care, 48*(12), 1080-1087.

Divi, C., Koss, R.G., Schmaltz, S.P., & Leob, J.M. (2007). Language proficiency and adverse events in US hospitals: A pilot study. *International Journal for Quality in Healthcare, 19*(2), 60-67.

Dower, C. (2003). *Health Care Interpreters in California.* San Francisco: University of California San Francisco Center for the Health Professions.

Downing, B., & Roat, C.E. (2002). Models for the provision of language access in health care settings. Washington, DC: National Council on Interpreting in Health Care.

ECRI Institute and ISMP. (2011). Managing patients with Limited English Proficiency. *Pennsylvania Patient Safety Advisory*, *8*(1), 26-33.

Eneriz-Wiemer, M., Sanders, L.M., Barr, D.A., & Mendoza, F.S. (2014). Parental limited English proficiency and health outcomes for children with special healthcare needs: A systematic review. *Academic Pediatrics, 14*(2), 128-136.

Eugenides, J. (2002). *Middlesex*. New York, New York: Macmillan.

European Study Group on Heterosexual Transmission of HIV. (1992). Comparison of female to male and male to female transmission of HIV in 563 stable couples. *British Medical Journal, 304*(6830), 809-813.

Fiscella, K., Franks, P., Doescher, M.P., & Saver, B.G. (2002). Disparities in health care by race, ethnicity, and language among the insured: Findings from a national sample. *Medical Care, 40,* 52-59.

Forna, F.M., Fitzpatrick, L., Adimora, A.A., McLellan-Lemal, E., Leone, P., Brooks, J.T., Marks, G., & Greenberg, A. (2006). A case-control study of factors associated with HIV infection among black women. *Journal of teh National Medical Association, 98*(11), 1798-1804.

Flores, G., Abreu, M., Pizzo Barone, C., Bachur, R., & Lin, H. (2012). Errors in medical interpretation and their potential clinical consequences: A comparison of professional versus ad hoc versus no interpreters. *Annals of Emergency Medicine, 60*(5), 545-553.

Flores, G., Laws, M.B., Mayo, S.J., Zuckerman, B., Abreu, M., Medina, L., & Hardt, E.J. (2003). Errors in medical interpretation and their potential clinical consequences in pediatric encounter. *Pediatrics, 111*(1), 6-14.

Fox, S.A., & Stein, J.A. (1991). The effect of physician–patient communication on mammography utilization by different ethnic groups. *Medical Care, 11,* 1065-1082.

Freire, P. (1970, 2000). *Pedagogy of the Oppressed*. New York, New York: Bloomsbury Academic.

Gandhi, T.K., Burstin, H.R., Cook, E.F., Puopolo, A.L., Haas, J.S., Brennan, T.A., & Bates, D.W. (2000). Drug complications in outpatients. *Journal of General Internal Medicine, 15,* 149-154

Grandin, G. (2014). *The Empire of Necessity Slavery, Freedom, and Deception in the New World*. New York: Metropolitan.

Green, D. (2009). *The economics of language services: Or how to save healthcare in Texas.* (slide presentation). Retrieved from www.slideshare.net/DouglasGreen/the-economics-of-language-services-in-healthcarefinal

Hardt, E. (1999). Comments to MA Healthcare Committee, April 9, 1999, from E. Hardt, MD, clinical director of geriatrics and medical consultant to interpreter services at Boston Medical Center. Retrieved from www.slideshare.net/DouglasGreen/the-economics-of-language-services-in-healthcarefinal

HHS. (2016). *Nondiscrimination in health programs and activities.* Washington, DC: The U.S. Department of Health and Human Services. See www.federalregister.gov/articles/2016/05/18/2016-11458/nondiscrimination-in-health-programs-and-activities#sec-92-201%20

HIN. (2007). *National Standards Guide for Community Interpreting Services.* Toronto, Ontario: Healthcare Interpretation Network.

Hua, V. (2006). Alameda County non-English speakers find ERs hard to reach: More than half of testers in study didn't get help. *San Francisco Chronicle*. February 17.

Institute of Medicine. (2000). *To Err Is Human: Building a Safer Health System.* Washington, DC: The National Academies Press.

Jacobs, E.A., Agger-Gupta. N., Chen, A.H., Piotrowski, A., & Hardt, E.J. (2003) *Language Barriers in Health Care Settings: An Annotated Bibliography of the Research Literature.* Woodland Hills, California: The California Endowment.

James, J.T. (2013). A new, evidence-based estimate of patient harms associated with hospital care. *Journal of Patient Safety, 9*(3), 122-128.

John-Baptiste, A., Naglie, G., Tomlinson, G., Alibhai, S.M.H., Etchells, E., Cheung, A., Kapral, M., Gold, W.L., Abrams, H., Bacchus, M., & Krahn, M. (2004). The effect of English language proficiency on length of stay and in-hospital mortality. *Journal of General Internal Medicine, 19*(3), 221-228.

Juckett, G., & Unger, K. (2014). Appropriate use of medical interpreters. *American Family Physician, 90*(7), 476-480.

Karliner, L.S., Auerbach, A., Nápoles A., Schillinger, D., Nickleach, D., & Pérez-Stable, E.J. (2012). Language barriers and understanding of hospital discharge instructions. *Medical Care*, *50*, 283-289.

Karliner, L.S., Jacobs, E.A., Chen, A.H., & Mutha, S. (2007). Do professional interpreters improve clinical care for patients with limited English proficiency? A systematic review of the literature. *Health Services Research, 42*(2), 727-754.

Karliner, L.S., Perez-Stable E.J., & Gildengorin, G. (2004). The language divide. The importance of training in the use of interpreters for outpatient practice. *Journal of General Internal Medicine, 19*(2),175-183.

Kelly, N. (2008). The voice on the other end of the phone. *Health Affairs, 27*(6), 1701-1706.

Kirkman-Liff, B., Mondragón, D. (1991) Language of interview: Relevance for research of southwest Hispanics. *American Journal of Public Health, 81,* 1399-1404.

Kristof, N.D., & WuDunn, S. (2009). *Half the Sky: Turning Oppression into Opportunity for Women Worldwide.* New York: Alfred A. Knopf.

Ku, L., & Flores, G. (2005) Pay now or pay later: providing interpreter services in healthcare. *Health Affairs, 24*(2), 435-444.

Kuo, D., & Fagan, M. (1991). Satisfaction with methods of Spanish interpretation in an ambulatory care clinic. *Journal of General and Internal Medicine, 14*(9), 547-550.

Lee, K.C., Winickoff, J.P., & Kim, M.K. (2006). Resident physicians' use of professional and nonprofessional interpreters: a national survey. *Journal of the American Medical Association, 296*(9), 1050-1053.

Lewis-Thornton, R. (2012). *The horror of HIV/AIDS: The murder of Cicely*. Retrieved from www.thebody.com/content/69080/the-horror-of-hivaids-the-murder-of-cicely.html?ic=700100

Ludden, J. (2009). Patient interpreters save money, but who pays? National Public Radio, July 27. Retrieved from www.npr.org/templates/story/story.php?storyId=111066555&sc=emaf

Manson, A. (1988). Language concordance as a determinant of patient compliance and emergency room use in patients with asthma. *Medical Care, 26,* 1119-1128.

Martín del Campo, M. (1999). *Amor y Conquista: La novela de Malinalli mal llamada la Malinche.* México, DF: Editorial Planeta Mexicana.

Mikkelson, H. (2003). Telephone interpreting: Boon or bane? In González, L.P. (Ed.). *Speaking in Tongues: Language Across Contexts and Users.* Valencia, Spain, Universitat de València. pp. 251-269.

MMIA. (1995). *Medical interpreting standards of practice.* Boston, Massachusetts: Medical Interpreters Association (now the International Medical Interpreters Association).

Moser-Mercer, B. (2003). *Remote interpreting: Assessment of human factors and performance parameters.* Geneva: Joint project International Telecommunication Union (ITU)-Ecole de Traduction et d'Interpretation, Université de Genève.

Nápoles, A.M., Santoyo-Olsson, J., Karliner, L.S., O'Brien, H., Gregorich, S.E., & Pérez-Stable, E.J. (2010). Clinician ratings of interpreter mediated visits in underserved primary care settings with ad hoc, in-person professional, and video conferencing modes. *Journal of Healthcare for the Poor and Underserved, 21*(1), 301-317.

Narrigan, D. (2003). Examining an ethical dilemma; a case study in clinical practice. *Journal of Midwifery & Women's Health, 49*(3), 243-249.

NCIHC. (2004). *A National Code of Ethics for Interpreters in Health Care*. Washington, DC: National Council on Interpreting in Health Care.

NCIHC. (2005). *National Standards of Practice for Interpreters in Health Care.* Washington, DC: National Council on Interpreting in Health Care.

Njeru, J.W., St. Sauver, J.L., Jacobsen, D.J., Ebbert, J.O., Takahashi, P.Y., Fan, C., & Wieland, M.L. (2015). Emergency department and inpatient healthcare utilization among patients who require interpreter services. *BMC Health Services Research, 15*, 214.

Ochoa, K.C., Evans, M.A., & Kaiser, S.A. (2003). Negotiating care: The teaching and practice of cultural competence in medical school. A student perspective. *Medical Education Online*. Retrieved from www.med-ed-online.org/pdf/l0000001.pdf

Perkins, J., & Youdelman, M. (2008). *Summary of State Law Requirements Addressing Language Needs in Healthcare*. Washington, DC: National Health Law Program.

Pöchhacker, F. (2007). Critical linking up: Kinship and convergence in interpreting studies. *The Critical Link 4: Professionalism of Interpreting in the Community.* (C. Wadensjö, B. Englund Dimitrova, & A-L. Nilsson, Eds.). Philadelphia, Pennsylvania: John Benjamins Publishing Company.

Reiss-Končar, S. (2010). *Language access advocacy in medical interpreter training curricula*. (Unpublished master's thesis. San Francisco State University, San Francisco, California).

Riera, A., Navas-Nazario, A., Shabanova, V., & Vaca, F.E. (2014). The impact of limited English proficiency on asthma action plan use. *The Journal of Asthma, 51*, 178-184.

Roat, C.E. (2010). *Healthcare Interpreting in Small Bites: 50 Nourishing Selections from the "Pacific Interpreters Newsletter," 2002-2010.* Victoria, British Columbia, Canada: Trafford.

Schenker, Y., Lo, B., Ettinger, K.M., & Fernendez, A. (2008). Navigating language barriers under difficult circumstances. *Annals of Internal Medicine, 149*(4), 264-269.

Schenker, Y., Wang, F., Selig, S.J., Ng, R., & Fernandez, A. (2007). The impact of language barriers on documentation of informed consent at a hospital with on-site interpreter Services. Journal of *General Internal Medicine, 22*(S2), 294-299.

Schiaffino, M.K., Nara, A., & Mao, L. (2016). Language services in hospitals vary by ownership and location. *Health Affairs*, *35*(8), 1399-1403.

Sidibé, M. (2010). Families on the front line of AIDS. Speech of M. Sidibé, executive director, United Nations Program on Aids (UNAIDS) at the Colloquium on the Empowerment of the Family in the Modern World: Challenges and Promises Ahead. Doha, Qatar, 2010. Retrieved from www.unaids.org/sites/default/files/media_asset/20100127_sp_doha_families_en_0.pdf

Smith, A.K., Sudore, R.L., & Pérez-Stable, E. (2009). Palliative care for Latino patients and their families: Whenever we prayed, she wept. *The Journal of the American Medical Association*, *301*(10), 1047-1057.

Smith, D.L. (2010). Health care disparities for persons with Limited English Proficiency: Relationships from the 2006 Medical Expenditure Panel Survey (MEPS). *Journal of Health Disparities Research and Practice, 3*(3), 57-67.

UCSF (University of California at San Francisco). (2008). *Frontiers in medicine: News from the UCSF Department of Medicine, 7*.

U.S. Office of Management and Budget. (2002). *Report to Congress. Assessment of the Total Benefits and Costs of Implementing Executive Order No. 13166: Improving Access to Services for Persons with Limited English Proficiency*. Washington, DC: U.S. White House.

Woloshin, S., Schwartz, L.M., Katz, S.J., & Welch, H.G. (1997). Is language a barrier to the use of preventive services? *Journal of General Internal Medicine*, *12*(8), 472-477.

Wyatt, G. (2012) Presentation at 2012 International AIDS Conference. Retrieved from http://abcnews.go.com/Health/hivaids-infection-rates-rise-us-rare-conference-opens/story?id=16831699#.UEomsLJmT8k)

Yawman, D., McIntosh, S., Fernandez, D., Auinger, P., Allan, M., & Weitzman, M. (2006). The use of Spanish by medical students and residents at one university hospital. *Academic Medicine, 81*(5), 468-473.

Youdelman, M. (2009). Good interpreters can save lives and limbs. Retrieved from http://ccf.georgetown.edu/2009/04/30/good_interpreters_can_save_lives_and_limbs/